T0226489

Breast Cancer: Uses and Opportunities for Molecular Imaging

Editors

ELIZABETH S. MCDONALD
GARY A. ULANER

PET CLINICS

www.pet.theclinics.com

Consulting Editor
ABASS ALAVI

July 2018 • Volume 13 • Number 3

ELSEVIER

1600 John F. Kennedy Boulevard • Suite 1800 • Philadelphia, Pennsylvania, 19103-2899

http://www.pet.theclinics.com

PET CLINICS Volume 13, Number 3
July 2018 ISSN 1556-8598, ISBN-13: 978-0-323-61062-9

Editor: John Vassallo (j.vassallo@elsevier.com)
Developmental Editor: Casey Potter

PET Clinics (ISSN 1556-8598) is published quarterly by Elsevier Inc., 360 Park Avenue South, New York, NY 10010-1710. Months of issue are January, April, July, and October. Periodicals postage paid at New York, NY, and additional mailing offices. Subscription prices per year are $232.00 (US individuals), $396.00 (US institutions), $100.00 (US students), $263.00 (Canadian individuals), $446.00 (Canadian institutions), $140.00 (Canadian students), $268.00 (foreign individuals), $446.00 (foreign institutions), and $140.00 (foreign students). To receive student and resident rate, orders must be accompanied by name of affiliated institution, date of term, and the signature of program/residency coordinator on institution letterhead. Orders will be billed at individual rate until proof of status is received. Foreign air speed delivery is included in all Clinics subscription prices. All prices are subject to change without notice. POSTMASTER: Send address changes to PET Clinics, Elsevier Health Sciences Division, Subscription Customer Service, 3251 Riverport Lane, Maryland Heights, MO 63043. **Customer Service: 1-800-654-2452 (U.S. and Canada); 314-447-8871 (outside U.S. and Canada). Fax: 314-447-8029. E-mail: journalscustomerservice-usa@elsevier.com (for print support); journalsonlinesupport-usa@elsevier.com (for online support).**

Reprints. For copies of 100 or more of articles in this publication, please contact the Commercial Reprints Department, Elsevier Inc., 360 Park Avenue South, New York, NY 10010-1710. Tel.: 212-633-3874; Fax: 212-633-3820; E-mail: reprints@elsevier.com.

PET Clinics is covered in MEDLINE/PubMed (Index Medicus).

Contributors

CONSULTING EDITOR

ABASS ALAVI, MD, MD (Hon), PhD (Hon), DSc (Hon)
Professor of Radiology and Neurology, Department of Radiology, Division of Nuclear Medicine, Hospital of the University of Pennsylvania, University of Pennsylvania Perelman School of Medicine, Philadelphia, Pennsylvania, USA

EDITORS

ELIZABETH S. McDONALD, MD, PhD, FSBI
Fellow of the Society of Breast Imaging, Assistant Professor of Radiology, Perelman School of Medicine, University of Pennsylvania, Philadelphia, Pennsylvania, USA

GARY A. ULANER, MD, PhD, FACNM
Fellow of the American College of Nuclear Medicine, Associate Member, Department of Radiology, Memorial Sloan Kettering Cancer Center, Associate Professor, Department of Radiology, Weill Cornell Medical School, New York, New York, USA

AUTHORS

ABASS ALAVI, MD, MD (Hon), PhD (Hon), DSc (Hon)
Professor of Radiology and Neurology, Department of Radiology, Division of Nuclear Medicine, Hospital of the University of Pennsylvania, University of Pennsylvania Perelman School of Medicine, Philadelphia, Pennsylvania, USA

SANDIP BASU, MD
Consultant Physician, Department of Nuclear Medicine, Head, Nuclear Medicine Academic Programme, Radiation Medicine Centre, Bhaba Atomic Research Centre, Mumbai, India

WENDIE A. BERG, MD, PhD
Department of Radiology, University of Pittsburgh School of Medicine, Magee-Womens Hospital of UPMC, Pittsburgh, Pennsylvania, USA

DHRITIMAN CHAKRABORTY, MD
Department of Nuclear Medicine, All India Institute of Medical Sciences, New Delhi, India

SUET-FEUNG CHIN, BSc, PhD
Senior Research Associate, Cancer Research UK Cambridge Institute, University of Cambridge, Li Ka Shing Centre, Cambridge, United Kingdom

CHAU DANG, MD
Chief, Westchester Medical Oncology, Memorial Sloan Kettering Cancer Center, Associate Professor of Medicine, Weill Cornell Medical College, New York, New York, USA

AZADEH ELMI, MD
Department of Radiology, Perelman School of Medicine, University of Pennsylvania, Philadelphia, Pennsylvania, USA

AMY M. FOWLER, MD, PhD
Assistant Professor, Department of Radiology, University of Wisconsin-Madison, School of Medicine and Public Health, Madison, Wisconsin, USA

DAVID GROHEUX, MD, PhD
Department of Nuclear Medicine, Saint-Louis Hospital, Paris, France

KELLY E. HENRY, PhD
Research Fellow, Department of Radiology, Memorial Sloan Kettering Cancer Center, New York, New York, USA

ANDREI IAGARU, MD
Division of Nuclear Medicine and Molecular Imaging, Stanford University, Stanford, California, USA

MAXINE S. JOCHELSON, MD
Attending, Department of Radiology, Memorial Sloan Kettering Cancer Center, New York, New York, USA

RAKESH KUMAR, MD, PhD
Professor and Head, Department of Nuclear Medicine, Diagnostic Nuclear Medicine Division, All India Institute of Medical Sciences, New Delhi, India

LIZZA LEBRON-ZAPATA, MD
Assistant Attending, Department of Radiology, Memorial Sloan Kettering Cancer Center, New York, New York, USA

JASON S. LEWIS, PhD
Radiochemist (with tenure, Professor equivalent), Department of Radiology, Program in Molecular Pharmacology and Chemistry, Radiochemistry and Molecular Imaging Probes Core, Memorial Sloan Kettering Cancer Center, Departments of Radiology and Pharmacology, Weill Cornell Medical College, New York, New York, USA

HANNAH M. LINDEN, MD
Professor, Department of Medical Oncology, Seattle Cancer Care Alliance, UW Medical Center, Seattle, Washington, USA

DAVID MANKOFF, MD, PhD
Department of Radiology, Perelman School of Medicine, University of Pennsylvania, Philadelphia, Pennsylvania, USA

ELIZABETH S. McDONALD, MD, PhD, FSBI
Fellow of the Society of Breast Imaging, Assistant Professor of Radiology, Perelman School of Medicine, University of Pennsylvania, Philadelphia, Pennsylvania, USA

RYOGO MINAMIMOTO, MD, PhD
Division of Nuclear Medicine, National Center for Global Health and Medicine, Tokyo, Japan

TRACY-ANN MOO, MD
Assistant Attending Surgeon, Breast Service, Department of Surgery, Memorial Sloan Kettering Cancer Center, Assistant Member, Memorial Hospital for Cancer and Allied Diseases, Assistant Professor of Surgery, Weill Cornell Medical College, New York, New York, USA

MONICA MORROW, MD
Chief, Breast Service, Department of Surgery, Anne Burnett Windfohr Chair of Clinical Oncology, Memorial Sloan Kettering Cancer Center, Professor of Surgery, Weill Cornell Medical College, New York, New York, USA

DEEPA NARAYANAN, MS
National Cancer Institute, Rockville, Maryland, USA

LANELL M. PETERSON, BA
Research Scientist, Department of Medical Oncology, Seattle Cancer Care Alliance, UW Medical Center, Seattle, Washington, USA

ELENA PROVENZANO, MBBS, PhD, FRCPath
Lead Breast Histopathologist, Cambridge Experimental Cancer Medicine Centre (ECMR), NIHR Cambridge Biomedical Research Centre, Cambridge University Hospitals NHS Foundation Trust, Department of Histopathology, Addenbrookes Hospital, Cambridge, United Kingdom

RACHEL SANFORD, MD
Assistant Attending, Breast Medicine Service, Department of Medicine, Memorial Sloan Kettering Cancer Center, New York, New York, USA

DAVID M. SCHUSTER, MD
Associate Professor, Department of Radiology and Imaging Sciences, Division of Nuclear Medicine and Molecular Imaging, Emory University Hospital, Atlanta, Georgia, USA

GARY A. ULANER, MD, PhD, FACNM
Fellow of the American College of Nuclear Medicine, Associate Member, Department of Radiology, Memorial Sloan Kettering Cancer Center, Associate Professor, Department of Radiology, Weill Cornell Medical School, New York, New York, USA

Contents

Section 1: Principles of Breast Cancer

Screening mammography saves lives. The mainstay of screening has been mammography. Multiple alternative options, however, for supplemental imaging are now available. Some are just improved anatomic delineation, whereas others include physiology added to anatomy. The third group (molecular imaging) is purely physiologic. This article describes and compares the available options and for which patient populations they should be used.

Breast cancer is a heterogeneous disease, observed traditionally by morphology and protein expression but more recently, with the advent of modern molecular technologies, at the genomic and transcriptomic level. This article describes the association between the different molecular subtypes with the histologic subtypes of breast cancer alongside some of their major genomic characteristics and illustrates how these subtypes may affect the appearance of tumors on imaging studies. The authors aim to show how molecular stratification can be used to augment traditional methods to improve the understanding of breast cancers and their clinical management.

Breast cancer treatment is multidisciplinary. Most women with early-stage breast cancer are candidates for breast-conserving surgery with radiotherapy or mastectomy. The risk of local recurrence and the chance of survival do not differ with these approaches. Sentinel node biopsy is used for axillary staging, and individualized approaches are minimizing the need for axillary dissection in women with positive sentinel nodes. Adjuvant systemic therapy is used in most women based on proven survival benefit, and molecular profiling to individualize treatment based on risk is now a clinical reality for patients with hormone receptor–positive cancers.

Section 2: Current Concepts in Molecular Imaging of Breast Cancer

Histologic subtype, receptor status, and other biologic factors greatly affect the avidity of breast malignancy on fluorodeoxyglucose (FDG) PET. FDG PET/computed tomography (CT) has demonstrated excellent value in the evaluation of extra-axillary nodal and distant metastases. Patients with early-stage breast cancers do not benefit from FDG PET/CT; however, unsuspected distant metastases may be revealed by systemic staging of locally advanced breast cancers by FDG PET/CT, and this has substantial impact on patient management. FDG PET/CT has demonstrated value in the evaluation of treatment response and in detection of disease recurrence.

Section 3: Innovative Radiotracers for Molecular Imaging of Breast Cancer

therapy response. The current multicenter trial of FES-PET imaging will help bring this radiotracer closer to clinical use. There is tremendous potential for these tracers to advance drug development, enhance the understanding of estrogen receptor–positive tumor biology, and personalize treatment.

Increased expressions of the human epidermal growth factor receptor (HER) protein family are targets in breast cancer for imaging and therapy. Imaging modalities targeting HER2 and HER3 can diagnose breast cancer with a specific, biologically relevant target. Repeat biopsies do not address heterogeneity intratumorally or between primary disease and metastasis. HER2- and HER3-targeted PET is an important tool to diagnose disease in breast cancer and evaluate response to targeted therapies. PET and single-photon emission computed tomography with radiolabeled biomolecules can be used to detect and quantify specific targets, conferring a better understanding of the behavior and effectiveness of treatments.

Amino acids are an alternate energy source to glucose, and amino acid metabolism is upregulated in multiple malignancies, including breast cancers. Multiple amino acid radiotracers have been used to image breast cancer, with unique strengths and weaknesses. ^{11}C-methionine uptake correlates with S-phase fraction in breast cancer and may be useful for the evaluation of treatment response. Invasive lobular breast cancers may demonstrate greater avidity for ^{18}F-fluciclovine than for ^{18}F-fluorodeoxyglucose. Thus, different histologic subtypes of breast cancer may use diverse metabolic pathways and may be better imaged by different tracers.

Uncontrolled growth is a hallmark of cancer; imaging cell proliferation provides an early indicator of therapeutic response. This capability is especially well matched to the emerging cell cycle–specific chemotherapeutics with the goal of identifying patients who benefit from these treatments early in the course of treatment to guide personalized therapy. This article focuses on investigational cell proliferation imaging PET radiotracers to evaluate tumor proliferation in the setting of cell cycle–targeted chemotherapy and endocrine therapy for metastatic breast cancer.

PET CLINICS

THE CLINICS ARE AVAILABLE ONLINE!
Access your subscription at:
www.theclinics.com

PROGRAM OBJECTIVE

The goal of the *PET Clinics* is to keep practicing radiologists and radiology residents up to date with current clinical practice in positron emission tomography by providing timely articles reviewing the state of the art in patient care.

TARGET AUDIENCE

Practicing radiologists, radiology residents, and other health care professionals who provide patient care utilizing radiologic findings.

LEARNING OBJECTIVES

Upon completion of this activity, participants will be able to:
1. Review the role of FDG in breast cancer treatment response.
2. Discuss the molecular classification of breast cancer.
3. Recognize current and emerging predictive imaging biomarkers in breast cancer.

ACCREDITATION

The Elsevier Office of Continuing Medical Education (EOCME) is accredited by the Accreditation Council for Continuing Medical Education (ACCME) to provide continuing medical education for physicians.

The EOCME designates this enduring material for a maximum of 15 *AMA PRA Category 1 Credit*(s)™. Physicians should claim only the credit commensurate with the extent of their participation in the activity.

All other health care professionals requesting continuing education credit for this enduring material will be issued a certificate of participation.

DISCLOSURE OF CONFLICTS OF INTEREST

The EOCME assesses conflict of interest with its instructors, faculty, planners, and other individuals who are in a position to control the content of CME activities. All relevant conflicts of interest that are identified are thoroughly vetted by EOCME for fair balance, scientific objectivity, and patient care recommendations. EOCME is committed to providing its learners with CME activities that promote improvements or quality in healthcare and not a specific proprietary business or a commercial interest.

The planning committee, staff, authors and editors listed below have identified no financial relationships or relationships to products or devices they or their spouse/life partner have with commercial interest related to the content of this CME activity:

Abass Alavi, MD, MD (Hon), PhD (Hon), DSc (Hon); Sandip Basu, MD; Wendie A. Berg, MD, PhD; Dhritiman Chakraborty, MD; Suet-Feung Chin, BSc, PhD; Azadeh Elmi, MD; Amy M. Fowler, MD, PhD; David Groheux, MD, PhD; Kelly E. Henry, PhD; Andrei Iagaru, MD; Maxine S. Jochelson, MD; Alison Kemp; Rakesh Kumar, MD; Lizza Lebron-Zapata, MD; Jason S. Lewis, PhD; Hannah M. Linden, MD; Elizabeth S. McDonald, MD, PhD, FSBI; Ryogo Minamimoto, MD, PhD; Tracy-Ann Moo, MD; Deepa Narayanan, MS; Lanell M. Peterson, BA; Elena Provenzano, MBBS, PhD, FRCPath; Rachel Sanford, MD; Gary A. Ulaner, MD, PhD, FACM; John Vassallo; Vignesh Viswanathan.

The planning committee, staff, authors and editors listed below have identified financial relationships or relationships to products or devices they or their spouse/life partner have with commercial interest related to the content of this CME activity:

Chau Dang, MD: has received research support from Genentech, Inc. and Puma Biotechnology, Inc.
David Mankoff, MD, PhD: is a consultant/advisor for Blue Earth Diagnostics Limited and General Electric Company; has received research support from Siemens Medical Solutions USA, Inc.; and has been a consultant/advisor and owns stock in Reflexion Medical
Monica Morrow, MD: has been a consultant/advisor for Genomic Health
David M. Schuster, MD: has participated in a speaker's bureau for PETNET Solutions, Inc. and has been a consultant/advisor for Syncona

UNAPPROVED/OFF-LABEL USE DISCLOSURE

The EOCME requires CME faculty to disclose to the participants:
1. When products or procedures being discussed are off-label, unlabelled, experimental, and/or investigational (not US Food and Drug Administration [FDA] approved); and
2. Any limitations on the information presented, such as data that are preliminary or that represent ongoing research, interim analyses, and/or unsupported opinions. Faculty may discuss information about pharmaceutical agents that is outside of FDA-approved labelling. This information is intended solely for CME and is not intended to promote off-label use of these medications. If you have any questions, contact the medical affairs department of the manufacturer for the most recent prescribing information.

TO ENROLL

To enroll in the *PET Clinics* Continuing Medical Education program, call customer service at 1-800-654-2452 or sign up online at http://www.theclinics.com/home/cme. The CME program is available to subscribers for an additional annual fee of USD $235.

METHOD OF PARTICIPATION

In order to claim credit, participants must complete the following:

1. Complete enrolment as indicated above.
2. Read the activity.
3. Complete the CME Test and Evaluation. Participants must achieve a score of 70% on the test. All CME Tests and Evaluations must be completed online.

CME INQUIRIES/SPECIAL NEEDS

For all CME inquiries or special needs, please contact elsevierCME@elsevier.com

Preface

Uses and Opportunities for Molecular Imaging in Patients with Breast Cancer

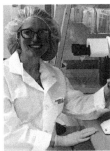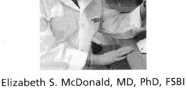

Elizabeth S. McDonald, MD, PhD, FSBI   Gary A. Ulaner, MD, PhD, FACNM

Editors

PET has established itself as a clinically valuable imaging method for patients with breast cancer, particularly as hybrid PET/computed tomography (CT) and now as PET/MR. Given the substantial impact of FDG PET and the growing numbers of novel PET radiotracers in development for patients with breast cancer, it is timely for *PET Clinics* to review the status of current and future PET imaging modalities for breast malignancy.

This issue of *PET Clinics* is divided into three sections. The first section covers the principles of breast cancer detection and characterization, which are important for interpretation of PET and other imaging studies. Lebron-Zapata and Jochelson begin the issue with an overview of current breast cancer screening and diagnosis, describing the anatomic and molecular techniques currently in use and the opportunities for molecular and PET techniques to aid in this important aspect of patient care. Next, Provenzano and colleagues summarize the important molecular and histologic subtypes of breast cancer and illustrate how these differences impact the interpretation of PET examinations. Moo and colleagues then summarize the principles of breast cancer therapy, highlighting that while MR has been shown to be effective for surveillance within the breast, other imaging modalities have not demonstrated effective surveillance for recurrence of metastatic disease in asymptomatic patients. This represents an area of tremendous opportunity for PET and other molecular techniques to develop and provide clinical value.

The second section of this issue emphasizes current concepts and successful clinical applications of PET and molecular imaging in patients with breast cancer. FDG is the PET radiotracer that has by far played the most valuable role in PET imaging of breast cancer, including important contributions for the initial systemic staging of patients with locally advanced breast cancer and monitoring of treatment response. These clinical applications of FDG PET are reviewed by Chakraborty and colleagues and Groheux. Dedicated imaging of the breasts by gamma and PET techniques has led to improved molecular imaging of primary breast malignancies. These techniques, their potential clinical applications, and the barriers to widespread adoption of these technologies are summarized by Narayanan and Berg. Bone is the most common site of metastatic disease from breast cancer. Minamimoto and Iagaru appraise the roles of molecular and PET imaging for the detection and monitoring of osseous metastases. Sentinel lymph node mapping is an important molecular imaging technique, but as PET imaging does not yet contribute to sentinel node imaging, it was not included as an article in this issue. For a discussion of sentinel node imaging for patients with breast cancer, we suggest a separate excellent recent review by Kim and Zukotynski.[1]

PET Clin 13 (2018) xi–xii
https://doi.org/10.1016/j.cpet.2018.05.001
1556-8598/18/© 2018 Published by Elsevier Inc.

The third and final section of this issue addresses the tremendous recent advances in the development of novel PET radiotracers for patients with breast cancer. Hormone receptor-targeted PET has a growing range of applications in breast cancer, including assisting early-phase clinical trials of new estrogen receptor (ER)-targeted drug therapies and predicting clinical benefit from these targeted therapies. The developing applications of hormone receptor-targeted PET imaging are discussed by Linden and colleagues. Human epidermal growth factor receptor (HER) family members are the targets of some of the most successful systemic therapies for patients with breast cancer. This makes the potential of HER2- and HER3-targeted imaging an area of considerable interest. These developing applications, including evaluation of heterogeneity of HER2 expression within an individual patient, are presented by Henry and colleagues. Amino acids are an alternate energy source to glucose in multiple malignancies, including breast cancer. Ulaner and Schuster discuss the potential of amino acid tracers for breast cancer, including the finding that lobular breast cancers are more avid for an amino acid tracer than for FDG. Finally, imaging cell proliferation may be valuable as an early indicator of cancer therapy response. Elmi and colleagues review the development of investigational PET imaging agents for cell proliferation.

We hope this issue of *PET Clinics* provides an overview of the principles of breast cancer and applications of PET imaging in these patients that will improve your interpretation of PET studies and challenge the field to develop new solutions to unanswered questions.

Elizabeth S. McDonald, MD, PhD, FSBI
University of Pennsylvania
3400 Spruce Street
Philadelphia, PA 19104-4283, USA

Gary A. Ulaner, MD, PhD, FACNM
Department of Radiology
Memorial Sloan Kettering Cancer Center
1275 York Avenue, Box 77
New York, NY, 10065, USA

Department of Radiology
Weill Cornell Medical School
New York, NY, 10065, USA

E-mail addresses:
Elizabeth.Mcdonald@uphs.upenn.edu
(E.S. McDonald)
ulanerg@mskcc.org (G.A. Ulaner)

REFERENCE

1. Kim CK, Zukotynski KA. Desirable properties of radiopharmaceuticals for sentinel node mapping in patients with breast cancer given the paradigm shift in patient management. Clin Nucl Med 2017;42(4): 275–9.

Section 1: Principles of Breast Cancer

Overview of Breast Cancer Screening and Diagnosis

Lizza Lebron-Zapata, MD*, Maxine S. Jochelson, MD

KEYWORDS

- Screening mammography • Tomosynthesis • Whole-breast ultrasound
- Contrast-enhanced mammography • Breast MR imaging • Breast imaging with sestamibi
- Positron emission mammography

KEY POINTS

- Screening mammography remains the only examination to reduce breast cancer mortality. Among the guidelines, annual screening from ages 40 to 84 has the highest mortality reduction.
- Physiologic plus anatomic imaging is superior to purely anatomic imaging in both sensitivity and specificity for breast cancer detection.
- Molecular imaging of the breasts can detect mammographically occult breast cancers, but the high total body dose of the tracers precludes yearly screening.

INTRODUCTION

Breast cancer is a leading cause of death among women worldwide. Over the past several decades there has been significant improvement in survival. New treatment strategies, including better chemotherapy and targeted therapies (precision medicine), are partially responsible for this improvement. Even in this era of precision medicine, however, it remains true that smaller, node-negative cancers have better outcomes than larger node-positive cancers. The ability to detect smaller cancers is the result of breast cancer screening.

SCREENING MAMMOGRAPHY

Mammographic breast cancer screening (**Fig. 1**) continues to be a controversial issue. Numerous prospective randomized screening trials in the 1970s, however, prove that early diagnosis of breast cancer translates into a survival benefit, which also implies that breast cancer is not necessarily a primary systemic disease. Clinical studies since then consistently show an approximately 30% decrease in breast cancer–specific mortality.[1–3] Additionally, in women from ages 40 years to 49 years, those who are screened are less likely to require chemotherapy or mastectomy compared with those who are not screened.[4]

Routine mammographic screening continues to be highly recommended by many professional organizations. These organizations, however, offer competing guidelines for women at average risk (**Box 1**). The current standard recommendation in the United States is annual screening beginning at age 40 years until life expectancy is less than 5 years. This recommendation is supported by the Society of Breast Imaging (SBI), American College of Radiology (ACR), National Comprehensive Cancer Network (NCCN), National Consortium of Breast Centers, and the American Congress of Obstetricians and Gynecologists (ACOG). In 2009, the United States Preventive Services Task Force (USPSTF) alternatively recommended biennial screening from ages 50 years to 74 years. The USPSTF concluded that evidence was insufficient for screening beyond 74 years. In 2016, USPSTF recommendations as part of updated guidelines remained unchanged but they noted that women between ages 40 years and 50 years may discuss

Disclosure Statement: The authors have nothing to disclose.
Department of Radiology, Memorial Sloan Kettering Cancer Center, 1275 York Avenue, New York, NY 10065, USA
* Corresponding author.
E-mail address: lebronzl@mskcc.org

PET Clin 13 (2018) 301–323
https://doi.org/10.1016/j.cpet.2018.02.001
1556-8598/18/Published by Elsevier Inc.

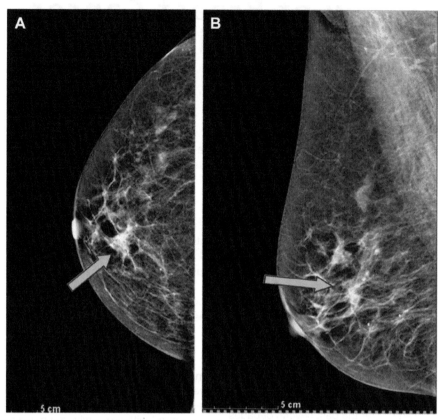

Fig. 1. Screening mammogram. (*A*) Craniocaudal view demonstrating a spiculated suspicious mass (*arrow*) in the medial breast, anterior third depth. (*B*) Mediolateral view demonstrating the partially obscured suspicious mass (*arrow*) in the superior breast, anterior third depth. This was subsequently biopsied and proved to be invasive carcinoma.

Box 1
Summary of the current guidelines for average-risk woman

Screening guidelines 2016: average risk

SBI, ACR, ACOG: current standard

- Annual mammography beginning at age 40 years until life expectancy less than 5 years
- Yearly clinical breast examinations

ACS

- Annual mammography from ages 45 years to 54 years but can begin at age 40
- Transition to every 2 years after age 55 years until life expectancy less than 10 years but can do yearly
- No breast examination by physician, no self-examination

USPSTF

- Ages 40 years to 49 years, discuss with MD
- Biennial mammography from ages 50 years to 74 years

the utility of mammograms with their doctors. This is also supported by American Association of Family Practice and the American College of Physicians. In 2015, the American Cancer Society (ACS) issued new guidelines, taking a middle road between the standard guidelines and USPSTF guidelines. The ACS recommended annual screening from ages 45 years to 54 years and biannual screening until life expectancy is less than 10 years. The American Society of Clinical Oncology and the American Society of Breast Surgeons support these recommendations.

To compare standard guidelines and USPTF guidelines, Arleo and colleagues[5] evaluated outcomes of the 3 screening paradigms using CISNET modeling. They found that the mean mortality reduction was greatest with annual screening from ages 40 years to 84 years (39.6%) compared with the ACS guidelines (30.8%) and the USPSTF guidelines (23.2%).

LIMITATIONS OF MAMMOGRAPHY

Despite substantial benefits, there are several valid criticisms and limitations of screening mammography. Although its general sensitivity ranges from 70% to 85%, screening mammography is much less sensitive in approximately 50% of women with dense breasts.[6,7] In these women, supplemental imaging is likely necessary.

In addition, screening mammography is said not to decrease the number of patients presenting with advanced disease, is associated with harms caused by anxiety from being called back for additional imaging or biopsy, and is criticized for leading to overdiagnosis. We describe the limitations of screening mammography below and elaborate upon supplemental screening after.

No Decrease in Advanced Cancers

Mammography preferentially detects slowly growing cancers.[8] This fact is well established in the scientific literature. Cancers detected mammographically are usually less aggressive and tend to have a better prognosis than cancers detected by other modalities, such as MR imaging.[9] Critics of mammography cite this effect as "length bias," which is a concept that mammographic screening is more apt to detect slower-growing cancers but tends to miss the faster-growing more aggressive tumors that may appear between screens as interval cancers.[8] A study by Sung and colleagues[9] agrees with this concept. Their study found that in women at high risk for breast cancer, cancers detected at screening with MR imaging were more likely to be invasive, whereas cancers detected at screening mammography were ductal carcinoma in situ (DCIS) or lower-grade tumors.

Anxiety from Call Backs

The specificity of screening mammography in randomized controlled trials is high, ranging from 93% to 99%.[10] Lehman and colleagues[11] showed a specificity of 88.9% as part of an update from the Breast Cancer Surveillance Consortium (BCSC). On the other hand, the positive predictive value (PPV) of mammography has been reported to range from 10% to 35%[12] and was 28.6% in the BCSC.[11]

Critics point to the harms related to the anxiety of being called back for additional imaging, image-guided biopsy, or surgery. In the writing of the ACS guidelines, it was determined that the risk of anxiety/benefit ratio stated by the USPSTF was overstated and that the actual benefit of mammography compared with the risks warranted the updated guidelines.

Overdiagnosis

Overdiagnosis is defined as screen-detected cancers that otherwise would not come to clinical attention due to the indolent nature of the cancer or comorbidities. Although there is little disagreement that overdiagnosis exists, the degree to which it exists is a major area of disagreement. Recent analyses suggest that 1% to 10% of mammographic detected cancers are clinically unimportant or overdiagnosed.[13,14] DCIS has been increasingly diagnosed by screening mammography and is often considered as an over-diagnosed cancer.

Because the benefit-to-risk ratio overwhelmingly favors the value of screening for detecting lesions that are clinically significant, concerns about overtreatment of the small number of nonprogressive lesions should be directed at choices regarding therapy, not screening. Prospective trials offering less treatment to patients with certain subtypes of cancer are under way to determine if there are accurate ways to determine which cancers do not need to be treated. Until those trials are completed, it is difficult to accurately withhold or reduce treatment in any one group.

Screening, even with overdiagnosis, has been shown to be valuable. In a study evaluating the utility of mammographic screening in English and Swedish women from ages 50 years to 69 years, Duffy and colleagues[15] compared the number of breast cancer deaths that were prevented to the tumors considered overdiagnosed by mammography. They confirmed that screening significantly reduced breast cancer mortality, with the absolute benefits estimated at 8.8 breast cancer deaths and 5.7 breast cancer deaths prevented per 1000 women screened for 20 years starting at age 50 from the Sweden Two-County Trial and the screening program in England, respectively. They found that between 2 lives and 2.5 lives are saved for every overdiagnosed case.

SUPPLEMENTAL SCREENING FOR BREAST CANCER IN WOMEN AT INCREASED RISK

Because of the inherent limitations of mammography described previously, supplemental imaging may be warranted in both average-risk women with dense breasts as well as women at increased risk.

Current Guidelines for Supplemental Screening

The 2007 ACS guidelines[16] are the current standard for supplemental screening in women at high risk. Their evidence-based recommendation is to add yearly screening MR imaging to mammography for women with a greater than 20% lifetime risk for developing breast cancer based on breast cancer risk models (eg, BRCAPRO or other models largely dependent on family history) (**Box 2**).

The ACS does not recommend for or against MR imaging screening for intermediate-risk women due to insufficient evidence. For example, the study by Sung and colleagues[17] found that MR imaging was a useful adjunct modality in women with a history of lobular carcinoma in situ (LICS), a high-risk marker: 17 cancers were detected in 14 patients; 12 cancers were detected with MR imaging alone; and 5 were detected with mammography alone. MR imaging resulted in a 4.5% incremental cancer detection rate. Finding additional cancers, however, does not always translate into improved outcomes. In a large prospectively maintained database comprising 776 women with LCIS, King and colleagues[18] did not find that MR imaging improved outcomes when comparing cancer detection rates with mammography alone versus mammography plus MR imaging. Cancer detection rates were 13% in both groups and MR imaging was not associated with earlier stage, smaller size, or node negativity. Thus, they concluded that routine MR imaging did not result in increased cancer detection rates (short-term) or earlier stage at diagnosis.

Another population at increased risk for developing breast cancer is that of breast cancer survivors, comprising greater than 3 million women in the United States. Current ACS and NCCN guidelines recommend yearly mammography for breast cancer survivors unless they have greater than 20% lifetime risk. This is in part due to concern over poor specificity of MR imaging leading to additional call backs and biopsies. Some investigators, however, demonstrated the value of MR imaging in breast cancer survivors. Brennan and colleagues[19] evaluated the cancer detection and biopsy rate of MR imaging among breast cancer survivors with no other risk factors and found that MR imaging was clinically valuable, finding malignancies in 12%, with a PPV of 39%. Similarly, Lehman and colleagues[20] evaluated screening MR imaging in women with personal history of breast cancer compared with those with genetic risk or

---

Box 2
Recommendations for breast MR imaging screening as an adjunct to mammography

Recommend annual MR imaging screening (based on evidence[a])

- BRCA mutation
- First-degree relative of BRCA carrier but untested
- Lifetime risk approximately 20%–25% or greater, as defined by BRCAPRO or other models that are largely dependent on family history

Recommend annual MR imaging screening (based on expert consensus opinion[b])

- Radiation to chest between ages 10 years and 30 years
- Li-Fraumeni syndrome and first-degree relatives
- Cowden and Bannayan-Riley-Ruvalcaba syndromes and first-degree relatives

Insufficient evidence to recommend for or against MR imaging screening[c]

- Lifetime risk 15% to 20%, as defined by BRCAPRO or other models that are largely dependent on family history
- Lobular carcinoma in situ or atypical lobular hyperplasia
- Atypical ductal hyperplasia
- Heterogeneously or extremely dense breast on mammography
- Women with a personal history of breast cancer, including DCIS

Recommend against MR imaging screening (based on expert consensus opinion)

- Women at 15% lifetime risk

[a] Evidence from nonrandomized screening trials and observational studies.
[b] Based on evidence of lifetime risk for breast cancer.
[c] Payment should not be a barrier. Screening decisions should be made on a case-by-case basis, because there may be particular factors to support MR imaging. More data on these groups are expected to be published soon.

family history of breast cancer and found that false-positive rates were lower in the former (12.3% vs 21.6%), specificity was higher (94.0% vs 86.0%), and sensitivity and cancer detection rate were not statistically different (*P*>.99). Therefore, in their analysis, MR imaging performance was superior and should be considered in breast cancer survivors.

Increased Breast Density

Increased breast density is a 2-fold problem for women: it is associated with an increased risk of breast cancer and may also make breast cancer more difficult to detect by mammography, thereby increasing the risk of interval cancers. Boyd and colleagues[21] demonstrated that women with dense breasts (mammographic density of 75% or more) had an increased risk of breast cancer (odds ratio, 4.7) compared with those who had less than 10% density. A meta-analysis found that 10% of women with extremely dense breasts have a 4-fold to 6-fold increase of breast cancer compared with 10% of women with predominantly fatty breast, in addition to leading to reduced sensitivity and specificity of mammography.[22] This reduced ability to detect breast cancers leads to an increase in interval cancers and cancers that are larger at presentation.

As discussed previously, dense breasts are an important limitation in breast cancer screening and affect approximately 50% of women. Breast density is currently classified by visual assessment according to the ACR Breast Imaging Reporting and Data System (BI-RADS) 4-category scale although development of more objective methods of assessing breast density is a significant area of research. The 2013 BI-RADS density terminology[23] is used to classify the levels of breast density and to standardize mammographic reporting. The categories are "a" to "d" rather than numbers (to avoid confusion with the BI-RADS classification system for determining the likelihood of cancer) (**Fig. 2**):

a. Breast tissue is almost entirely fatty 10%
b. Breast tissue with scattered areas of fibro-glandular density 40%
c. Breast tissue is heterogeneously dense, which may obscure small masses 40%
d. Breast tissue is extremely dense, which lowers the sensitivity of mammography 10%

The magnitude of the dense breast problem is both the number of women with dense breasts and the significant change in the accuracy of mammography as a result. The BCSC demonstrated that 43.3% of American women between ages 40 years and 74 years had dense breasts, approximately 27.6 million women.[24] A prospective cohort of 365,426 women with dense breasts ages 40 years to 74 years who had 831,455 digital screening mammography examinations showed that sensitivity decreased from 81% to 63% and specificity decreased from 94% to 89% in women ages 40 years to 49 years, and sensitivity decreased from 91% to 65% and specificity from 95% to 92% in women ages 50 years to 74 years.[25] Therefore, there needs to be a strategy for improved breast cancer detection for this large number of women.

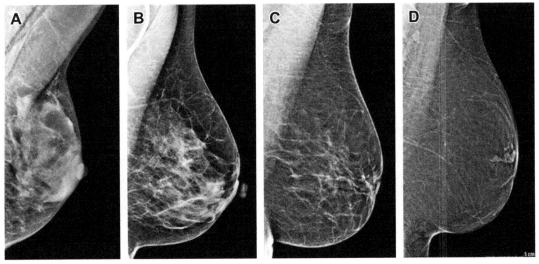

Fig. 2. Four categories of breast density: (*A*) extremely dense breast; (*B*) heterogeneously dense breast; (*C*) scattered fibroglandular densities; and (*D*) almost entirely fatty breast.

Supplemental screening of women with dense breasts or other increased risks will improve breast cancer detection rates. In the process, there will likely be an increase in the number of false-positive examinations and biopsies. It will, therefore, be critical to document that supplemental imaging findings will lead to improved survival and reduced morbidity. It is critical that good-quality prospective studies are done to both compare various supplemental modalities for their accuracy and demonstrate improved patient outcomes as a result.

ANATOMIC BREAST IMAGING MODALITIES
Digital Breast Tomosynthesis

Digital breast tomosynthesis (DBT) uses an x-ray source to acquire image data moving along an arc, and then thin slices are reconstructed in 3-D to decrease the effects of overlapping breast tissue, leading to improved conspicuity of lesions in the breast regardless of tissue density (Fig. 3).

In 2011, DBT was approved by the Food and Drug Administration (FDA) to be used in combination with standard digital mammography (DM) for breast cancer screening.[26] This combined mode (DM and

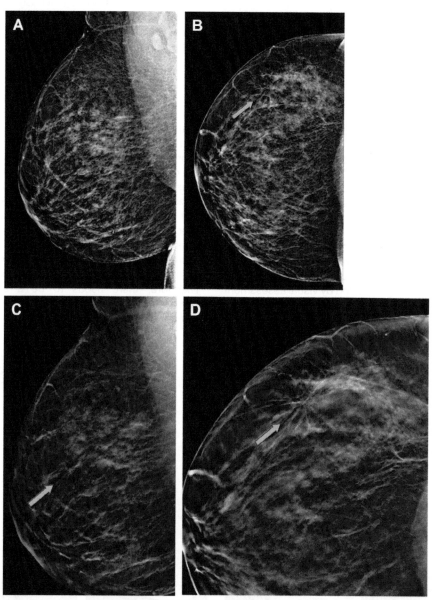

Fig. 3. Biopsy-proved invasive lobular carcinoma 2-D DBT craniocaudal (A) and (B) mediolateral views with subtle distortion in the right upper outer quadrant (arrow). 3-D mammogram confirms distortion on mediolateral (C) and craniocaudal (D) views, now more conspicuous (arrows) and not related to overlapping breast structures.

DBT) addresses the primary limitations of conventional screening mammography by increasing sensitivity without reducing specificity.[27–30]

Friedewald and colleagues[29] analyzed the added value of combining tomosynthesis to DM in 454,850 patients. DM alone detected cancer in 1207 patients, of the 5056 biopsies performed in 29,726 recalled patients. When DM was combined with tomosynthesis, 15,541 patients were recalled and 3,285 biopsies performed, yielding 950 cancers. Recall rates per 1000 screens were 107 women for DM and 91 women for DM combined with tomosynthesis, and cancer detection rates were 4.2 cancers versus 5.4 cancers, respectively. Tomosynthesis combined with DM increased the PPV for recall rate from 4.3% to 6.4%.

The prolonged effect of improved outcomes using DBT in addition to DM was assessed by McDonald and colleagues.[30] They analyzed 44,468 examinations in 23,958 women in 4 consecutive years. The number of cancers detected per recalled cases rose from 4.4% DM year 0 cohorts to 6.2%, 6.5%, and 6.7% for years 1, 2, and 3 of DBT, respectively. The recall rate for women who had DBT screening alone went from 130 women per 1000 women screened in year 1, to 78 women per 1000 women screened in year 2, to 59 women per 1000 women screened in year 3. Interval cancers rate was 0.7 per 1000 screened patients with DM compared with 0.5 per 1000 in those screened with DBT.

Total radiation dose when DBT is performed in addition to 2-D mammography is approximately 2 times the current DM dose but remains well below the limits defined by the FDA.[31] The reconstruction of a generated 2-D image from the tomosynthesis data set, a technology recently approved by the FDA, alleviates concerns regarding dose.[32] With the use of special software, 2-D images can be generated directly from the 3-D data set (eg, C-view (synthesized 2D image from the tomosynthesis image)), avoiding the need for the additional 2-D images. This keeps the radiation dose for DBT similar to that of DM.

Zuckerman and colleagues[33] compared synthesized 2-D DM (s2D) combined with DBT to DM with DBT in 15,571 women. The average glandular dose was 3% less in s2D/DBT versus DM/DBT, 4.88 mGy versus 7.97 mGy, respectively. Their data suggest that s2D could replace DM in DBT with less radiation dose but similar cancer detection rates.

In several studies, the addition of DBT to DM was associated with a reduction in recall rate.[29,34,35] For example, in a retrospective analysis[29] of 13 academic and nonacademic breast centers, DBT increased the detection of invasive cancer from 2.9 cancers per 1000 women to 4.1 cancers per 1000 women, a relative increase of 41%, whereas detection of DCIS was unchanged at 1.4 per 1000.

In a large prospective screening trial of more than 12,000 women, Skaane and colleagues[36] found a 27% increase in breast cancer detection rates when tomosynthesis was added to mammography with 8 per 1000 cancers found, with mammography plus tomosynthesis, compared with 6 per 1000 using only mammography. False-positive rates were lower when tomosynthesis was added to mammography, with a 15% decrease. There was a 40% increase in detection of invasive cancers when using combined modalities with 25 additional cancers detected.

Although most studies demonstrate a small additional detection rate of invasive cancers using DBT, it has not yet been demonstrated to improve survival. That said, in the United States, it is believed that DBT will become the standard method for mammographic screening rather than a supplemental examination particularly because of the significant reduction in the number of call backs without reduction in cancer detection.

The Tomosynthesis Mammographic Imaging Screening Trial (TMIST) Trial is the first randomized trial to compare the diagnostic accuracy of screening for breast cancer with 3-D DBT plus 2-D full-field DM (FFDM) versus FFDM alone. This is a multicenter study is currently enrolling patients, developed by the Eastern Cooperative Oncology Group (ECOG)–American College of Radiology Imaging Network (ACRIN) Cancer Research Group and the National Cancer Institute, part of the National Institutes of Health. This trial will attempt to better characterize the types of additional cancers and whether outcomes improve as a result.

Limitations of DBT that must be considered are increased radiation dose if not using reconstructed images, longer reading time, and increased expense.

Screening Ultrasound

Screening ultrasound is the most commonly used modality for supplemental imaging, particularly in women with dense breasts. Ultrasound is well tolerated, is relatively inexpensive, is widely available, and exposes patients to no radiation. Ultrasound detects approximately 1.9 to 4.2 additional cancers per 1000 women with negative mammograms, and its variability is in large part operator-dependant.[37] In the process of finding these additional cancers, however, it generates a large number of false-positive findings, leading to biopsies with a low PPV.[38]

Bilateral handheld screening ultrasound using a high-frequency transducer has been shown to detect early stage mammographically occult breast cancers (**Fig. 4**) in patients with dense

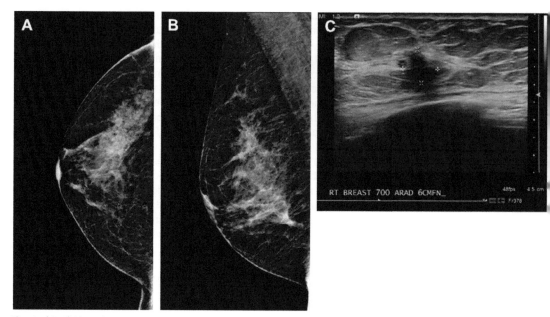

Fig. 4. (*A*, *B*) Negative screening mammogram in heterogeneously dense breast, craniocaudal (*A*) and mediolateral (*B*) views. (*C*) Subcentimeter invasive cancer found on screening ultrasound.

breast parenchyma.[39] Kaplan[40] evaluated 1862 asymptomatic women with dense breast tissue using bilateral whole-breast ultrasound as an adjunct examination to mammography. Ultrasounds were performed by a technologist and abnormal findings were corroborated by a fellowship-trained breast imaging radiologist. The average scanning time was 10 minutes and the cancer detection rate was 0.3%.

Several studies have assessed the clinical utility of ultrasound in women with dense breast as an adjunct study to mammography, often finding that cancers detected sonographically are mammographically occult even in retrospect. Bae and colleagues[41] reviewed 335 breast cancers seen only on screening ultrasound; 263 of 335 (78%) were mammographically occult due to dense breast tissue. In 72 patients (21%), cancer was not detected mammographically due to interpretive errors or because it was not included in the field-of-view due to location or positioning.

A randomized controlled trial by Ohuchi and colleagues[42] evaluated 72,998 asymptomatic women ages 40 to 49 years without a personal history of cancer in the Japan Strategic Anti-cancer Randomized Trial. They randomly assigned women in a 1:1 ratio into either an intervention group (mammography and ultrasonography) or a control group (mammography alone). The women underwent screening twice in 2 years. The intervention group was associated with a higher sensitivity (91% vs 77%) but lower specificity (87% vs 91%). Cancers detected in the intervention group

were more frequently stages 0 and I (144 [71%] vs 79 [52%]). In the future, this study will assess for changes in survival as a result of the ultrasound screening.

In a population of 935 women with dense breast tissue, Hooley and colleagues[38] evaluated the performance and utility of additional screening breast ultrasound. The false-positive rate was 5% and the overall PPV for interventions performed in patients with BI-RADS category 4 results was 6.5% (3 of 46). Three cancers were detected per 1000 women screened. Although technologist-performed handheld screening breast ultrasound offered to women in the general population with dense breasts can aid detection of small mammographically occult breast cancers, this analysis again demonstrated a low PPV for screening breast ultrasound.

In Connecticut, where dense breast legislation was first implemented, Weigert[43] retrospectively reviewed the addition of screening breast ultrasound in women with mammographically normal but dense breasts for 4 consecutive years. In the first year, they performed 151 biopsies in 2706 patients who underwent ultrasound and found 11 cancers, with a PPV of 7.3% and 4 cancers per 1000 women screened detection rate. In the second year, they detected 11 cancers and high-risk lesions after performing 180 biopsies in 3351 patients who underwent ultrasound, with a PPV of 6.1% and a detection rate of 3 cancers per 1000 women screened. In the third year, they performed 148 biopsies on 4128 patients and found 13 cancers and high-risk lesions with a PPV of 8.8% and a cancer detection rate of 3.1 cancers per 1000 women screened. The fourth year, the PPV increased to 20.1%, 11 cancers were detected in 3331 patients with a detection rate of 3.3 cancers per 1000 women screened. The detection rate was maintained at the same level, whereas the PPV doubled in 4 years.

In an effort to prospectively compare the additional value of DBT to ultrasound, Tagliafico and colleagues[44] conducted a trial evaluating 3231 mammography-negative women. They found that in women with dense breast and negative mammograms, sonography has a higher cancer detection rate compared with tomosynthesis (7.1 vs 4.0), with a similar recall rate.

A study by Nam and colleagues[45] evaluated the percentage of cancers detected by screening ultrasonography compared with FFDM and DBT in women with negative mammograms and sonographically detected breast cancers; 25 of the 41 cases (61.0%) were visible on FFDM and 34 cancers (82.9%) were seen on DBT. 54% of the cancers were detectable by screening using DBT but not evident on 2-D mammography.

In the ACRIN 6666 trial, screening ultrasound in approximately 3000 women with dense breasts and at least 1 other risk factor produced an increased detection of approximately 4 cancers per 1000 women screened.[46] The cancers detected were primarily invasive and node negative; 8% of these patients, however, were recommended to have biopsies and the PPV of these recommendations was less than 10%. Additionally, 612 of these women were offered screening MR imaging after 2 years of negative combined ultrasound and mammography and 16 cancers were detected. Of the 16 cancers detected, 9 (56%) were only seen on MR imaging. Therefore, a combination of a negative mammogram plus ultrasound may give a patient a false sense of security. This finding confirmed the idea that no matter how good the anatomic imaging is, physiologic imaging trumps purely anatomic imaging.

BREAST MR IMAGING

MR imaging is the most sensitive imaging method for breast cancer detection. Sensitivities range from 71% to 100% compared with 35% to 50% for mammography in high-risk women with dense breasts.[47] The sensitivity of MR imaging is in large part due to its ability to image neovascularity. Aggressive breast tumors maintain rapid growth by increasing the supply of oxygen and nutrients. The tumors achieve this by releasing peptides that promote angiogenesis. Angiogenesis then

leads to changes in the tumor's microvascular architecture, including development of new vessels and differentiation of endothelial cells. These changes tend to increase vascular permeability. Detection of these changes is possibly due to rapid enhancement and washout of contrast material on MR imaging, which is a characteristic finding of breast cancer[48,49] (**Fig. 5**). If tumor growth rate exceeds angiogenesis, hypoxia may occur. On diagnostic contrast-enhanced MR imaging, centrally hypoxic tumors may have rim enhancement.[50]

The specificity of MR imaging has been demonstrated to be lower than that of mammography in many studies, resulting in more recalls and biopsies.[51–54] MR imaging specificity improves with the interpreting radiologist's experience, and recall and false-positive rates decrease when prior MR images are available for comparison.[51,55]

One study comparing the sensitivity and specificity of mammography, ultrasound, MR imaging, and clinical breast examination in 278 BRCA1-positive or BRCA2-positive women detected 11 cancers in the first round of screening and 7 in the second round (14 invasive and 4 DCIS) Of these, 6 of 18 (33%) were found by MR imaging alone. The sensitivity was 94% for MR imaging, 59% for mammography, 65% for ultrasound, and 50% for clinical breast examination. PPV was 63% for MR imaging, 77% for mammography, 65% for ultrasound and 82% for clinical breast examination.

Follow-up of a large prospective Dutch multicenter study (MRI Screening [MRISC])[56,57] was performed to determine whether the increased screening accuracy of MR imaging over mammography would prevail on subsequent screening sessions. After analyzing 2157 women with hereditary breast cancer, including 599 mutation carriers, they confirmed that MR imaging was more sensitive for invasive cancers but not DCIS. Results were inferior for BRCA1 patients compared with BRCA2 patients and those women at moderate risk. Patients diagnosed by MR imaging had lower-stage disease when compared with age-matched symptomatic controls. Cumulative distant metastasis-free and overall 6-year survival rates of 42 mutation carriers with invasive carcinoma were 83.9% for those with BRCA1 patients and 92.7% for BRCA2 patients. Survival was 100% in patients with familial breast cancer without an identified mutation. In a later comparison, 2308 women were matched with screened and unscreened women. Cancers in MRISC patients were smaller and more likely to be node negative. They demonstrated that annual screening with mammography and MR imaging

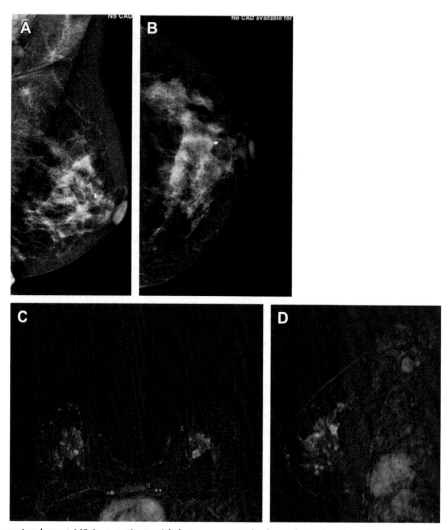

Fig. 5. Screening breast MR in a patient with heterogeneously dense breast and negative screening mammography. Axial (*C*) and sagittal (*D*) fat-saturated T1-weighted image demonstrating a mammographically occult enhancing irregular mass in the left upper inner breast (*arrows*), with subsequently biopsy yielding invasive carcinoma.

improved metastasis-free survival in BRCA1 carriers and those with familial histories of breast cancer (**Fig. 6**).

MR imaging screening in mutation carriers has also been demonstrated to detect smaller cancers that are theoretically associated with better outcomes. A study by Warner and colleagues[58] evaluated 1275 mutation carriers. They demonstrated that patients screened with MR imaging were significantly more likely to present with DCIS or early-stage cancers than those not screened with MR imaging.

Lastly, a prospective multicenter cohort by Kuhl and colleagues[59] investigated the cancer yield and stage at diagnosis of clinical breast examination, mammography, ultrasound, and quality-assured breast MR imaging, to determine the superiority of MR imaging used alone or in a different combination for screening women at elevated risk for breast cancer. They found 27 women with breast cancer: 11 DCIS (41%) and 16 invasive cancers (59%). Mammography detected 5.4 cancers per 1000 women, ultrasound 6 cancers per 1000 women, and combined mammography and ultrasound 7.7 cancers per 1000 women whereas MR imaging alone detected 14.9 cancers per 1000 women. The detection rate of MR imaging was not significantly improved by adding mammography (MR imaging plus mammography: 16.0 cancers per 1000 women) and did not change by adding ultrasound (MR imaging plus ultrasound: 14.9 cancers per 1000 women). PPV was 39% for mammography, 36% for ultrasound, and 48% for MR imaging.

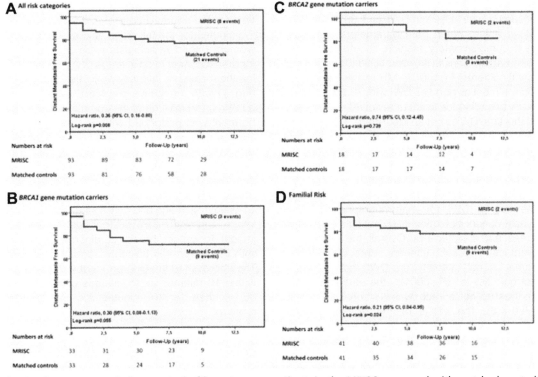

Fig. 6. Distant metastasis-free survival of breast cancer patients in the MRISC compared with matched controls per risk category. MRISC patients were screened with annual mammography and MR imaging. Controls received no screening if younger than 50 years or were screened with biennial mammography in the Dutch National Population Breast Cancer Screening Program if age 50 years or older. Controls were matched on risk category, age of diagnosis, and year of diagnosis. Distant metastasis-free survival was defined as time from histologic diagnosis until breast cancer specific distant metastasis. Differences in breast cancer specific distant metastasis free survival were compared by means of a log-rank test. The unadjusted hazard ratio for breast cancer–specific distant metastasis of the MRISC patients in comparison to the controls is shown. (*A*) All risk categories. (*B*) BRCA1 gene mutation carriers. (*C*) BRCA2 gene mutation carriers. (*D*) Familial risk. (*From* Saadatmand S, Obdeijn IM, Rutgers EJ, et al. Survival benefit in women with BRCA1 mutation or familial risk in the MRI screening study (MRISC). Int J Cancer 2015;137(7):1735; with permission.)

Diffusion-Weighted Imaging

Diffusion-weighted imaging (DWI) is a method of tissue characterization based on the different freedom of movement of water molecules (diffusion) along multiple spatial directions, quantified via the measurement of the mean diffusivity and the apparent diffusion coefficient (ADC). Malignant breast tissues show restricted diffusion and significantly lower ADC values compared with those of normal and benign breast tissues. For instance, Bogner and colleagues[60] compared the diagnostic quality of DWI schemes and found that an ADC threshold level of 1.25×10^{-3} mm^2/s allowed discrimination between malignant and benign lesions with a diagnostic accuracy of 95%. The best contrast-to-noise ratio for tumors was identified at 850 mm^2/s.

An advantage of DWI is that it does not require contrast administration. At a time when repeated use of gadolinium has been shown to cause deposition of gadolinium in brain tissue, there is great interest in performing highly accurate MR imaging without contrast. Pinker and colleagues (Pinker K, Moy L, Sutton EJ, et al. DWI with apparent diffusion coefficient mapping for breast cancer detection: comparison with dynamic contrast-enhanced and multiparametric magnetic resonance imaging. Submitted for publication.) analyzed whether DWI could be used as a stand-alone parameter for breast cancer detection and compared it with dynamic contrast-enhanced (DCE)–MR imaging and multiparametric MR imaging. Of the 110 detected breast tumors, 42 were benign and 58 were malignant. DCE–MR imaging was the most sensitive test for breast cancer detection with sensitivity of 100%. DWI as a stand-alone parameter was significantly less sensitive with 80% but more specific, 78.6%, compared with DCE–MR imaging, with 66.7%. Diagnostic accuracy was 80% for DWI and 86% for DCE–MR imaging. When both parameters were used in a complementary fashion as multiparametric MR imaging, sensitivity was still 96.7%, not significantly different from DCE–MR imaging and specificity almost as good as DWI with 76.2%, resulting in the best diagnostic accuracy of 88%. Therefore, at this time DWI is not an ideal stand-alone parameter for breast cancer detection. Many investigators, however, are working on improving DWI techniques with the hope of improving sensitivity further without sacrificing specificity.

A group led by Elizabeth McDonald[61] analyzed the use of DWI for mammographically occult breast cancer detection in 48 patients with dense breast and elevated-risk. Overall, the 24 mammographically occult cancers detected showed higher signal intensity on DWI than ipsilateral normal tissue (P<.0001); the median lesion contrast-to-noise ratio was 1.4 on DWI (range, -0.6–4.6). The ADCs of the lesions (median, 1.31×10^{-3} mm^2/s; range, 0.49–2.24 $\times$ 10^{-3} mm^2/s) were lower than the ADCs of the ipsilateral normal tissue (median, 1.79×10^{-3} mm^2/s; range, 1.33–2.39 $\times$ 10^{-3} mm^2/s; P<.0001). Therefore, their conclusion was that DWI can detect mammographically occult cancers with a low false-positive rate.

Abbreviated MR imaging

Because of the superb sensitivity of MR imaging, it would be ideal to perform MR imaging on larger populations of women than just those with greater than 20% risk. MR imaging is expensive, however, and not uniformly available to all women. Abbreviated breast MR imaging protocols are an attempt to address these issues. Kuhl and colleagues[62] prospectively evaluated 606 screening MR images in high-risk patients with a 3-minute acquisition time for the abbreviated protocol (compared with 17 minutes for the full diagnostic protocol) in 443 women. Expert radiologists were able to screen for breast cancer in an average of 2.8 seconds using the maximum intensity projection (MIP) image (**Fig. 7**) with a negative predictive value (NPV) of 99.8%. Interpretation of the complete abbreviated protocol was performed with an average time of 28 seconds and all cancers were diagnosed; sensitivity was 100% and specificity 94.3%. Similarly, a study by Mango and colleagues[63] evaluated breast cancer detection with an abbreviated breast MR imaging protocol using precontrast T1-weighted image and only a single postcontrast image (and single early postcontrast T1-weighted image) to detect breast carcinoma in patients with biopsy proven unicentric breast carcinoma. The abbreviated imaging protocol was performed within 10 minutes to 15 minutes compared with 30 minutes to 40 minutes for the standard protocol.

CONTRAST-ENHANCED MAMMOGRAPHY

Even with abbreviated MR imaging, it may not be feasible to perform MR imaging on all women who require supplemental imaging. Additionally, claustrophobia, gadolinium allergies, and metallic implants limit the number of women who are able to undergo MR imaging.

Contrast-enhanced DM (CEDM) or contrast-enhanced spectral mammography (CESM) is a novel technique based on the same principle as MR imaging by imaging blood flow associated with neovascularity. It uses the platform of DM. Two nearly simultaneous images are performed with each exposure: a low-energy image below the K-edge of iodine (33 keV) and a high-energy

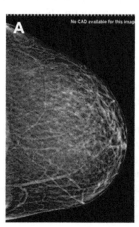
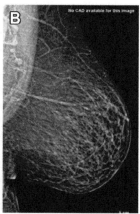
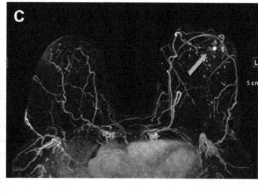

Fig. 7. Craniocaudal (*A*) and mediolateral (*B*) negative screening mammogram. (*C*) MIP single image of abbreviated screening MR imaging detecting a subcentimeter invasive carcinoma in the left breast (*arrow*).

image above the K-edge of iodine. Postprocessing subtracts out nonenhancing tissue, yielding an iodine image meant to enhance any cancers. Iodinate-based contrast, such as that used with CT at a dose of 1.5 mL/kg, is typically injected via power injector at 3 mL/s, The first image is acquired approximately 3 minutes postinjection. The standard craniocaudal and mediolateral oblique views are obtained within 5 minutes of completed injection and additional views can also be obtained because the contrast remains present for up to 10 minutes. Kinetic information, however, is not provided. The low-energy images are the equivalent of a routine mammogram so no additional mammogram is necessary. The radiation dose is approximately 20% more than routine screening mammogram or the equivalent of 1 extra image.[64]

In the diagnostic setting, multiple studies have demonstrated a higher sensitivity for CEDM compared with conventional mammography. Data have been consistent among all investigators. Jochelson and colleagues[64] demonstrated that the CEDM index cancer detection rate in a population with known cancer was both comparable to that of MR imaging and significantly better than mammography. Tumor visualization was independent of the order in which images were obtained. Overall, MR imaging and CEDM both depicted 50 (96%) of 52 index tumors, whereas conventional mammography depicted 42 (81%). CEDM depicted 14 (56%) of 25 additional ipsilateral cancers compared with 22 (88%) of 25 for MR imaging. There were 2 false-positive findings with CEDM and 13 false-positive findings with MR imaging. Thus, CEDM had a lower sensitivity for detecting additional ipsilateral cancers than did MR imaging, but the specificity of CEDM was significantly higher. Similarly, a study by Fallenberg and colleagues[65] compared standard mammography, CESM, and MR imaging in the detection and size estimation of newly diagnosed breast cancers in 80 women. Contrast mammography detected all 80 cancers whereas mammography only detected 66. MR imaging detected 77 of 79 examinations. Of the 14 cancers missed on mammography but seen on CESM, 13 were in women with dense breasts. No significant difference was found between lesion size measurement on MR imaging and contrast mammography compared with histopathology.

Preliminary results for the use of CEDM as a screening tool (**Fig. 8**) in women with intermediate risk or dense breasts are promising. In a prospective trial comparing CEDM to MR imaging, Jochelson and colleagues[66] assessed 307 heavily pre-screened patients and found no cancers on

mammography and 2 invasive lobular carcinomas on both CEDM and MR imaging. One patient had atypia on MR imaging not seen on CEDM, which was upgraded at surgery. After 1-year follow-up, 2 additional cancers were detected. Sung and colleagues[67] prospectively compared CEDM versus ultrasound in 250 intermediate-risk patients and found 5 cancers; of these 5 cancers, 1 was detected on conventional mammography, 2 were detected on ultrasound, and all 5 were detected on CEDM. These early data suggest that CEDM may be more sensitive than ultrasound in the screening setting.

As with MR imaging, calcifications on CEDM warrant biopsy, regardless of lack enhancement. Cheung and colleagues[68] evaluated 256 studies to determine the clinical utility of CEDM. They found 59 cases with suspicious malignant microcalcifications. Lesion enhancement was seen in 20 (76.9%) of 22 cancers, 3 (11.55%) of 19 atypical lesions, and 3 (11.55%) of 18 benign lesions. Overall, the diagnostic sensitivity of enhancement was 90.9%, with 83.78% specificity, 76.92% PPV, 93.94% NPV, and 86.4% accuracy.

Patient experience is also an important factor when comparing and deciding which modality is preferable. Hobbs and colleagues[69] compared patient experience of CEDM to contrast-enhanced MR imaging during preoperative breast cancer staging in 49 patients. They evaluated comfort of breast compression, comfort of intravenous contrast injection, anxiety, and overall preference. They demonstrated a significantly higher overall preference toward CEDM (n = 49, $P < .001$), with faster procedure time, greater comfort, and lower noise level cited as the most common reasons leading to lower anxiety.

CEDM also has limitations. A small number of patients are allergic to iodinated contrast material requiring screening prior to injection. Patients who are allergic to iodine should not undergo CEDM. Patients with compromised renal function should also not be given iodine for routine breast imaging examinations. Radiation dose is 20% higher than routine mammography but well within accepted Mammography Quality Standards Act guidelines. CEDM currently lacks biopsy capability. Lesions seen on low energy images or ultrasound can undergo biopsy using those stereotactic biopsy or ultrasound core biopsies but if suspicious enhancing lesions cannot be visualized, MR imaging is necessary.

MOLECULAR IMAGING OF THE BREAST

Mammography requires mass formation, tissue distortion, or calcium precipitation for cancer detection, which explains why the average size of cancer at detection by mammography is

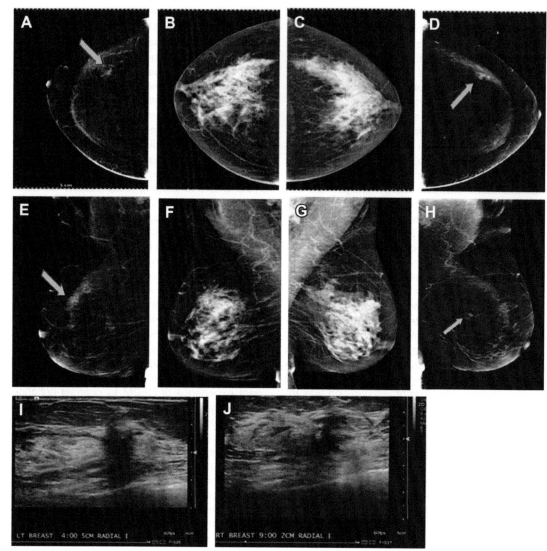

Fig. 8. Negative screening mammogram of heterogeneously dense breast, craniocaudal (*B, C*) and mediolateral views (*F, G*). CEDM craniocaudal (*A, D*) and mediolateral (*E, H*) views, demonstrating bilateral irregular enhancing masses (*arrows*). Bilateral ultrasound (*I, J*) demonstrating irregular hypoechoic masses; patient underwent ultrasound-guided biopsies yielding carcinomas.

1.5 cm. Ultrasound requires mass formation, with an average size of the detected tumors at 0.9 cm.[70] MR imaging and CEDM use enhancement of neovascularity in cancerous lesions to detect them at a smaller stage/size. Compared with these modalities, molecular imaging offers the advantage of being independent of either anatomic changes or capillary growth for detection. Physiologic changes are the earliest manifestations of cancer. Radiotracers can diffuse into the interstitial space and be taken up by the abnormal cells before the presence of a distinct mass or neovascularity, unaffected by breast density.

There are 2 broad categories of molecular breast imaging (MBI) using radionuclide tracers: techniques using sestamibi and those using PET tracers, primarily fludeoxyglucose F 18 (18F-FDG).

Techniques Using Sestamibi: Breast-Specific Gamma Imaging and Molecular Breast Imaging

Technetium (Tc99m)-sestamibi is a 140-keV gamma emitter with a half-life of 6 hours. Originally, it was a cationic lipophilic cardiac perfusion agent taken up by mitochondria. It entered into oncologic imaging when Hassan and colleagues first reported its use for lung cancer in 1989.[71] In 1990, it was subsequently approved by the FDA for imaging cardiac perfusion. Because of standard whole-body collimators, however, sensitivity was limited for small cancers. A prospective multicenter trial reported a sensitivity of only 48.2% for cancers smaller than 1 cm compared with 74.2% for larger tumors.[72] As such, this technique was abandoned until better breast imaging techniques could be developed.

Since 1990, 2 new imaging techniques have allowed the use of Tc99m-sestamibi for breast imaging: breast-specific gamma imaging (BSGI) and MBI. Both techniques use gentle compression for stabilizing the breast between a compression paddle and their detector(s), and similar positioning to that of mammography. The typical procedure is as follows: imaging begins 5 minutes after intravenous injection and involves 10-minute acquisitions for each of the 4 routine projections used in mammography. Additional views may also be required especially in women with larger breasts.

BSGI uses a single-detector scintillating NaI crystal. The potential impact of BSGI was evaluated in a multicenter study[73]; 1042 patients with equivocal conventional breast imaging or clinical finding were included found that BSGI was positive in 408 patients (227 malignant or high-risk lesions), negative in 634 patients (23 with malignant or high-risk lesions), and indeterminate in 69 patients (all benign). The overall sensitivity was 91% and specificity was 77%. A limitation of this analysis was that high-risk lesions were included as true positives, therefore increasing the specificity, whereas on standard breast imaging studies, high-risk lesions are considered false positives. The most prominent limitation of BSGI is the low sensitivity for small lesions. Park and colleagues[74] evaluated 56 breast cancers, 48 of which (85.7%) were positive on BSGI. Although the sensitivity of BSGI was 90.7% for tumors larger than 1 cm, however, it was only 55.6% when tumors were smaller than 1 cm. Seven cancers were not detected on mammography and 8 were not seen on BSGI.

MBI confers an advantage over BSGI, including improved sensitivity, spatial resolution, and lesion detection.[75,76] MBI uses 2 cadmium zinc telluride detectors.

Patient preparation is not required before imaging with sestamibi. Recent studies, however, show improved uptake of Tc99m-sestamibi if patients are in a fasting, resting, and warm state at the time of injection.[77]

Hruska and colleagues[78] evaluated 150 patients with BI-RADS category 4 (suspicious for cancer) or category 5 (highly suspicious for cancer) lesions smaller than 2 cm, identified on mammography or sonography and scheduled for biopsy, who underwent MBI with Tc99m-sestamibi. A total of 128 cancers were confirmed in 88 patients. The sensitivity of dual-head MBI was 90% (115/128), whereas the sensitivity from review of only single-head MBI was 80% (102/128). The overall sensitivity was 69% for lesions smaller than 5 mm, 88% invasive ductal carcinoma all sizes, 79% invasive lobular carcinoma all sizes, and 89% for all DCIS. For the detection of cancers less than or greater to 10 mm in diameter, the overall sensitivity was 82% (50/61) for dual-head MBI and 68% (41/61) for single-head MBI. On average, 13 additional cancers were seen on dual-head images.

MBI has been studied for its utility as a supplemental screening tool. Rhodes and colleagues[79] prospectively evaluated the diagnostic performance of supplemental screening MBI in women with mammographically dense breasts in 1585 participants with a complete reference standard. Of these, 21 were diagnosed with cancer: 2 were detected by mammography only, 14 by MBI only, 3 by both modalities, and 2 by neither. The cancers detected only by MBI were all invasive with a median size of 0.9 cm. The overall cancer detection rate (per 1000 women screened) increased from 3.2 to 12.0 by using MBI (supplemental yield 8.8). The combination of MBI and mammography yielded a sensitivity of 91%; specificity, 83%; and PPV3, 28%. These rates were much higher than mammography alone, which yielded a sensitivity of 24%; specificity, 89%; and PPV3, 25%. The cancer yield of 3.2 cancers per 1000 women screened and the sensitivity of 24% for mammography are well below those cited in any other study, limiting the applicability of these results.

MBI has been shown superior to BSGI.[80] It identifies 76% of cancers sized 6 to 10 mm and 71% less than or equal to 5 mm.

Similarly, Shermis and colleagues[81] retrospectively assessed the clinical performance of MBI as a supplementary screening tool for women with dense breast tissue in 1696 average risk women. They detected 13 mammographically occult malignancies, of which 11 were invasive, 1 was node positive, and 1 had unknown node positivity. The lesion size ranged from 0.6 cm to 2.4 cm, with a mean of 1.1 cm. The incremental cancer detection rate was 7.7%, the recall rate was 8.4%, and the biopsy rate was 3.7%. The PPV for biopsy was 19.4%.

Several small studies have compared BSGI to MR imaging for the detection of cancer. Kim and colleagues[82] demonstrated higher sensitivity for the detection of DCIS with MR imaging

(91.4%) compared with BSGI (68.6%) in 35 women with pathologically proved DCIS whereas Keto and colleagues[83] demonstrated equal sensitivity in a prospective trial of 18 patients. Brem and colleagues[84] demonstrated no significant difference in sensitivity between BSGI (89%) and MR imaging (100%) for the detection of invasive cancer in 8 patients with 9 cancers. In a recent meta-analysis of 10 studies with 517 patients, Zhang and colleagues[85] compared BSGI to MR imaging and demonstrated no significant difference in sensitivity (84% vs 89%) but superiority in specificity (82% vs 39%). They note, however, that for the detection of smaller lesions, imaging modalities using morphologic detection, such as MR imaging, are superior to BSGI because of their superior spatial resolution. Additionally, the sensitivity and specificity quoted for MR imaging are less than those actually seen in the literature.

Sestamibi imaging has also been evaluated for defining extent of disease in women with known cancer (Fig. 9). Zhou and colleagues[86] showed that BSGI detected additional disease in 10.9% of women with newly diagnosed breast cancer.

Sestamibi detects additional 7 mammographically occult cancers per 1000 women compared with ultrasound, which historically detects 3.5

cancers per 1000 women, and tomosynthesis 2 cancers per 1000 women.

A persistent barrier to use of MBI is concern about radiation exposure. Although the dose to the breast is low, the colon receives 40 mGy to 55.5 mGy.[87,88] Investigators have studied the possibility of reducing the dose of tracer and have demonstrated that it is possible to cut it in half without reducing sensitivity. The whole-body dose, however, remains a concern when considering it a yearly screening tool in normal-risk patients. BSGI and MBI are not currently standard screening modalities. Hendrick and Tredennick[89] demonstrated that even using lower doses of sestamibi (300 MBq), the benefit-to-risk ratio of BSGI is inferior to that of mammography.

Lack of biopsy capability and nonvalidated BI-RADS–like lexicon are important limitations for MBI.

Techniques Using Fluorodeoxyglucose: Breast PET and Positron Emission Mammography

Molecular imaging of breast cancer with fluoro-deoxyglucose (FDG) takes advantage of differences in metabolic activity between the tumor and normal tissue and, therefore, has the potential to improve detection of cancer in

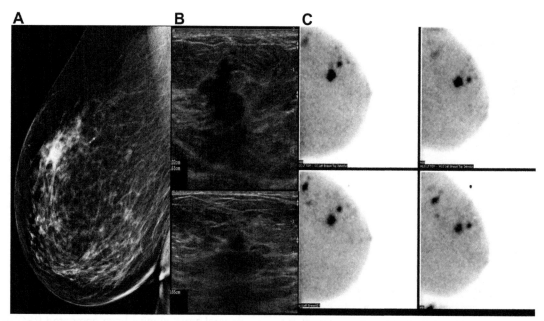

Fig. 9. (A) Mediolateral view on a mammogram showing an irregular mass (2 cm) in the left superior outer quadrant of the breast. (B) Two sonographically detected masses(larger one in the left 1:00 position, 2 × 1.6 cm and the smaller one in the left 2:00 position, 0.7 × 0.9 cm; the larger one is the correlate for mass seen on mammogram. (C) Craniocaudal and mediolateral molecular breast imaging views with multicentric disease detected.

mammographically dense breasts, distinguish recurrent cancer from scar tissue,[90] and depict the extent of disease for surgical planning.[91]

PET has been demonstrated to be an extremely sensitive and specific method of staging and following many cancers, including breast carcinoma. Many radiotracers are available but ^{18}F-FDG is currently the most commonly used, in part because of its relatively long half-life and in part because it uses the ever-present glycolytic pathway to visualize even small cancers: 18F-FDG is a 511-keV positron-emitting glucose analog with a half-life of 120 minutes. Imaging with FDG requires a 4-hour to 6-hour fasting period and 1 hour of resting after the tracer injection, prior to imaging. Just as with sestamibi imaging, however, early data regarding utility of FDG-PET for the detection of breast cancers showed poor sensitivity due to the distance of the breasts from the whole-body collimators. Again, newer techniques have been developed for breast PET imaging.

Positron emission mammography (PEM) of the breast can result in higher spatial resolution (1–2 mm) compared with whole-body PET (4–6 mm) by having the breasts in direct contact with the detectors and immobilizing the breast gently. PEM also minimizes the radiation dose by reducing breast thickness.[92] For each view (craniocaudad and mediolateral oblique of each breast), PEM requires 10 minutes and produces 12 essentially tomographic images.[92] PEM has shown greater sensitivity to small cancers than whole-body PET and sestamibi imaging due to higher spatial resolution. Eo and colleagues[93] analyzed 113 breast lesions in 101 patients who underwent 18F-FDG PEM and whole-body PET/CT before surgical resection. Overall, tumor size was 2.2 cm ± 1.1 cm. PEM showed significantly higher imaging sensitivity than PET/CT (95% vs 87), especially in the group with smaller tumors.

PEM has high diagnostic accuracy (**Fig. 10**) when interpreted with mammographic and clinical findings. A prospective multicenter trial[94] assessed 94 women with known breast cancer or suspicious breast lesions who received intravenous 18F-FDG prior to PEM. PEM detected 10 of 11 (91%) DCIS and 33 of 37 (89%) invasive cancers. Excluding 16 women (8 who were diabetic and 8 who had clearly benign lesions at conventional imaging), sensitivity was 91%, specificity

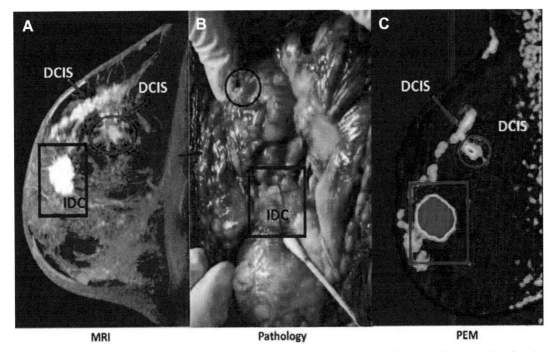

MRI   Pathology   PEM

Fig. 10. Radiopathologic correlation for invasive and in situ carcinomas. (*A*) MR imaging MIP projection showing an irregular enhancing mass consistent with invasive ductal carcinoma (IDC), linear clumped and nonmass enhancement at sites of DCIS. (*B*) Macroscopic pathologic specimen and (*C*) PEM mediolateral view correlation. (*Adapted from* MacDonald L, Edwards J, Lewellen T, et al. Clinical imaging characteristics of the positron emission mammography camera: PEM Flex Solo II. J Nucl Med 2009;50(10):1672; with permission.)

93%, PPV 95%, NPV 88%, and accuracy 92%. Additionally, compared with MR imaging, Berg and colleagues[95] showed that in 388 women with known cancer undergoing preoperative staging, the combination of PEM and MR imaging led to an increase in breast cancers detected versus MR imaging alone: 61/80 (74%) and 49/80 (60%), respectively.

Pros and cons of breast fluorodeoxyglucose PET and positron emission mammography

Dedicated breast PET is sensitive and specific, detecting malignancy regardless of density or hormone status. A smooth learning curve and short image interpretation time are 2 important advantages of PEM. A study by Narayanan and colleagues[96] showed that experienced breast imagers interpreted PEM images with high performance after minimal training. The major limitations of PEM are the very high radiation dose and inconveniently long fasting, uptake, and scan times. With biopsy capability, PEM can be a useful tool when used in the diagnostic setting.[88]

The major limitations of PEM for screening are radiation dose, and inconveniently long fasting, uptake, and scan times.

PET/MR Imaging

Advances in technology in recent years have led to the development of PET/MR imaging systems. This dual modality combines the specificity of the metabolic data from PET with the structural information from MR imaging to improve diagnostic accuracy. This dual-technique allows for a decreased total number of separate imaging examinations as well as a reduction in ionizing radiation exposure from CT. The cumulative lifetime radiation dose reduction afforded by PET/MR imaging in a patient requiring serial imaging examinations as part of their management is potentially significant.

Grueneisen and colleagues[97] compared integrated PET/MR imaging, PET/CT, and MR imaging of the breast for lesion detection and local tumor staging of patients with primary breast cancer. PET/MR imaging and MR imaging identified 47/49 (96%) patients with breast cancer, whereas PET/CT identified 46/49 (94%) patients. The investigators concluded that integrated PET/MR imaging has no advantage for local tumor staging of breast cancer patients compared with MR imaging alone. Both PET/MR imaging and MR imaging performed better for determining local tumor extent compared with PET/CT. All evaluated imaging modalities were comparable for identifying axillary disease. PET/MR imaging has proved useful in local tumor staging, but its utility for screening has yet to be validated.

Although radionuclide imaging has been demonstrated extremely useful in the diagnostic setting, its use for yearly screening mammography is limited by the total-body radiation exposure. No screening guidelines include it at this time, and unless the total body dose can be significantly lowered, it is unlikely to become a routine screening examination. Its use in the diagnostic setting could be more likely with more data. These examinations could in theory be used for problem solving, staging known cancers, or following patients receiving neoadjuvant chemotherapy.

Other PET Tracers for Detecting Breast Cancer

Although FDG is the most validated radiotracer for breast cancer staging in molecular imaging, other available tracers have proved useful for detecting some cancer subtypes.

18F-fluciclovine

18F-fluciclovine, a leucine analog radiotracer, depicts amino acid transport into cells. It is upregulated in some cancers and has been used to visualize invasive ductal and invasive lobular breast cancers. Ulaner and colleagues[98] evaluated 21 patients with locally advanced breast cancer and demonstrated strong concordance for metabolic tumor volume between 18F-FDG–PET and 18F-fluciclovine. In patients with invasive lobular cancers, however, a group often not very avid with 18F-FDG, there was greater avidity with 18F-fluciclovine, median standardized uptake value (SUV) 6.1 compared with 3.7 median SUV with 18F-FDG (**Fig. 11**).

16α-[18F]-fluoro-17β-estradiol

16α-[18F]-fluoro-17β-estradiol PET/CT is a validated and accurate method for localizing estrogen receptor–expressing tumors. Although it is a potentially useful biomarker of estrogen receptor occupancy and/or down-regulation, it has no validity for breast cancer screening at the present time.

18F-fluoromisonidazole

Pinker and colleagues[99] assessed 8 consecutive patients with suspicious breast lesions using combined 3T 18F-FDG/18F-fluoromisonidazole (FMISO) PET–MR imaging for detection of increased glycolysis and tumor hypoxia. Imaging results were correlated with pathologic features, such as tumor grading and ki-67 proliferation rate, and immunohistochemistry. The clinical endpoints were metastases and death. Tumor size range was 9 mm to 170 mm (median, 56.6 mm). On contrast-enhanced MR imaging, 6 malignant tumors were detected as masses

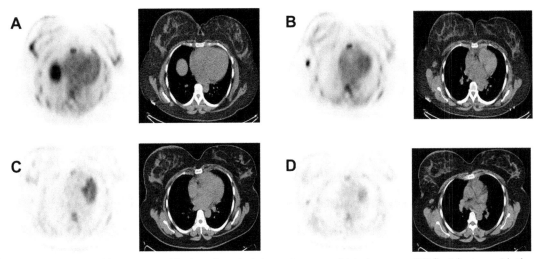

Fig. 11. A 43-year-old woman with invasive ductal carcinoma, which is more 18F-fluciclovine-avid than 18F-FDG–avid. (*A*) Axial 18F-fluciclovine PET/CT demonstrates an 18F-fluciclovine–avid (SUV 4.9) primary right breast malignancy. (*B*) Axial 18F-fluciclovine PET/CT demonstrates an 18F-fluciclovine–avid (SUV 5.8) right axillary nodal metastasis. (*C*) Axial 18F-FDG PET/CT demonstrates near background 18F-FDG avidity (SUV 1.8) in the right breast malignancy. (*D*) Axial 18F-FDG PET/CT demonstrates only mild 18F-FDG avidity (SUV 2.8) in the right axillary nodal metastasis.

and 1 as nonmass enhancement. One area of nonmass enhancement had benign histology. 18F-FDG maximum SUV values were in the range of 2.7 to 19.6 (median, 11.1); for 18F-FMISO, maximum SUV range was 1.26 to 3.47 (median, 1.8). Whole-tumor 18F-FMISO is never completely avid but confined areas were indicative of hypoxia.

Radiation dose for multiple imaging modalities		
Imaging Modality	**Whole-Body Effective Dose (mSv)**	**Organ Dose (mGy)**
Analog mammography	0.60	4.98 breast
DM	0.47	3.91 breast
DBT	0.48–0.96[33]	4–8 breast
MBI and BSGI (1100 MBq Tc99m)	8.9–9.4	50 large intestine, 20 kidney/ bladder wall, gallbladder, 2 breast
PEM (370 MBq 18F-FDG)	6.2–7.1	59 bladder wall, 8 uterus, 5 ovaries, 4.8 colon, 2.5 breast

SUMMARY

In conclusion, although controversial, screening mammography reduces mortality from breast cancer by at least 30%. Improved technologies, such as DBT and ultrasound, find more cancers than mammography, with potential mortality reduction from early detection. Vascular modalities, such as CEDM and MR imaging, improve cancer detection even further. Each has its limitations, including contrast allergies for CEDM and MR imaging and gadolinium deposition in the brain for MR imaging. MR imaging is also expensive. DWI also has potential to detect mammographically occult cancers without contrast or radiation but is currently less sensitive than contrast-enhanced MR imaging and, therefore, not yet recommended for that purpose Pinker and colleagues[100] Molecular imaging of the breast detects a significant number of mammographically occult breast cancers, particularly in women with dense breasts. Despite decreasing tracer doses, however, the magnitude of total body radiation remains prohibitive for yearly use of these technologies. At this time, therefore, they are not recommended for screening by the ACR appropriateness criteria or any other screening recommendation. For now, they can be used for problem solving, staging known cancers, and possibly assessing chemotherapy response.

Going forward, better individual risk-assessment tools may help stratify which type of imaging study might benefit which patients and, most importantly, as new examinations are added, with their risks and costs, it is imperative to design studies to determine if the newer technology reduces morbidity and mortality for screened women.

REFERENCES

1. Shapiro S. Screening: assessment of current studies. Cancer 1994;74(1 Suppl):231–8.
2. Tabar L, Fagerberg CJ, Gad A, et al. Reduction in mortality from breast cancer after mass screening with mammography. Randomised trial from the breast cancer screening working group of the Swedish National board of Health and Welfare. Lancet 1985;1(8433):829–32.
3. Andersson I, Aspegren K, Janzon L, et al. Mammographic screening and mortality from breast cancer: the Malmo mammographic screening trial. BMJ 1988;297(6654):943–8 (Clinical research ed).
4. Plecha D, Salem N, Kremer M, et al. Neglecting to screen women between 40 and 49 years old with mammography: what is the impact on treatment morbidity and potential risk reduction? AJR Am J Roentgenol 2014;202(2):282–8.
5. Arleo EK, Hendrick RE, Helvie MA, et al. Comparison of recommendations for screening mammography using CISNET models. Cancer 2017; 123(19):3673–80.
6. Buist DS, Porter PL, Lehman C, et al. Factors contributing to mammography failure in women aged 40-49 years. J Natl Cancer Inst 2004;96(19):1432–40.
7. Carney PA, Miglioretti DL, Yankaskas BC, et al. Individual and combined effects of age, breast density, and hormone replacement therapy use on the accuracy of screening mammography. Ann Intern Med 2003;138(3):168–75.
8. Wishart GC, Greenberg DC, Britton PD, et al. Screen-detected vs symptomatic breast cancer: is improved survival due to stage migration alone? Br J Cancer 2008;98(11):1741–4.
9. Sung JS, Stamler S, Brooks J, et al. Breast cancers detected at screening MR imaging and mammography in patients at high risk: method of detection reflects tumor histopathologic results. Radiology 2016;280(3):716–22.
10. Mushlin AI, Kouides RW, Shapiro DE. Estimating the accuracy of screening mammography: a meta-analysis. Am J Prev Med 1998;14(2):143–53.
11. Lehman CD, Arao RF, Sprague BL, et al. National performance benchmarks for modern screening digital mammography: update from the breast cancer surveillance Consortium. Radiology 2017; 283(1):49–58.
12. Humphrey LL, Ballard DJ. Early detection of breast cancer in women. Prim Care 1989;16(1):115–32.
13. Etzioni R, Xia J, Hubbard R, et al. A reality check for overdiagnosis estimates associated with breast cancer screening. J Natl Cancer Inst 2014;106(12) [pii:dju315].
14. Puliti D, Duffy SW, Miccinesi G, et al. Overdiagnosi in mammographic screening for breast cancer i Europe: a literature review. J Med Screen 2012 19(Suppl 1):42–56.
15. Duffy SW, Tabar L, Olsen AH, et al. Absolut numbers of lives saved and overdiagnosis i breast cancer screening, from a randomized tria and from the Breast Screening Programme in En gland. J Med Screen 2010;17(1):25–30.
16. Saslow D, Boetes C, Burke W, et al. American Can cer Society guidelines for breast screening wit MRI as an adjunct to mammography. CA Cance J Clin 2007;57(2):75–89.
17. Sung JS, Malak SF, Bajaj P, et al. Screening breas MR imaging in women with a history of lobular car cinoma in situ. Radiology 2011;261(2):414–20.
18. King TA, Muhsen S, Patil S, et al. Is there a role fo routine screening MRI in women with LCIS? Breas Cancer Res Treat 2013;142(2):445–53.
19. Brennan S, Liberman L, Dershaw DD, et al. Breas MRI screening of women with a personal history o breast cancer. AJR Am J Roentgenol 2010;195(2) 510–6.
20. Lehman CD, Lee JM, DeMartini WB, et al Screening MRI in women with a personal history of breast cancer. J Natl Cancer Inst 2016;108(3 [pii:djv349].
21. Boyd NF, Guo H, Martin LJ, et al. Mammographic density and the risk and detection of breast cancer N Engl J Med 2007;356(3):227–36.
22. McCormack VA, dos Santos Silva I. Breast density and parenchymal patterns as markers of breas cancer risk: a meta-analysis. Cancer Epidemio Biomarkers Prev 2006;15(6):1159–69.
23. Sickles EA, D'Orsi CJ, Bassett LW, et al. ACR BI-RADS® mammography. ACR BI-RADS® atlas, breast imaging reporting and data system. Reston (VA): American College of Radiology; 2013.
24. Sprague BL, Gangnon RE, Burt V, et al. Prevalence of mammographically dense breasts in the United States. J Natl Cancer Inst 2014;106(10) [pii:dju255].
25. Kerlikowske K, Zhu W, Tosteson AN, et al. Identifying women with dense breasts at high risk for interval cancer: a cohort study. Ann Intern Med 2015; 162(10):673–81.
26. US Food and Drug Administration. Premarket Approval (PMA) Selenia Dimensions 3D System–P080003. 2011. Available at: https://www. accessdata.fda.gov/scrIpts/cdrh/cfdocs/cfpma/ pma.cfm?id=P080003. Accessed November 15, 2017.
27. Andersson I, Ikeda DM, Zackrisson S, et al. Breast tomosynthesis and digital mammography: a comparison of breast cancer visibility and BIRADS classification in a population of cancers with subtle

mammographic findings. Eur Radiol 2008;18(12): 2817–25.

28. Gur D, Abrams GS, Chough DM, et al. Digital breast tomosynthesis: observer performance study. AJR Am J Roentgenol 2009;193(2):586–91.

29. Friedewald SM, Rafferty EA, Rose SL, et al. Breast cancer screening using tomosynthesis in combination with digital mammography. JAMA 2014; 311(24):2499–507.

30. McDonald ES, Oustimov A, Weinstein SP, et al. Effectiveness of digital breast tomosynthesis compared with digital mammography: outcomes analysis from 3 years of breast cancer screening. JAMA Oncol 2016;2(6):737–43.

31. US Food and Drug Administration. Mammography Quality Standards Act regulations. Available at: https://www.fda.gov/Radiation-EmittingProducts/ MammographyQualityStandardsActandProgram/ Regulations/ucm110906.htm. Accessed November 15, 2017.

32. US Food and Drug Administration. PMA P080003/ S001: summary of safety and effectiveness data (SSED). 2013. Available at: https://www.accessdata. fda.gov/cdrh_docs/pdf8/P080003S001B.pdf. Accessed November 15, 2017.

33. Zuckerman SP, Conant EF, Keller BM, et al. Implementation of synthesized two-dimensional mammography in a population-based digital breast tomosynthesis screening program. Radiology 2016;281(3):730–6.

34. Rose SL, Tidwell AL, Bujnoch LJ, et al. Implementation of breast tomosynthesis in a routine screening practice: an observational study. AJR Am J Roentgenol 2013;200(6):1401–8.

35. Haas BM, Kalra V, Geisel J, et al. Comparison of tomosynthesis plus digital mammography and digital mammography alone for breast cancer screening. Radiology 2013;269(3):694–700.

36. Skaane P, Bandos AI, Gullien R, et al. Comparison of digital mammography alone and digital mammography plus tomosynthesis in a population-based screening program. Radiology 2013;267(1):47–56.

37. Houssami N, Ciatto S. The evolving role of new imaging methods in breast screening. Prev Med 2011;53(3):123–6.

38. Hooley RJ, Greenberg KL, Stackhouse RM, et al. Screening US in patients with mammographically dense breasts: initial experience with Connecticut Public Act 09-41. Radiology 2012;265(1):59–69.

39. Kolb TM, Lichy J, Newhouse JH. Occult cancer in women with dense breasts: detection with screening US–diagnostic yield and tumor characteristics. Radiology 1998;207(1):191–9.

40. Kaplan SS. Clinical utility of bilateral whole-breast US in the evaluation of women with dense breast tissue. Radiology 2001;221(3):641–9.

41. Bae MS, Moon WK, Chang JM, et al. Breast cancer detected with screening US: reasons for nondetection at mammography. Radiology 2014;270(2):369–77.

42. Ohuchi N, Suzuki A, Sobue T, et al. Sensitivity and specificity of mammography and adjunctive ultrasonography to screen for breast cancer in the Japan Strategic Anti-cancer Randomized Trial (J-START): a randomised controlled trial. Lancet 2016;387(10016):341–8.

43. Weigert JM. The Connecticut experiment; the third installment: 4 years of screening women with dense breasts with bilateral ultrasound. Breast J 2017;23(1):34–9.

44. Tagliafico AS, Calabrese M, Mariscotti G, et al. Adjunct screening with tomosynthesis or ultrasound in women with mammography-negative dense breasts: interim report of a prospective comparative trial. J Clin Oncol 2016;34(16):1882–8.

45. Nam KJ, Han BK, Ko ES, et al. Comparison of full-field digital mammography and digital breast tomosynthesis in ultrasonography-detected breast cancers. Breast 2015;24(5):649–55.

46. Berg WA, Zhang Z, Lehrer D, et al. Detection of breast cancer with addition of annual screening ultrasound or a single screening MRI to mammography in women with elevated breast cancer risk. JAMA 2012;307(13):1394–404.

47. Lehman CD. Role of MRI in screening women at high risk for breast cancer. J Magn Reson Imaging 2006;24(5):964–70.

48. Kuhl CK, Mielcareck P, Klaschik S, et al. Dynamic breast MR imaging: are signal intensity time course data useful for differential diagnosis of enhancing lesions? Radiology 1999;211(1):101–10.

49. Kuhl CK, Schild HH. Dynamic image interpretation of MRI of the breast. J Magn Reson Imaging 2000; 12(6):965–74.

50. Liu M, Guo X, Wang S, et al. BOLD-MRI of breast invasive ductal carcinoma: correlation of R2* value and the expression of HIF-1alpha. Eur Radiol 2013; 23(12):3221–7.

51. Kriege M, Brekelmans CT, Boetes C, et al. Efficacy of MRI and mammography for breast-cancer screening in women with a familial or genetic predisposition. N Engl J Med 2004;351(5):427–37.

52. Kuhl CK, Schrading S, Leutner CC, et al. Mammography, breast ultrasound, and magnetic resonance imaging for surveillance of women at high familial risk for breast cancer. J Clin Oncol 2005;23(33): 8469–76.

53. Leach MO, Boggis CR, Dixon AK, et al. Screening with magnetic resonance imaging and mammography of a UK population at high familial risk of breast cancer: a prospective multicentre cohort study (MARIBS). Lancet 2005; 365(9473):1769–78.

54. Sardanelli F, Podo F. Breast MR imaging in women at high-risk of breast cancer. Is something changing in early breast cancer detection? Eur Radiol 2007;17(4):873–87.

55. Warner E, Causer PA. MRI surveillance for hereditary breast-cancer risk. Lancet 2005;365(9473):1747–9.

56. Kriege M, Brekelmans CT, Boetes C, et al. Differences between first and subsequent rounds of the MRISC breast cancer screening program for women with a familial or genetic predisposition. Cancer 2006;106(11):2318–26.

57. Saadatmand S, Obdeijn IM, Rutgers EJ, et al. Survival benefit in women with BRCA1 mutation or familial risk in the MRI screening study (MRISC). Int J Cancer 2015;137(7):1729–38.

58. Warner E, Hill K, Causer P, et al. Prospective study of breast cancer incidence in women with a BRCA1 or BRCA2 mutation under surveillance with and without magnetic resonance imaging. J Clin Oncol 2011;29(13):1664–9.

59. Kuhl C, Weigel S, Schrading S, et al. Prospective multicenter cohort study to refine management recommendations for women at elevated familial risk of breast cancer: the EVA trial. J Clin Oncol 2010;28(9):1450–7.

60. Bogner W, Gruber S, Pinker K, et al. Diffusion-weighted MR for differentiation of breast lesions at 3.0 T: how does selection of diffusion protocols affect diagnosis? Radiology 2009;253(2):341–51.

61. McDonald ES, Hammersley JA, Chou SH, et al. Performance of DWI as a rapid unenhanced technique for detecting mammographically occult breast cancer in elevated-risk women with dense breasts. AJR Am J Roentgenol 2016;207(1):205–16.

62. Kuhl CK, Schrading S, Strobel K, et al. Abbreviated breast magnetic resonance imaging (MRI): first postcontrast subtracted images and maximum-intensity projection-a novel approach to breast cancer screening with MRI. J Clin Oncol 2014;32(22):2304–10.

63. Mango VL, Morris EA, David Dershaw D, et al. Abbreviated protocol for breast MRI: are multiple sequences needed for cancer detection? Eur J Radiol 2015;84(1):65–70.

64. Jochelson MS, Dershaw DD, Sung JS, et al. Bilateral contrast-enhanced dual-energy digital mammography: feasibility and comparison with conventional digital mammography and MR imaging in women with known breast carcinoma. Radiology 2013;266(3):743–51.

65. Fallenberg EM, Dromain C, Diekmann F, et al. Contrast-enhanced spectral mammography versus MRI: initial results in the detection of breast cancer and assessment of tumour size. Eur Radiol 2014;24(1):256–64.

66. Jochelson MS, Pinker K, Dershaw DD, et al. Comparison of screening CEDM and MRI for women at increased risk for breast cancer: a pilot study. Eur J Radiol 2017;97:37–43.

67. Sung JS, Jochelson MS, Lee CH, et al. SSJ01–05 comparison of contrast enhanced digital mammography and whole breast screening ultrasound for supplemental breast cancer screening. Chicago: RSNA; 2016.

68. Cheung YC, Tsai HP, Lo YF, et al. Clinical utility of dual-energy contrast-enhanced spectral mammography for breast microcalcifications without associated mass: a preliminary analysis. Eur Radiol 2016;26(4):1082–9.

69. Hobbs MM, Taylor DB, Buzynski S, et al. Contrast-enhanced spectral mammography (CESM) and contrast enhanced MRI (CEMRI): patient preferences and tolerance. J Med Imaging Radiat Oncol 2015;59(3):300–5.

70. Buchberger W, Niehoff A, Obrist P, et al. Clinically and mammographically occult breast lesions: detection and classification with high-resolution sonography. Semin Ultrasound CT MR 2000;21(4):325–36.

71. Hassan IM, Sahweil A, Constantinides C, et al. Uptake and kinetics of Tc-99m hexakis 2-methoxy isobutyl isonitrile in benign and malignant lesions in the lungs. Clin Nucl Med 1989;14(5):333–40.

72. Khalkhali I, Villanueva-Meyer J, Edell SL, et al. Diagnostic accuracy of 99mTc-sestamibi breast imaging: multicenter trial results. J Nucl Med 2000;41(12):1973–9.

73. Weigert JM, Bertrand ML, Lanzkowsky L, et al. Results of a multicenter patient registry to determine the clinical impact of breast-specific gamma imaging, a molecular breast imaging technique. AJR Am J Roentgenol 2012;198(1):W69–75.

74. Park JY, Yi SY, Park HJ, et al. Breast-specific gamma imaging: correlations with mammographic and clinicopathologic characteristics of breast cancer. AJR Am J Roentgenol 2014;203(1):223–8.

75. Hruska CB, O'Connor MK, Collins DA. Comparison of small field of view gamma camera systems for scintimammography. Nucl Med Commun 2005;26(5):441–5.

76. Long Z, Conners AL, Hunt KN, et al. Performance characteristics of dedicated molecular breast imaging systems at low doses. Med Phys 2016;43(6):3062–70.

77. O'Connor MK, Hruska CB, Tran TD, et al. Factors influencing the uptake of 99mTc-sestamibi in breast tissue on molecular breast imaging. J Nucl Med Technol 2015;43(1):13–20.

78. Hruska CB, Phillips SW, Whaley DH, et al. Molecular breast imaging: use of a dual-head dedicated gamma camera to detect small breast tumors. AJR Am J Roentgenol 2008;191(6):1805–15.

79. Rhodes DJ, Hruska CB, Conners AL, et al. Journal club: molecular breast imaging at reduced radiation dose for supplemental screening in mammographically dense breasts. AJR Am J Roentgenol 2015;204(2):241–51.

80. Conners AL, Jones KN, Hruska CB, et al. Direct-conversion molecular breast imaging of invasive breast cancer: imaging features, extent of invasive disease, and comparison between invasive ductal and lobular histology. AJR Am J Roentgenol 2015;205(3):W374–81.

81. Shermis RB, Wilson KD, Doyle MT, et al. Supplemental breast cancer screening with molecular breast imaging for women with dense breast tissue. AJR Am J Roentgenol 2016;207(2):450–7.

82. Kim JS, Lee SM, Cha ES. The diagnostic sensitivity of dynamic contrast-enhanced magnetic resonance imaging and breast-specific gamma imaging in women with calcified and non-calcified DCIS. Acta Radiol 2014;55(6):668–75.

83. Keto JL, Kirstein L, Sanchez DP, et al. MRI versus breast-specific gamma imaging (BSGI) in newly diagnosed ductal cell carcinoma-in-situ: a prospective head-to-head trial. Ann Surg Oncol 2012;19(1):249–52.

84. Brem RF, Petrovitch I, Rapelyea JA, et al. Breast-specific gamma imaging with 99mTc-Sestamibi and magnetic resonance imaging in the diagnosis of breast cancer–a comparative study. Breast J 2007;13(5):465–9.

85. Zhang A, Li P, Liu Q, et al. Breast-specific gamma camera imaging with 99mTc-MIBI has better diagnostic performance than magnetic resonance imaging in breast cancer patients: a meta-analysis. Hell J Nucl Med 2017;20(1):26–35.

86. Zhou M, Johnson N, Gruner S, et al. Clinical utility of breast-specific gamma imaging for evaluating disease extent in the newly diagnosed breast cancer patient. Am J Surg 2009;197(2):159–63.

87. Brem RF, Tabar L, Duffy SW, et al. Assessing improvement in detection of breast cancer with three-dimensional automated breast US in women with dense breast tissue: the SomoInsight Study. Radiology 2015;274(3):663–73.

88. Hendrick RE. Radiation doses and cancer risks from breast imaging studies. Radiology 2010; 257(1):246–53.

89. Hendrick RE, Tredennick T. Benefit to radiation risk of breast-specific gamma imaging compared with mammography in screening asymptomatic women with dense breasts. Radiology 2016;281(2):583–8.

90. Kamel EM, Wyss MT, Fehr MK, et al. [18F]-Fluorodeoxyglucose positron emission tomography in patients with suspected recurrence of breast cancer. J Cancer Res Clin Oncol 2003;129(3):147–53.

91. Eubank WB, Mankoff D, Bhattacharya M, et al. Impact of FDG PET on defining the extent of disease and on the treatment of patients with recurrent or metastatic breast cancer. AJR Am J Roentgenol 2004;183(2):479–86.

92. Glass SB, Shah ZA. Clinical utility of positron emission mammography. Proc (Bayl Univ Med Cent) 2013;26(3):314–9.

93. Eo JS, Chun IK, Paeng JC, et al. Imaging sensitivity of dedicated positron emission mammography in relation to tumor size. Breast 2012;21(1):66–71.

94. Berg WA, Weinberg IN, Narayanan D, et al. High-resolution fluorodeoxyglucose positron emission tomography with compression ("positron emission mammography") is highly accurate in depicting primary breast cancer. Breast J 2006;12(4): 309–23.

95. Berg WA, Madsen KS, Schilling K, et al. Breast cancer: comparative effectiveness of positron emission mammography and MR imaging in pre-surgical planning for the ipsilateral breast. Radiology 2011;258(1):59–72.

96. Narayanan D, Madsen KS, Kalinyak JE, et al. Interpretation of positron emission mammography and MRI by experienced breast imaging radiologists: performance and observer reproducibility. AJR Am J Roentgenol 2011;196(4):971–81.

97. Grueneisen J, Nagarajah J, Buchbender C, et al. Positron emission tomography/magnetic resonance imaging for local tumor staging in patients with primary breast cancer: a comparison with positron emission tomography/computed tomography and magnetic resonance imaging. Invest Radiol 2015;50(8):505–13.

98. Ulaner GA, Goldman DA, Gonen M, et al. Initial results of a prospective clinical trial of 18F-fluciclovine PET/CT in newly diagnosed invasive ductal and invasive lobular breast cancers. J Nucl Med 2016;57(9):1350–6.

99. Pinker K, Baltzer P, Andrzejewski P, et al. Dual tracer PET/MRI of breast tumors: insights into tumor biology. Honolulu (HI): WMIC; 2015.

100. Pinker K, Bogner W, Baltzer P, et al. Improved diagnostic accuracy with multiparametric magnetic resonance imaging of the breast using dynamic contrast-enhanced magnetic resonance imaging, diffusion-weighted imaging, and 3-dimensional proton magnetic resonance spectroscopic imaging. Invest Radiol 2014;49(6):421–30.

Molecular Classification of Breast Cancer

Elena Provenzano, MBBS, PhD, FRCPath[a,b], Gary A. Ulaner, MD, PhD[c,d],
Suet-Feung Chin, BSc, PhD[e,*]

KEYWORDS

• Breast cancer • Molecular classification • Genes • Mutations • Copy number alterations

KEY POINTS

• Breast cancer is a heterogeneous disease.
• It can be classified based on its molecular profiles.
• These molecular subtypes have different prognostic indices and may require different clinical management.

INTRODUCTION

Breast cancer is not a single entity but a heterogeneous group of diseases with highly variable clinical behavior[1]. Pathologists have long recognized this diversity at the morphologic level, and it is reflected in the various special histologic types of breast cancer with their distinct microscopic appearances and associated clinical outcomes. However, 70% to 80% of breast cancers fall into the ductal/no-special-type category (invasive ductal carcinoma [IDC]), which, rather than representing a unique entity, show marked heterogeneity with respect to tumor morphology, underlying molecular biology, and prognosis.[2]

Cancer is driven by DNA alterations, including chromosomal rearrangements, mutations, and epigenetic changes, such as promoter hypermethylation resulting in activation of growth-promoting genes (oncogenes) or suppression of growth-inhibiting genes (tumor suppressor genes). The advent of array-based technologies enabled quantification of DNA copy number changes and global expression profiling of tens of thousands of genes in a single experiment. Recent advances, for example, next-generation sequencing allowed detection of mutations, chromosomal rearrangements, and copy number alterations across the entire genome, including those only present within minor subclones of tumor cells.[3,4] These high-throughput (HT) technologies have changed how we conceptualize and classify breast cancer as well as provide a new level of insight into the complexity of genetic changes and the existence of intratumoural heterogeneity.[5–7]

Historically, patient management decisions have been based on traditional histologic features, including tumor size, histologic grade, lymph node status, and hormone and human epidermal growth factor receptor 2 (HER2) receptor status in conjunction with patient characteristics, such as age.[8,9] These variables show a strong association with survival outcomes but, even when combined in algorithms, such as Nottingham Prognostic Index, Predict, or Adjuvant! Online, are a crude measure of risk in individual patients.[10–15] Accurate prediction of tumor behavior is key to oncological decision-making, avoiding overtreatment with

a Cambridge Experimental Cancer Medicine Centre (ECMR), NIHR Cambridge Biomedical Research Centre, Cambridge University Hospitals NHS Foundation Trust, Cambridge CB2 0QQ, UK; b Department of Histopathology, Addenbrookes Hospital, Box 235, Hills Road, Cambridge CB2 0QQ, UK; c Department of Radiology, Memorial Sloan Kettering Cancer Center, 1275 York Avenue, Box 77, New York, NY 10065, USA; d Department of Radiology, Weill Cornell Medical School, New York, NY 10065, USA; e Cancer Research UK Cambridge Institute, University of Cambridge, Li Ka Shing Centre, Robinson Way, Cambridge CB2 0RE, UK
* Corresponding author.
E-mail address: suet-feung.chin@cruk.cam.ac.uk

PET Clin 13 (2018) 325–338
https://doi.org/10.1016/j.cpet.2018.02.004

harmful drugs in patients with a good prognosis, and more aggressive intervention with first-line chemotherapy in patients with a poor prognosis.[16–18] However, use of algorithms based on these histologic variables result in a significant number of patients being overtreated, with as many as 85% of patients deriving no benefit from chemotherapy. At the other extreme, 20% of patients still die despite receiving maximum therapy.[19]

The ultimate goal of modern oncological management is personalized medicine, with a more precise determination of patient prognosis based on tumor biology and the opportunity for targeted treatment directed at the underlying molecular aberrations driving individual tumor growth. HT molecular techniques offer the potential to revolutionize patient management in this way. But these techniques are currently expensive compared with standard methods, such as immunohistochemistry (IHC); the vast amounts of data generated require complex bioinformatic analyses limiting their clinical use currently.[20]

Intrinsic Subtypes

The mainstays of breast cancer characterization are still histologic subtype, tumor grade, and stage, which provide a basic reflection of the degree of tumor differentiation (tubule formation) and growth rate (size and mitotic count). The seminal article that led to the identification of 5 intrinsic subtypes was published by Perou and colleagues[5] in 2000. The investigators took a series of 38 invasive breast cancers (36 ductal and 2 lobular), 1 case of ductal carcinoma in situ (DCIS), and 4 benign samples and undertook complementary DNA microarray gene expression analysis followed by hierarchical clustering of differentially expressed genes and identified 5 subtypes primarily separated by estrogen receptor (ER) expression; 2 ER-positive luminal subtypes, and 3 ER-negative subtypes (HER2 enriched, basal and normal-like). A follow-up study showed that these subtypes were associated with differences in survival.[21]

These 5 intrinsic subtypes have been validated in other series and have changed how we think about the taxonomy of breast cancer.[22,23] The separation into good and poor prognosis ER-positive, HER2-positive, and triple-negative (ER, progesterone receptor [PR], and HER2 negative: triple-negative breast cancer [TNBC]) groups is highly clinically relevant, given that current therapeutic regimens are centered on antiestrogen therapy, chemotherapy, and HER2-targeted agents. The normal-like subtype has subsequently been dropped, as it is thought to represent contamination by normal glands. Classification of cohorts of breast cancers into the intrinsic subtypes seems robust across studies; however, assignment of individual tumors to a subgroup shows only moderate reproducibility depending on the array platform used, composition of the entire tumor population, and setting of gene expression thresholds.[24–26] Identification of the basal-like group is most reproducible, with the luminal B and HER2 groups the most poorly reproducible.[26,27] The commercially available Prediction Analysis of Microarray 50(PAM50) classifier (Prosigna),[28,29] based on expression of 50 genes that can separate tumors into the intrinsic subtypes, has been shown to be an independent marker of prognosis.[30–33] Attempts to replicate these groups using IHC-based panels, including ER, PR, HER2, Ki67, and basal cytokeratins, have produced modest concordance between gene expression and IHC-defined intrinsic subtypes at best.[22,34]

Luminal Breast Cancer

Luminal breast cancers are enriched for ER-positive tumors and include special type cancers, such as tubular, cribriform, lobular, and mucinous carcinomas. Luminal cancers form a continuous spectrum that can be arbitrarily divided into 2 subgroups based on the expression of proliferation-related genes. Luminal A tumors are typically low grade with an excellent prognosis, ER/PR positive and HER2 negative, with high expression of ER-related genes and low expression of proliferation-related genes.[23,35] In contrast, luminal B tumors are higher grade with worse prognosis and may be PR negative and/or HER2 positive with high expression of proliferation-related genes.[36,37] Clinically, the luminal A group is likely to benefit from hormonal therapy alone, whereas luminal B tumors with their increased proliferation may be candidates for chemotherapy.

Molecular signatures that separate ER-positive tumors into good and poor prognosis subgroups form the basis for many of the multi-gene assays that are currently available for clinical use, such as Oncotype Dx, Mammaprint, and EndoPredict.[38–40] Although there is little overlap in the specific genes that make up these signatures, they all include genes involved in proliferation and ER signaling.[27,41] In studies whereby multiple signatures are applied to the same patient cohort, they all identify low- and high-risk groups with a significantly different prognosis; however, there is disagreement at the individual patient level in many cases.[42–46]

Because of the present high cost of these commercial multi-gene assays, attempts have been made to recapitulate the luminal A and B subtypes using IHC markers of proliferation, such as Ki67. Cheang and colleagues[37] looked at a series of 357 cancers with known gene expression profiling and identified an optimum Ki67 cut point of 13.25% for distinguishing luminal A from B tumors, with a sensitivity of 72% and a specificity of 77%. This cut point was rounded to 14% for clinical use. Hence, the surrogate IHC definition of luminal A tumors was ER positive and HER2 negative with a Ki67 index less than 14% and of luminal B tumors was ER positive and HER2 negative with a Ki67 index of greater than 14% or HER2 positive. In 2 large clinical trial using this IHC surrogate definition, 81% to 85% of luminal A tumors were correctly classified, whereas 35% to 52% of luminal B tumors were misclassified as IHC luminal A.[35] The IHC definition of luminal A tumors was subsequently modified to include PR expression of greater than 20% to better identify a good prognosis subgroup akin to the luminal A tumors defined by gene expression profiling. Despite the initial enthusiasm, Ki67 is not currently accepted as a routine prognostic marker in breast cancer by the American Society of Clinical Oncology because of disagreement as to the best scoring method and suboptimal reproducibility in scoring.[47]

Human Epidermal Growth Factor Receptor 2–Positive Breast Cancer

ER-negative cancers comprise biologically distinct entities with different drivers that can be divided into 2 main groups: HER2 enriched and basal-like/TNBC. The HER2-enriched group is driven by overexpression of HER2 and genes associated with related pathways or with the HER2 amplicon on chromosome 17q12. Before the introduction of HER2-targeted therapies, they had the worst prognosis of all breast cancer subtypes. Although most tumors within this subgroup (>80%) show HER2 gene amplification or HER2 protein overexpression on IHC, not all clinically defined HER2-positive tumors fall into this subgroup; many ER-positive/HER2-positive tumors fall into the luminal B group mentioned earlier.[23,48] In one series looking at clinically HER2-positive breast cancers, 47% were of the HER2-enriched subtype, whereas conversely only 65% of HER2-enriched subtype cancers were clinically HER2 positive.[49] In a retrospective analysis of the NeoAdjuvant Herceptin (NOAH) clinical trial looking at neoadjuvant therapy with or without trastuzumab for clinically HER2-positive breast cancer, on PAM50 testing only 55% of the cancers were classed as HER2 enriched; 21% were luminal, 7% basal-like, and 18% normal-like. Of note, the HER2-enriched tumors had a significantly higher pathologic complete response (pCR) rate versus HER2-luminal tumors (53% vs 29% respectively) and had a larger improvement in event-free survival with the addition of trastuzumab.[50]

Basal-Like/Triple-Negative Breast Cancers

The basal-like breast cancers are typically high-grade TNBC that are characterized by upregulation of genes expressed by basal/myoepithelial cells, including high-molecular-weight cytokeratins (CK5 and 14), P-cadherin, and epidermal growth factor receptor.[23] The basal-like group includes diverse histologic types of breast cancer; although most are high-grade IDC, they also include medullarylike cancers with a prominent lymphocytic infiltrate; metaplastic cancers, which may show squamous or spindle cell differentiation; and rare special type cancers like adenoid cystic carcinoma (AdCC), which carry a good prognosis.[51–55]

Breast cancers arising in BRCA1 mutation carriers are typically basal-like; BRCA1 dysfunction mediated by alternative mechanisms, such as methylation, has been identified in non-BRCA1 mutated basal-like tumors.[51,56,57] The terms basal-like and TNBC have been used interchangeably; however, not all TNBC are of the basal type. On gene expression profiling, TNBCs have been subdivided into 6 subgroups with different molecular drivers and variable clinical outcomes and response to neoadjuvant chemotherapy, although this has subsequently been revised to 4 groups.[58–60]

An important subgroup is the luminal androgen receptor (LAR) group, characterized by high expression of androgen receptor and hormonally regulated pathways with similarities to the molecular apocrine group of breast cancers.[61] They have a relatively good prognosis and show a lower pCR rate following neoadjuvant chemotherapy (10%) more akin to ER-positive tumors.[60] As well as expressing androgen receptor, LAR tumors frequently have PIK3CA mutations and may be candidates for antiandrogenic agents and/or phosphatidylinositide 3-kinase (P13K) pathway inhibitors.[62]

There are 2 basal-like subgroups, BL1 and BL2, enriched for genes involved in proliferation, DNA damage response (BL1), and growth factor receptor signaling pathways (BL2). The BL1 group shows high pCR rates following neoadjuvant chemotherapy (52%), whereas the BL2 group shows poor response.[60] The immune modulatory group is enriched for genes involved in immune cell processes, such as B- and T-cell receptor signaling, cytokine signaling, and antigen presentation, and is now thought to reflect infiltration by immune cells rather than represent a true TNBC subtype.[59] The mesenchymal (M) group shows enrichment for genes involved in cell motility, differentiation, growth signaling pathways, and extracellular matrix interactions, with low expression of proliferation-related genes and high expression of genes associated with stem cells. The last group was associated with worse 5-year distant recurrence-free survival consistent with upregulation of pathways involved in motility and metastasis; the M group also showed the poorest disease-free survival and overall survival following neoadjuvant chemotherapy.[60]

TNBCs demonstrate particularly elevated uptake of fluorodeoxyglucose (FDG) on PET.[63,64] They are also known to result in early metastatic disease and have a propensity for extraskeletal metastases,[65] increasing the importance of imaging for systemic staging.

Integrative Clusters

Breast cancer is a copy number disease.[66] Recently, a classifier based on integrated analysis of both genomic and transcriptomic data from 2000 primary breast tumors MolEcular TAxonomy of BReast cancer International Consortium (METABRIC) was produced, which revealed 10 groups termed *integrative clusters* (IntClusts) with a distinct clinical outcome[67] further refining the existing expression-based subgroups (Table 1). IntClust 5 is composed of HER2-positive tumors; TNBCs predominantly fall in IntClust 10 with some in IntClust 4, which is characterized by immune infiltration. The remaining 7 IntClusts are predominantly composed of ER-positive/HER2-negative cancers highlighting the heterogeneity present within this subtype includes an ER-positive group (IntClust2) with a prognosis worse than ER-negative disease characterized by *CCND1* amplification.

Special Histologic Subtypes

There are more than 20 special histologic subtypes of breast cancer, each associated with a distinct histologic appearance and clinical behavior.[2] New genomic techniques have led to considerable interest in interrogating the molecular profiles of these special-type tumors to help understand them.[68] Although some special-type tumors have been associated with characteristic genetic changes, there is also considerable genetic heterogeneity within many special-type cancers despite their distinct morphology. Some of

these special-type cancers are described in more detail later.

Invasive Lobular Carcinoma

The most common special-type cancer is invasive lobular carcinoma (ILC), accounting for 5% to 15% of breast cancers (Fig. 1).[2] ILC is composed of small, monotonous cells with round nuclei that lack cohesion, infiltrating as cords and single files around existing normal breast structures. There is often minimal stromal reaction; this absence of disruption to background breast architecture is what results in the difficulties in radiological detection of these tumors, with up to 43% being occult on standard mammography.[69] ILCs are typically ER positive (95%–99%) and HER2 negative (>95%), and most fall into luminal subtypes with 30% to 85% being luminal A and 20% to 64% luminal B.[70] A small subset show more aggressive histologic features, such as a solid growth pattern and/or severe nuclear pleomorphism. The latter group are referred to as pleomorphic ILC and can have a more aggressive biological phenotype with ER negativity in up to 25% and *HER2* gene amplification in 15% to 35%.[71,72]

The characteristic molecular feature of ILC is downregulation of the *CDH1* gene on 16q that encodes the E-cadherin protein. E-cadherin is a cell adhesion molecule that forms part of the cadherin-catenin complex and is responsible for the glandular architecture of the breast.[73] However, 12% to 16% of classic ILC retain expression of the E-cadherin protein on IHC and 25% to 50% of IDCs may show reduced or absent E-cadherin expression, so ILC is defined by morphology and not by absent E-cadherin staining alone.[74–76]

Clinically, ILC have a similar prognosis to stage-matched IDC in most series, although long-term prognosis may be poorer with higher rates of late relapse after 10 years.[77] Grade is a significant prognostic factor, with grade 3 tumors showing a worse outcome. ILC show a poor response to neoadjuvant chemotherapy, with low pCR rates and a lower rate of tumor downsizing and conversion to breast-conservation therapy.[78,79] On Oncotype Dx testing, most fall into the low- (32%–77%) and intermediate-risk (23%–57%) groups, with only 1% to 10% having a high-risk recurrence score, consistent with the limited benefit of chemotherapy in these patients.[80]

Historically, ILC and IDC were thought to develop via separate pathways, with ILC originating in the lobules and IDC originating from ducts; it is now known that most breast cancers arise in the terminal duct lobular units, which is also the location of the stem cell niche.[81] ILC and

Table 1
Description of the 10 integrative cluster subtypes

IntClust	Frequency (%)	Prognosis	Distinguishing Molecular Features	Histologic Features	ER/HER2 (Intrinsic Subtype)
1	7	Intermediate	17q23 amplification GATA3 mutations High genomic instability	High grade, NST	85% ER+ 15% HER2+ (Lum B)
2	4	Poor	11q13–14 amplification (CCND1) High genomic instability	—	94% ER+ 8% HER2+ (Lum B)
3	15	Good	Low genomic instability with few copy number changes PIK3CA and CDH1 mutations	Low grade, tubular, lobular, mixed NST/ special types	94% ER+ 0% HER2+ (Lum A)
4	17	Good	Low genomic instability Upregulation immune response genes	Non–grade 3, lymphocytic infiltrate	70% ER+ 8% HER2 +
5	10	Poor	ERBB2 amplification	Grade 3	51% ER+ 85% HER2+ (HER2E)
6	4	Intermediate	8p12 amplification (ZNF703) High genomic instability	Non–low grade	98% ER+ 4% HER2+ (Lum B)
7	10	Good	16p gain, 16q loss, 8q amplification MAP3K1 mutations	Non–grade 3	97% ER+ 0.5% HER2+ (Lum A)
8	15	Good	1q gain, 16q loss PIK3CA and GATA3 mutations	Low grade	96% ER+ 1% HER2+ (Lum A)
9	7	Intermediate	8q gain, 20q amplification High genomic instability TP53 mutations	Grade 3	87% ER+ 12% HER2+ (Lum B)
10	11	Poor	5q loss, 8q gain, 10p gain, 12p gain Impaired DNA checkpoint regulation TP53 mutations	Grade 3, medullarylike	14% ER+ 3% HER2+ (basal)

Abbreviations: Lum, luminal; NST, no special type.

low-grade ER-positive IDC share many genetic similarities, including gain on chromosome 1q and 16p and loss of 16q, and are now thought to share common precursor lesions, such as atypical lobular hyperplasia, atypical ductal hyperplasia, LCIS, and low-grade DCIS, that together form the low-grade ER-positive breast neoplasia pathway.[82] In a comparison with grade-matched ER-positive IDC, ILC showed differential expression of CDH1 and other genes involved in cell assembly and cell-cell interactions as well as reduced expression of cell cycle genes.[83] Other genes commonly mutated in ILC include PIK3CA (35%–48%), PTEN (14%), and ERBB2 (4%–18%).[70]

Gene expression profiling of ILC has identified 2 subtypes: one is hormone related with upregulation of ESR1 and cell cycle and ER target genes and the other is immune related with activation of immune signaling and cytokine pathways and associated with an increased lymphocytic infiltrate on histology.[84] In the METABRIC study, ILC fell across several intrinsic clusters, with approximately one-third in IntClust 3 associated with CDH1 and PIK3CA mutations[85,86]; in fact, it was the increased number of ILC in IntClust 3 that largely accounted for the CDH1 mutations[87]. The second largest group fell in IntClust 4, with low genome instability and increased expression of immune signatures. Given the generally poor

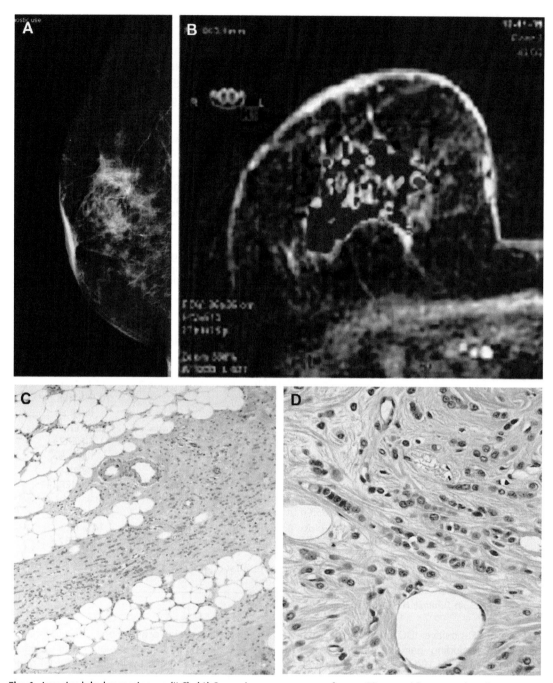

Fig. 1. Invasive lobular carcinoma (ILC). (*A*) Screening mammogram from a 69-year-old woman showing a 20-mm area of architectural distortion in the upper outer quadrant. (*B*) On MR imaging, the tumor was much larger than apparent on the mammogram. (*C*) Core biopsy revealed ILC, with the characteristic single-file growth pattern and minimal stromal reaction (H&E, original magnification x 10). (*D*) Higher power showing cells with regular round nuclei and occasional mucin vacuoles, which demonstrates the potential limitations, including undermeasurement of the malignancy, when imaging ILC by mammography (H&E, original magnification x 20).

response to traditional chemotherapy, these genetic profiles may offer new treatment opportunities, such as PI3K pathway and immune checkpoint inhibitors.

The lobular subtype has important implications for imaging studies (**Fig. 1**). Primary ILC lesions of the breast are more difficult to detect than ductal/IDC on all current imaging modalities, including mammography, ultrasound, magnetic resonance, and FDG PET.[88–93] On FDG PET, ILC demonstrates lower FDG avidity than comparable IDC malignancies in both primary[88,89,91,92] and metastatic lesions.[94,95] In addition, ILC differs in its patterns of metastatic spread, including a propensity for infiltrative growth along the peritoneum, retroperitoneum, gastrointestinal and genitourinary viscera, and the leptomeninges.[96–99] This infiltrative growth often makes detection of metastatic lesions more difficult on imaging[95] (**Figs. 2 and 3**). Unique molecular alterations in ILC may make this breast cancer subtype more amenable to imaging with novel PET radiotracers targeting specific metabolic pathways.[100,101]

Tubular Carcinoma

Invasive tubular carcinoma is an excellent prognosis special-type cancer that is often screen detected.[102] As the name suggests, it is characterized by prominent tubule formation (>90%) and is almost universally ER positive and HER2 negative of the luminal A subtype. They typically have the 1q gain and 16q loss seen in members of the low-grade neoplasia family. On gene expression profiling, tubular cancers cluster together with matched low-grade ER-positive IDC; however, on hierarchical analysis, they show a relative increase in expression of ER and PI3K signaling pathways.[103]

Within the METABRIC study, tubular cancers fell across several good prognosis subtypes, indicating that despite their distinct morphology and clinical behavior they have diverse molecular drivers. The largest group fell into IntClust 3 and harbored *PIK3CA* mutations, although as expected they lacked the *CDH1* mutations also seen in this cluster, whereas others fell into IntClusts 4, 7, and 8.[87]

Mucinous Carcinoma

Invasive mucinous carcinomas are composed of islands of tumor cells floating in pools of extracellular mucin.[2] Mucinous carcinomas can be difficult to diagnose, as the lack of an associated stromal response can give an indeterminate appearance on mammography and ultrasound[104] (**Fig. 4**). Clinically, pure mucinous carcinomas tend to occur in older patients and have a favorable prognosis. They are almost always ER positive and HER2 negative and fall into the luminal subtypes with most being luminal A.[105,106] At the genomic level, mucinous carcinomas are distinct from IDC, with low genomic instability and absence of the 1q gain and 16q loss seen in other low-grade ER-positive tumors and a relative paucity of PIK3CA mutations.[106,107]

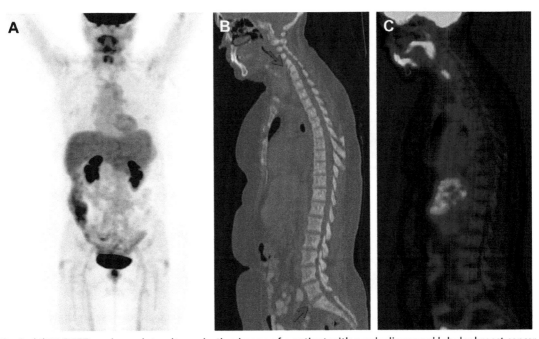

Fig. 2. (*A*) FDG PET maximum-intensity-projection image of a patient with newly diagnosed lobular breast cancer demonstrates physiologic FDG avidity, without abnormal foci. (*B*) Sagittal computed tomography (CT) on bone window demonstrates widespread sclerotic osseous metastases (*arrows*). Biopsy-confirmed osseous metastases. (*C*) Fused FDG PET/CT demonstrates the widespread osseous metastases are not appreciably FDG avid. This finding demonstrates the potential for substantial ILC malignancy with little or no FDG avidity on PET.

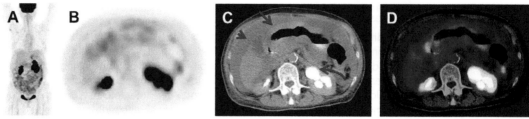

Fig. 3. (*A*) FDG PET maximum-intensity-projection image of a patient with newly diagnosed lobular breast cancer demonstrates physiologic FDG avidity, without abnormal foci. (*B*) Axial PET. (*C*) Axial CT. (*D*) Axial fused FDG PET/CT demonstrates gastric wall thickening (*arrow*), peritoneal free fluid (*arrowhead*), and hydronephrosis (*curved arrow*), better appreciated on CT than FDG PET. Endoscopy and biopsy confirmed ILC metastases to the stomach. Hydronephrosis is probably from ILC metastases to the retroperitoneum obstructing the ureters. This image is an example of widespread, multi-organ system ILC metastases with little or no FDG avidity.

Within the METABRIC cohort, mucinous carcinomas fell within the ER-positive IntClusts but were relatively evenly distributed across clusters and did not associate with any one cluster; hence, despite their unique morphology, as a group mucinous carcinomas show considerable heterogeneity in terms of underlying genetic drivers.[87]

Basal-like breast cancers are typically associated with aggressive clinical behavior and a poor outcome, but there is a subset of special-type cancers that fall within the basal group but has an excellent prognosis. This subset includes low-grade variants of spindle cell metaplastic carcinoma (fibromatosislike metaplastic carcinoma), low-grade adenosquamous carcinoma, and rare salivary glandlike tumors that occur in the breast, including AdCC and secretory carcinoma, both characterized by the presence of specific fusion genes.[53,55,108,109]

Adenoid Cystic Carcinoma

AdCCs are composed of a dual population of luminal and basaloid cells that form islands with

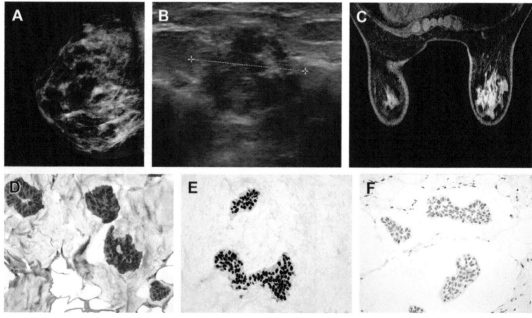

Fig. 4. A 49-year-old woman presented with a breast mass. (*A*) Mammogram showed dense breast tissue with no apparent focal lesions. (*B*) Ultrasound showed a circumscribed lobulated lesion with heterogeneous echogenicity. (*C*) MR imaging showed a 15-mm ring-enhancing lesion that did not reach threshold, with increased signal on T2 and low signal on T1. (*D*) Core biopsy showed an invasive mucinous carcinoma, with islands of tumor cells floating in background mucin. (*E*) The tumor cells stained strongly positive for estrogen receptor but were negative for HER2 (*F*). This finding demonstrates the potential limitations, including nonvisualization of the malignancy, when imaging mucinous tumors by mammography.

a cribriform or sievelike architecture with spaces filled with bluish mucin and pink basement membranelike material, although solid and tubular patterns can also be seen.[53,110] They were originally described in the salivary gland but can occur in the breast or lung. In the breast, AdCCs usually occur in older women and are low-grade with an excellent prognosis with adequate local therapy; lymph node and distant metastases are rare.[2] Regardless of site, AdCCs harbor a chromosomal rearrangement involving the MYB gene, typically resulting in a t(6;9)(q22–23;p23–24) translocation with the formation of a MYB-NFIB fusion gene. This translocation has been detected in 23% to 100% of breast AdCCs.[53] Apart from this translocation, the genome is stable and they lack copy number changes, such as 8q gain and 5q loss or mutations in TP53 and PIK3CA that are commonly seen in other TNBCs.[111] Rare cases with progression to poorly differentiated basaloid carcinoma accompanied by accumulation of additional genetic alterations have been described.[112]

Secretory Carcinoma

Secretory carcinoma is a very rare tumor that was originally described in children and adolescents but can occur in patients of all ages and in men.[2,113] It is composed of cells with abundant granular eosinophilic to foamy cytoplasm forming microcystic, tubular and solid patterns, with periodic acid–Schiff–positive intracellular and extracellular secretory material that gives it its name. Despite being triple negative, they are low grade and have an excellent prognosis. Secretory carcinoma has a characteristic t(12;15) translocation that produces a ETV6-NTRK3 fusion gene; this translocation is unique to secretory carcinoma in the breast but has been described in other tumors, such as infantile fibrosarcoma and congenital mesoblastic nephroma.[53,109] Similar to AdCC, the genome is otherwise stable with few copy number alterations. Interestingly, a salivary gland counterpart to secretory carcinoma has now been recognized, in part because it harbors the same t(12;15) translocation.

Medullarylike Carcinoma

In contrast, medullarylike carcinomas are TNBCs characterized by marked nuclear pleomorphism, a high mitotic rate, syncytial growth pattern, and pushing margins with a prominent lymphocytic inflammatory infiltrate. Despite the aggressive histologic features, the presence of pushing margins means that they are well circumscribed and can appear deceptively innocuous on imaging, particularly in young women.[53,104]

Classic medullary carcinoma is defined by strict histologic criteria that are poorly reproducible, and it is now thought that the relatively favorable prognosis compared with other grade-3 TNBCs is due to the associated immune response, so medullary, atypical medullary, and medullarylike IDC are grouped together in the most recent World Health Organization classification as carcinoma with medullary features.[2] These tumors show high levels of genomic instability with complex copy number aberrations and structural gene rearrangements. Structural gene rearrangements resulting in the creation of neo-antigens, which then activate the host immune response.[114,115] The cancers that arise in BRCA1 mutation carriers often have medullary features with a very high mitotic rate, although conversely only 13% of women diagnosed with medullarylike cancers have BRCA1 mutations.[116,117] Alternative mechanisms, such as promoter hypermethylation, may be responsible for BRCA1 downregulation in cases lacking a germline mutation.[118] Medullarylike carcinomas also frequently contain TP53 mutations; this was the only high-frequency mutation seen in medullary carcinomas within the METABRIC cohort, present in more than 80% of cases.[86]

In conclusion, new HT genetic technologies have enhanced our understanding of breast cancer biology and changed the way we conceptualize breast cancer classification. However, the traditional histologic subtypes of breast cancer retain their value because of their clinical and radiological correlations and provide some clues as to the underlying molecular biology. Hence, the two are complementary; both play an important role at present in determining patient management. The histologic and molecular subtypes of breast cancer have important implications for how tumors are visualized on imaging studies. Several subtypes of breast cancer are more difficult to image on mammography. Basal-like/TNBCs tend to be highly FDG avid on PET, whereas the lobular histologic subtype may be less avid and less perceptible on FDG PET imaging.

ACKNOWLEDGMENTS

Dr S. Chin acknowledges Cancer Research UK. Dr G.A. Ulaner acknowledges the Department of Defense Breast Cancer Research Program Breakthrough Award BC132676 and the MSKCC Radiochemistry and Molecular Imaging Probe Core (NIH/NCI Cancer Center Support Grant P30 CA008748).

REFERENCES

1. Ali HR, Rueda OM, Chin SF, et al. Genome-driven integrated classification of breast cancer validated in over 7,500 samples. Genome Biol 2014;15(8):431.

2. Lakhani SR, Ellis IO, Schnitt SJ, et al. WHO classification of tumours of the breast. 4 edition. Lyon (France): International Agency for Research on Cancer (IARC) Press; 2012.

3. Cavallaro S, Paratore S, de Snoo F, et al. Genomic analysis: toward a new approach in breast cancer management. Crit Rev Oncol Hematol 2012;81(3): 207–23.

4. Rizzo JM, Buck MJ. Key principles and clinical applications of "next-generation" DNA sequencing. Cancer Prev Res (Phila) 2012;5(7):887–900.

5. Perou CM, Sorlie T, Eisen MB, et al. Molecular portraits of human breast tumours. Nature 2000; 406(6797):747–52.

6. Russnes HG, Navin N, Hicks J, et al. Insight into the heterogeneity of breast cancer through next-generation sequencing. J Clin Invest 2011; 121(10):3810–8.

7. Sotiriou C, Neo SY, McShane LM, et al. Breast cancer classification and prognosis based on gene expression profiles from a population-based study. Proc Natl Acad Sci U S A 2003;100(18): 10393–8.

8. Rakha EA, Reis-Filho JS, Baehner F, et al. Breast cancer prognostic classification in the molecular era: the role of histological grade. Breast Cancer Res 2010;12(4):207.

9. Schnitt SJ. Classification and prognosis of invasive breast cancer: from morphology to molecular taxonomy. Mod Pathol 2010;23(Suppl 2):S60–4.

10. Haybittle JL, Blamey RW, Elston CW, et al. A prognostic index in primary breast cancer. Br J Cancer 1982;45(3):361–6.

11. Olivotto IA, Bajdik CD, Ravdin PM, et al. Population-based validation of the prognostic model ADJUVANT! for early breast cancer. J Clin Oncol 2005;23(12):2716–25.

12. Ravdin PM. A computer program to assist in making breast cancer adjuvant therapy decisions. Semin Oncol 1996;23(1 Suppl 2):43–50.

13. Wishart GC, Azzato EM, Greenberg DC, et al. PREDICT: a new UK prognostic model that predicts survival following surgery for invasive breast cancer. Breast Cancer Res 2010;12(1):R1.

14. Wishart GC, Bajdik CD, Dicks E, et al. PREDICT Plus: development and validation of a prognostic model for early breast cancer that includes HER2. Br J Cancer 2012;107(5):800–7.

15. Wishart GC, Rakha E, Green A, et al. Inclusion of KI67 significantly improves performance of the PREDICT prognostication and prediction model for early breast cancer. BMC Cancer 2014;14:908.

16. Brenton JD, Carey LA, Ahmed AA, et al. Molecular classification and molecular forecasting of breast cancer: ready for clinical application? J Clin Oncol 2005;23(29):7350–60.

17. Sinn P, Aulmann S, Wirtz R, et al. Multigene assays for classification, prognosis, and prediction in breast cancer: a critical review on the background and clinical utility. Geburtshilfe Frauenheilkd 2013; 73(9):932–40.

18. Sonnenblick A, Fumagalli D, Azim HA Jr, et al. New strategies in breast cancer: the significance of molecular subtypes in systemic adjuvant treatment for small T1a,bN0M0 tumors. Clin Cancer Res 2014; 20(24):6242–6.

19. Early Breast Cancer Trialists' Collaborative Group (EBCTCG), Peto R, Davies C, Godwin J, et al. Comparisons between different polychemotherapy regimens for early breast cancer: meta-analyses of long-term outcome among 100,000 women in 123 randomised trials. Lancet 2012;379(9814):432–44.

20. Maia AT, Sammut SJ, Jacinta-Fernandes A, et al. Big data in cancer genomics. Curr Opin Syst Biol 2017;4:78–84.

21. Sorlie T, Perou CM, Tibshirani R, et al. Gene expression patterns of breast carcinomas distinguish tumor subclasses with clinical implications. Proc Natl Acad Sci U S A 2001;98(19):10869–74.

22. Prat A, Pineda E, Adamo B, et al. Clinical implications of the intrinsic molecular subtypes of breast cancer. Breast 2015;24(Suppl 2):S26–35.

23. Weigelt B, Baehner FL, Reis-Filho JS. The contribution of gene expression profiling to breast cancer classification, prognostication and prediction: a retrospective of the last decade. J Pathol 2010; 220(2):263–80.

24. Mackay A, Weigelt B, Grigoriadis A, et al. Microarray-based class discovery for molecular classification of breast cancer: analysis of interobserver agreement. J Natl Cancer Inst 2011;103(8):662–73.

25. Pusztai L, Mazouni C, Anderson K, et al. Molecular classification of breast cancer: limitations and potential. Oncologist 2006;11(8):868–77.

26. Weigelt B, Mackay A, A'Hern R, et al. Breast cancer molecular profiling with single sample predictors: a retrospective analysis. Lancet Oncol 2010;11(4): 339–49.

27. Zhao X, Rodland EA, Sorlie T, et al. Systematic assessment of prognostic gene signatures for breast cancer shows distinct influence of time and ER status. BMC Cancer 2014;14:211.

28. Parker JS, Mullins M, Cheang MC, et al. Supervised risk predictor of breast cancer based on intrinsic subtypes. J Clin Oncol 2009;27(8):1160–7.

29. Wallden B, Storhoff J, Nielsen T, et al. Development and verification of the PAM50-based Prosigna breast cancer gene signature assay. BMC Med Genomics 2015;8:54.

30. Dowsett M, Sestak I, Lopez-Knowles E, et al. Comparison of PAM50 risk of recurrence score with oncotype DX and IHC4 for predicting risk of distant recurrence after endocrine therapy. J Clin Oncol 2013;31(22):2783–90.

31. Filipits M, Nielsen TO, Rudas M, et al. The PAM50 risk-of-recurrence score predicts risk for late distant recurrence after endocrine therapy in postmenopausal women with endocrine-responsive early breast cancer. Clin Cancer Res 2014;20(5):1298–305.

32. Gnant M, Filipits M, Greil R, et al. Predicting distant recurrence in receptor-positive breast cancer patients with limited clinicopathological risk: using the PAM50 Risk of Recurrence score in 1478 postmenopausal patients of the ABCSG-8 trial treated with adjuvant endocrine therapy alone. Ann Oncol 2014;25(2):339–45.

33. Gnant M, Sestak I, Filipits M, et al. Identifying clinically relevant prognostic subgroups of postmenopausal women with node-positive hormone receptor-positive early-stage breast cancer treated with endocrine therapy: a combined analysis of ABCSG-8 and ATAC using the PAM50 risk of recurrence score and intrinsic subtype. Ann Oncol 2015;26(8):1685–91.

34. Prat A, Perou CM. Deconstructing the molecular portraits of breast cancer. Mol Oncol 2011;5(1):5–23.

35. Prat A, Cheang MC, Martin M, et al. Prognostic significance of progesterone receptor-positive tumor cells within immunohistochemically defined luminal A breast cancer. J Clin Oncol 2013;31(2):203–9.

36. Ades F, Zardavas D, Bozovic-Spasojevic I, et al. Luminal B breast cancer: molecular characterization, clinical management, and future perspectives. J Clin Oncol 2014;32(25):2794–803.

37. Cheang MC, Chia SK, Voduc D, et al. Ki67 index, HER2 status, and prognosis of patients with luminal B breast cancer. J Natl Cancer Inst 2009;101(10):736–50.

38. Filipits M, Rudas M, Jakesz R, et al. A new molecular predictor of distant recurrence in ER-positive, HER2-negative breast cancer adds independent information to conventional clinical risk factors. Clin Cancer Res 2011;17(18):6012–20.

39. Paik S, Shak S, Tang G, et al. A multigene assay to predict recurrence of tamoxifen-treated, node-negative breast cancer. N Engl J Med 2004;351(27):2817–26.

40. van de Vijver MJ, He YD, van't Veer LJ, et al. A gene-expression signature as a predictor of survival in breast cancer. N Engl J Med 2002;347(25):1999–2009.

41. Kittaneh M, Montero AJ, Gluck S. Molecular profiling for breast cancer: a comprehensive review. Biomark Cancer 2013;5:61–70.

42. Ebbert MT, Bastien RR, Boucher KM, et al. Characterization of uncertainty in the classification of multivariate assays: application to PAM50 centroid-based genomic predictors for breast cancer treatment plans. J Clin Bioinforma 2011;1:37.

43. Fan C, Oh DS, Wessels L, et al. Concordance among gene-expression-based predictors for breast cancer. N Engl J Med 2006;355(6):560–9.

44. Kelly CM, Bernard PS, Krishnamurthy S, et al. Agreement in risk prediction between the 21-gene recurrence score assay (Oncotype DX(R)) and the PAM50 breast cancer intrinsic classifier in early-stage estrogen receptor-positive breast cancer. Oncologist 2012;17(4):492–8.

45. Prat A, Parker JS, Fan C, et al. Concordance among gene expression-based predictors for ER-positive breast cancer treated with adjuvant tamoxifen. Ann Oncol 2012;23(11):2866–73.

46. Varga Z, Sinn P, Fritzsche F, et al. Comparison of EndoPredict and Oncotype DX test results in hormone receptor positive invasive breast cancer. PLoS One 2013;8(3):e58483.

47. Harris LN, Ismaila N, McShane LM, et al. Use of biomarkers to guide decisions on adjuvant systemic therapy for women with early-stage invasive breast cancer: American Society of Clinical Oncology clinical practice guideline. J Clin Oncol 2016;34(10):1134–50.

48. Rouzier R, Perou CM, Symmans WF, et al. Breast cancer molecular subtypes respond differently to preoperative chemotherapy. Clin Cancer Res 2005;11(16):5678–85.

49. Prat A, Carey LA, Adamo B, et al. Molecular features and survival outcomes of the intrinsic subtypes within HER2-positive breast cancer. J Natl Cancer Inst 2014;106(8) [pii:dju152].

50. Prat A, Bianchini G, Thomas M, et al. Research-based PAM50 subtype predictor identifies higher responses and improved survival outcomes in HER2-positive breast cancer in the NOAH study. Clin Cancer Res 2014;20(2):511–21.

51. Badve S, Dabbs DJ, Schnitt SJ, et al. Basal-like and triple-negative breast cancers: a critical review with an emphasis on the implications for pathologists and oncologists. Mod Pathol 2011;24(2):157–67.

52. Jacquemier J, Padovani L, Rabayrol L, et al. Typical medullary breast carcinomas have a basal/myoepithelial phenotype. J Pathol 2005;207(3):260–8.

53. Pareja F, Geyer FC, Marchio C, et al. Triple-negative breast cancer: the importance of molecular and histologic subtyping, and recognition of low-grade variants. NPJ Breast Cancer 2016;2:16036.

54. Weigelt B, Kreike B, Reis-Filho JS. Metaplastic breast carcinomas are basal-like breast cancers: a genomic profiling analysis. Breast Cancer Res Treat 2009;117(2):273–80.

55. Wetterskog D, Lopez-Garcia MA, Lambros MB, et al. Adenoid cystic carcinomas constitute a genomically distinct subgroup of triple-negative and basal-like breast cancers. J Pathol 2012;226(1):84–96.

56. Foulkes WD, Stefansson IM, Chappuis PO, et al. Germline BRCA1 mutations and a basal epithelial phenotype in breast cancer. J Natl Cancer Inst 2003;95(19):1482–5.

57. Severson TM, Peeters J, Majewski I, et al. BRCA1-like signature in triple negative breast cancer: molecular and clinical characterization reveals subgroups with therapeutic potential. Mol Oncol 2015;9(8):1528–38.

58. Lehmann BD, Bauer JA, Chen X, et al. Identification of human triple-negative breast cancer subtypes and preclinical models for selection of targeted therapies. J Clin Invest 2011;121(7):2750–67.

59. Lehmann BD, Jovanovic B, Chen X, et al. Refinement of triple-negative breast cancer molecular subtypes: implications for neoadjuvant chemotherapy selection. PLoS One 2016;11(6):e0157368.

60. Masuda H, Baggerly KA, Wang Y, et al. Differential response to neoadjuvant chemotherapy among 7 triple-negative breast cancer molecular subtypes. Clin Cancer Res 2013;19(19):5533–40.

61. Farmer P, Bonnefoi H, Becette V, et al. Identification of molecular apocrine breast tumours by microarray analysis. Oncogene 2005;24(29):4660–71.

62. Lehmann BD, Bauer JA, Schafer JM, et al. PIK3CA mutations in androgen receptor-positive triple negative breast cancer confer sensitivity to the combination of PI3K and androgen receptor inhibitors. Breast Cancer Res 2014;16(4):406.

63. Basu S, Chen W, Tchou J, et al. Comparison of triple-negative and estrogen receptor-positive/progesterone receptor-positive/HER2-negative breast carcinoma using quantitative fluorine-18 fluorodeoxyglucose/positron emission tomography imaging parameters: a potentially useful method for disease characterization. Cancer 2008;112(5):995–1000.

64. Groheux D, Giacchetti S, Moretti JL, et al. Correlation of high 18F-FDG uptake to clinical, pathological and biological prognostic factors in breast cancer. Eur J Nucl Med Mol Imaging 2011;38(3):426–35.

65. Groheux D, Hindie E, Delord M, et al. Prognostic impact of (18)FDG-PET-CT findings in clinical stage III and IIB breast cancer. J Natl Cancer Inst 2012;104(24):1879–87.

66. Ciriello G, Miller ML, Aksoy BA, et al. Emerging landscape of oncogenic signatures across human cancers. Nat Genet 2013;45(10):1127–33.

67. Curtis C, Shah SP, Chin SF, et al. The genomic and transcriptomic architecture of 2,000 breast tumours reveals novel subgroups. Nature 2012;486(7403):346–52.

68. Horlings HM, Weigelt B, Anderson EM, et al. Genomic profiling of histological special types of breast cancer. Breast Cancer Res Treat 2013;142(2):257–69.

69. Johnson K, Sarma D, Hwang ES. Lobular breast cancer series: imaging. Breast Cancer Res 2015;17:94.

70. Ciriello G, Gatza ML, Beck AH, et al. Comprehensive molecular portraits of invasive lobular breast cancer. Cell 2015;163(2):506–19.

71. Monhollen L, Morrison C, Ademuyiwa FO, et al. Pleomorphic lobular carcinoma: a distinctive clinical and molecular breast cancer type. Histopathology 2012;61(3):365–77.

72. Simpson PT, Reis-Filho JS, Lambros MB, et al. Molecular profiling pleomorphic lobular carcinomas of the breast: evidence for a common molecular genetic pathway with classic lobular carcinomas. J Pathol 2008;215(3):231–44.

73. Cowin P, Rowlands TM, Hatsell SJ. Cadherins and catenins in breast cancer. Curr Opin Cell Biol 2005;17(5):499–508.

74. Da Silva L, Parry S, Reid L, et al. Aberrant expression of E-cadherin in lobular carcinomas of the breast. Am J Surg Pathol 2008;32(5):773–83.

75. Doyle S, Evans AJ, Rakha EA, et al. Influence of E-cadherin expression on the mammographic appearance of invasive nonlobular breast carcinoma detected at screening. Radiology 2009;253(1):51–5.

76. Rakha EA, Patel A, Powe DG, et al. Clinical and biological significance of E-cadherin protein expression in invasive lobular carcinoma of the breast. Am J Surg Pathol 2010;34(10):1472–9.

77. Guiu S, Wolfer A, Jacot W, et al. Invasive lobular breast cancer and its variants: how special are they for systemic therapy decisions? Crit Rev Oncol Hematol 2014;92(3):235–57.

78. Balmativola D, Marchio C, Maule M, et al. Pathological non-response to chemotherapy in a neoadjuvant setting of breast cancer: an inter-institutional study. Breast Cancer Res Treat 2014;148(3):511–23.

79. Petruolo OA, Pilewskie M, Patil S, et al. Standard pathologic features can be used to identify a subset of estrogen receptor-positive, HER2 negative patients likely to benefit from neoadjuvant chemotherapy. Ann Surg Oncol 2017;24(9):2556–62.

80. Tsai ML, Lillemoe TJ, Finkelstein MJ, et al. Utility of oncotype DX risk assessment in patients with invasive lobular carcinoma. Clin Breast Cancer 2016;16(1):45–50.

81. Weigelt B, Geyer FC, Reis-Filho JS. Histological types of breast cancer: how special are they? Mol Oncol 2010;4(3):192–208.

82. Lopez-Garcia MA, Geyer FC, Lacroix-Triki M, et al. Breast cancer precursors revisited: molecular features and progression pathways. Histopathology 2010;57(2):171–92.

83. Weigelt B, Geyer FC, Natrajan R, et al. The molecular underpinning of lobular histological growth pattern: a genome-wide transcriptomic analysis of invasive lobular carcinomas and grade- and molecular subtype-matched invasive ductal carcinomas of no special type. J Pathol 2010;220(1):45–57.

84. Michaut M, Chin SF, Majewski I, et al. Integration of genomic, transcriptomic and proteomic data identifies two biologically distinct subtypes of invasive lobular breast cancer. Sci Rep 2016;6:18517.

85. Dawson SJ, Rueda OM, Aparicio S, et al. A new genome-driven integrated classification of breast cancer and its implications. EMBO J 2013;32(5):617–28.

86. Pereira B, Chin SF, Rueda OM, et al. The somatic mutation profiles of 2,433 breast cancers refines their genomic and transcriptomic landscapes. Nat Commun 2016;7:11479.

87. Abhik Mukherjee, Roslin Russell, Suet-Feung Chin, et al. Associations between genomic stratification of breast cancer and centrally reviewed tumour pathology in the METABRIC cohort. British Journal of Cancer (in press).

88. Avril N, Menzel M, Dose J, et al. Glucose metabolism of breast cancer assessed by 18F-FDG PET: histologic and immunohistochemical tissue analysis. J Nucl Med 2001;42(1):9–16.

89. Avril N, Rose CA, Schelling M, et al. Breast imaging with positron emission tomography and fluorine-18 fluorodeoxyglucose: use and limitations. J Clin Oncol 2000;18(20):3495–502.

90. Berg WA, Gutierrez L, NessAiver MS, et al. Diagnostic accuracy of mammography, clinical examination, US, and MR imaging in preoperative assessment of breast cancer. Radiology 2004;233(3):830–49.

91. Bos R, van Der Hoeven JJ, van Der Wall E, et al. Biologic correlates of (18)fluorodeoxyglucose uptake in human breast cancer measured by positron emission tomography. J Clin Oncol 2002;20(2):379–87.

92. Buck A, Schirrmeister H, Kuhn T, et al. FDG uptake in breast cancer: correlation with biological and clinical prognostic parameters. Eur J Nucl Med Mol Imaging 2002;29(10):1317–23.

93. Lopez JK, Bassett LW. Invasive lobular carcinoma of the breast: spectrum of mammographic, US, and MR imaging findings. Radiographics 2009;29(1):165–76.

94. Dashevsky BZ, Goldman DA, Parsons M, et al. Appearance of untreated bone metastases from breast cancer on FDG PET/CT: importance of histologic subtype. Eur J Nucl Med Mol Imaging 2015;42(11):1666–73.

95. Hogan MP, Goldman DA, Dashevsky B, et al. Comparison of 18F-FDG PET/CT for systemic staging of newly diagnosed invasive lobular carcinoma versus invasive ductal carcinoma. J Nucl Med 2015;56(11):1674–80.

96. Borst MJ, Ingold JA. Metastatic patterns of invasive lobular versus invasive ductal carcinoma of the breast. Surgery 1993;114(4):637–41 [discussion: 641–2].

97. He H, Gonzalez A, Robinson E, et al. Distant metastatic disease manifestations in infiltrating lobular carcinoma of the breast. AJR Am J Roentgenol 2014;202(5):1140–8.

98. Kane AJ, Wang ZJ, Qayyum A, et al. Frequency and etiology of unexplained bilateral hydronephrosis in patients with breast cancer: results of a longitudinal CT study. Clin Imaging 2012;36(4):263–6.

99. Lamovec J, Bracko M. Metastatic pattern of infiltrating lobular carcinoma of the breast: an autopsy study. J Surg Oncol 1991;48(1):28–33.

100. Ulaner GA, Goldman DA, Corben A, et al. Prospective clinical trial of (18)F-fluciclovine PET/CT for determining the response to neoadjuvant therapy in invasive ductal and invasive lobular breast cancers. J Nucl Med 2017;58(7):1037–42.

101. Ulaner GA, Goldman DA, Gonen M, et al. Initial results of a prospective clinical trial of 18F-fluciclovine PET/CT in newly diagnosed invasive ductal and invasive lobular breast cancers. J Nucl Med 2016;57(9):1350–6.

102. Rakha EA, Lee AH, Evans AJ, et al. Tubular carcinoma of the breast: further evidence to support its excellent prognosis. J Clin Oncol 2010;28(1):99–104.

103. Lopez-Garcia MA, Geyer FC, Natrajan R, et al. Transcriptomic analysis of tubular carcinomas of the breast reveals similarities and differences with molecular subtype-matched ductal and lobular carcinomas. J Pathol 2010;222(1):64–75.

104. Larribe M, Thomassin-Piana J, Jalaguier-Coudray A. Breast cancers with round lumps: correlations between imaging and anatomopathology. Diagn Interv Imaging 2014;95(1):37–46.

105. Caldarella A, Buzzoni C, Crocetti E, et al. Invasive breast cancer: a significant correlation between histological types and molecular subgroups. J Cancer Res Clin Oncol 2013;139(4):617–23.

106. Lacroix-Triki M, Suarez PH, MacKay A, et al. Mucinous carcinoma of the breast is genomically distinct from invasive ductal carcinomas of no special type. J Pathol 2010;222(3):282–98.

107. Buttitta F, Felicioni L, Barassi F, et al. PIK3CA mutation and histological type in breast carcinoma: high frequency of mutations in lobular carcinoma. J Pathol 2006;208(3):350–5.

108. Geyer FC, Lambros MB, Natrajan R, et al. Genomic and immunohistochemical analysis of

adenosquamous carcinoma of the breast. Mod Pathol 2010;23(7):951–60.

109. Krings G, Joseph NM, Bean GR, et al. Genomic profiling of breast secretory carcinomas reveals distinct genetics from other breast cancers and similarity to mammary analog secretory carcinomas. Mod Pathol 2017;30(8):1086–99.

110. Foschini MP, Morandi L, Asioli S, et al. The morphological spectrum of salivary gland type tumours of the breast. Pathology 2017;49(2):215–27.

111. Martelotto LG, De Filippo MR, Ng CK, et al. Genomic landscape of adenoid cystic carcinoma of the breast. J Pathol 2015;237(2):179–89.

112. Fusco N, Geyer FC, De Filippo MR, et al. Genetic events in the progression of adenoid cystic carcinoma of the breast to high-grade triple-negative breast cancer. Mod Pathol 2016;29(11):1292–305.

113. Li D, Xiao X, Yang W, et al. Secretory breast carcinoma: a clinicopathological and immunophenotypic study of 15 cases with a review of the literature. Mod Pathol 2012;25(4):567–75.

114. McGranahan N, Furness AJ, Rosenthal R, et al. Clonal neoantigens elicit T cell immunoreactivity and sensitivity to immune checkpoint blockade. Science 2016;351(6280):1463–9.

115. Turajlic S, Litchfield K, Xu H, et al. Insertion-and-deletion-derived tumour-specific neoantigens and the immunogenic phenotype: a pan-cancer analysis. Lancet Oncol 2017;18(8):1009–21.

116. Armes JE, Egan AJ, Southey MC, et al. The histologic phenotypes of breast carcinoma occurring before age 40 years in women with and without BRCA1 or BRCA2 germline mutations: a population-based study. Cancer 1998;83(11):2335–45.

117. Lakhani SR, Jacquemier J, Sloane JP, et al. Multifactorial analysis of differences between sporadic breast cancers and cancers involving BRCA1 and BRCA2 mutations. J Natl Cancer Inst 1998; 90(15):1138–45.

118. Osin P, Lu YJ, Stone J, et al. Distinct genetic and epigenetic changes in medullary breast cancer. Int J Surg Pathol 2003;11(3):153–8.

Overview of Breast Cancer Therapy

Tracy-Ann Moo, MD[a], Rachel Sanford, MD[b], Chau Dang, MD[b], Monica Morrow, MD[a],*

KEYWORDS

- Breast cancer therapy • Local therapy • Adjuvant therapy • Breast-conserving therapy
- Mastectomy • Neoadjuvant chemotherapy • Breast cancer surveillance • Endocrine therapy

KEY POINTS

- Breast-conserving therapy and mastectomy are well-established local therapies for early-stage invasive breast cancer and have equivalent survival and recurrence outcomes with multimodal therapy.
- Neoadjuvant chemotherapy is increasingly used to downstage disease in the breast and axilla, allowing breast conservation and avoiding axillary lymph node dissection, and is most likely to be successful in a unicentric, human epidermal growth factor receptor 2–positive or triple negative breast cancer.
- Adjuvant medical therapies are given after breast surgery to eradicate clinically and radiographically occult micrometastatic disease that may develop into frank metastases if untreated.
- Disease burden and biology determine patients' risk of recurrence, which guides the selection of appropriate adjuvant medical therapies.

The diagnosis and treatment of invasive breast cancer requires a collaborative effort among multiple subspecialties. Diagnostic imaging workup and biopsy play a key role in establishing a diagnosis and informing surgical decisions on management of the primary tumor, staging of the axilla, and the sequence of therapy. Once a diagnosis of breast cancer is established, the extent of disease is assessed, which, for the most part, determines whether or not preoperative (neoadjuvant) systemic therapy is indicated. Confirmed stage IV breast cancer is considered incurable; it is treated with systemic therapy alone unless there is an indication for palliative resection of the primary tumor and is not discussed further. An important part of the initial clinical evaluation of patients with nonmetastatic breast cancer is to identify clinical criteria of inoperability, which necessitate the use of neoadjuvant therapy. These criteria include inflammatory carcinoma, fixation of the tumor to the bony chest wall (ribs, sternum), extensive skin involvement with ulceration or satellite skin nodules, fixed/matted axillary lymphadenopathy, involvement of neurovascular structures of the axilla, or lymphedema of the ipsilateral arm. All of these findings are readily identifiable on physical examination and should prompt an imaging evaluation for distant metastases. In these cases, systemic therapy is administered as initial treatment to reduce tumor volume and will render approximately 80% of patients operable.[1] In those patients who present with operable disease, the sequence of surgical resection and systemic therapy is variable. Preoperative systemic therapy

Disclosure Statement: Dr M. Morrow is a consultant for Genomic Health. Dr C. Dang receives research funding from Roche, Genentech, and PUMA. The remaining authors have no disclosures.
[a] Breast Service, Department of Surgery, Memorial Sloan Kettering Cancer Center, 300 East 66th Street, New York, NY 10065, USA; [b] Breast Medicine Service, Department of Medicine, Memorial Sloan Kettering Cancer Center, 300 East 66th Street, New York, NY 10065, USA
* Corresponding author.
E-mail address: morrowm@mskcc.org

pet.theclinics.com

may be used to reduce tumor volume in the breast, allowing breast conservation when mastectomy would otherwise be necessary, and to decrease the need for axillary lymph node dissection (ALND). In most patients presenting with stage I and II disease, resection of the tumor is the initial step in management, and patients have the option of breast conservation or mastectomy (**Fig. 1**).

LOCAL THERAPY FOR INVASIVE BREAST CANCER: BREAST-CONSERVING THERAPY AND MASTECTOMY

Breast-conserving therapy (BCT) and mastectomy are both well-established local therapies for invasive breast cancer. Multiple randomized clinical trials with a follow-up of up to 20 years have demonstrated that BCT is safe and has survival outcomes equivalent to mastectomy in stage I and II breast cancer.[2–6] Although a few earlier trials reported higher rates of locoregional recurrence (LRR) following BCT than were seen after mastectomy (10%–22%),[2,4,7] much lower LRR rates are reported in contemporary studies. The decrease in LRR can be attributed to the implementation of microscopic confirmation of negative resection margins and the widespread use of systemic therapy. In a study of LRR in patients with node-negative and node-positive breast cancer receiving systemic therapy after BCT in 5 National Surgical Adjuvant Breast and Bowel Project protocols, 10-year local recurrence rates were 5.2% and 8.7%, respectively.[8,9] These rates are comparable with observed 10-year rates of isolated local recurrence after mastectomy of approximately 8%.[10] It is now understood that local control is not solely a function of disease burden and extent of surgery, but varies with tumor molecular subtype and administration of systemic therapy. Rates of local recurrence differ significantly among breast cancer subtypes, regardless of whether patients are treated with mastectomy or BCT. Local recurrence rates are highest among patients with hormone receptor (HR)–negative, human epidermal growth factor receptor 2 (HER2)–negative cancers (triple negative), and lowest among patients with HR-positive, HER2-negative cancers.[11,12] This understanding eliminates the rationale for treating biologically aggressive cancers with mastectomy, and most patients with stage I and II disease are candidates for BCT.

BREAST-CONSERVING THERAPY

BCT involves excision of the tumor (lumpectomy) followed by adjuvant whole-breast irradiation (WBI). In order to perform BCT, it must be possible to excise the tumor to negative margins with an acceptable cosmetic outcome, patients must be able to receive radiotherapy, and the breast must be suitable for follow-up to allow prompt detection of local recurrence. The contraindications to BCT arise logically from these requirements. Contraindications to BCT include the presence of diffuse suspicious or malignant-appearing calcifications, disease that cannot be resected to negative margins with a satisfactory cosmetic result, and the presence of contraindications to delivery of radiation, such as prior treatment of the breast field or active scleroderma.[13] A negative margin is defined as "no ink on the tumor."[13,14] More widely clear margins do not improve local control in invasive breast cancer and are not required for BCT.[15] If negative margins can be achieved with an acceptable cosmetic outcome, then lumpectomy can be performed irrespective of tumor size. In women with large tumors relative to breast size, neoadjuvant chemotherapy (NAC) can be used to downstage the tumor (see later discussion). Young age, aggressive tumor subtype (HER2-positive and triple negative), and lobular histology are not contraindications to BCT. In patients with BRCA1/2 mutations, bilateral mastectomy is a consideration, as the risk of a new primary breast cancer development can range from 26% to 40% over the 20 years following diagnosis depending on the age of onset of the initial cancer, performance of oophorectomy, and use of endocrine therapy.[16] Despite this higher risk, a BRCA mutation is not an absolute contraindication to breast conservation, and patient preference must also be considered.

Physical examination, mammography, and diagnostic ultrasound are the imaging modalities in standard use to select patients for BCT. In a population-based study of 1984 women with ductal carcinoma in situ and stage I and II invasive cancers, 88% of those attempting BCT successfully had the procedure. This figure is probably an underestimate of the number of women eligible for BCT because many were converted to mastectomy without an attempt at reexcision.[17] The use of MR imaging in the preoperative setting is controversial. MR imaging is more sensitive than mammography or ultrasound, detecting additional disease in 16% of patients in a meta-analysis.[18] It was hoped that MR imaging would improve selection of lumpectomy candidates and decrease rates of reoperation. However, multiple studies of preoperative MR imaging have demonstrated an increase in both ipsilateral mastectomy for the index tumor and contralateral prophylactic mastectomy rates without an accompanying reduction in reoperation and recurrence rates.[19–26]

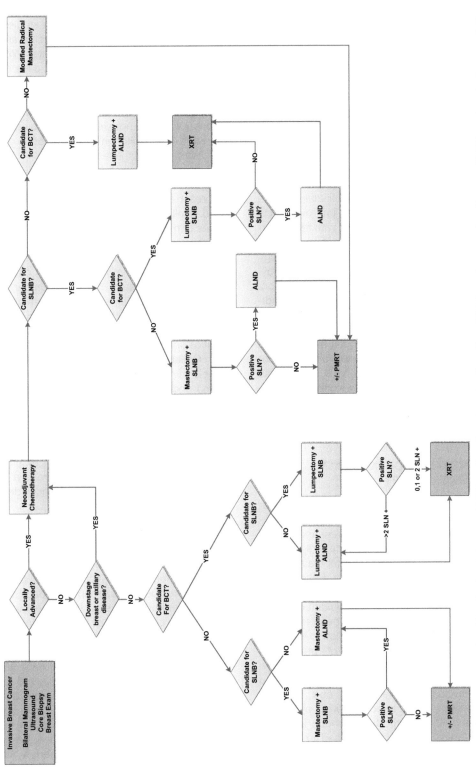

Fig. 1. Invasive breast cancer: algorithm for local therapy. ALND, axillary lymph node dissection; BCT, breast-conserving therapy; PMRT, postmastectomy radiation therapy; SLN, sentinel lymph node; SLNB, sentinel lymph node biopsy; XRT, breast radiation.

A systematic review that included 85,975 patients examined the association between preoperative MR imaging and surgical outcomes. MR imaging was associated with an increased likelihood of undergoing ipsilateral mastectomy (odds ratio [OR] 1.39; 95% confidence interval [CI] 1.23–1.57; $P < .001$) and contralateral prophylactic mastectomy (OR 1.9; 95% CI 1.25–2.91; $P = .003$) after adjusting for patient age. The use of preoperative MR imaging did not significantly reduce the rate of positive margins, reoperation, or reexcision.[27] Additionally, an individual patient-level meta-analysis of the impact of MR imaging on local recurrence rates after BCT observed no differences in patients selected with and without MR imaging.[24] The failure of detection of subclinical disease with MR imaging to translate into improved local recurrence outcomes is consistent with the understanding that local recurrence is determined not only by tumor burden but also by tumor biology and the use of effective adjuvant systemic therapy. In the absence of a specific clinical question, routine use of preoperative MR imaging is not indicated. Specific instances whereby preoperative MR imaging might be clinically useful include mammographically and/or sonographically occult tumors, Paget disease, evaluation of the extent of residual disease following NAC in patients desiring conservation, and when significant differences in the assessment of tumor size by physical examination, mammography, and ultrasound are seen.

ADJUVANT RADIATION IN BREAST-CONSERVING THERAPY

It is important to determine preoperatively whether or not patients are candidates for adjuvant radiation. Prior chest wall irradiation, pregnancy at the time of diagnosis, and the presence of a connective tissue/collagen vascular disorder may be contraindications to radiation treatment. Patients with a history of mantle radiation delivered for Hodgkin lymphoma may be ineligible for adjuvant radiation if the radiation threshold dose has been exceeded during prior therapy. Delivery of radiation is contraindicated during all trimesters of pregnancy. However, in a woman presenting with invasive breast cancer in the second or third trimester, a lumpectomy can be performed and adjuvant chemotherapy administered followed by breast irradiation in the postpartum period. In cases whereby breast cancer is diagnosed in the first trimester without an indication for adjuvant chemotherapy, mastectomy is the preferred procedure. Connective tissue/collagen vascular disorders, including scleroderma, Sjögren

syndrome, systemic lupus erythematosus, and dermatomyositis/polymyositis, are considered relative contraindications to the delivery of breast irradiation due to small retrospective studies suggesting an increased incidence of acute and late radiation toxicities in these patients. With the exception of scleroderma, matched case control studies have not consistently demonstrated an increase in risk; however, these were very small retrospective studies in which patients with severe disease were likely not selected for radiation.[28–30] Preoperative consultation with a radiation oncologist is warranted in these patients.

WBI is given following lumpectomy to eliminate residual microscopic disease that may remain in the breast even when negative margins are obtained. Holland and colleagues,[31] in pathologic studies of mastectomy specimens in 282 patients with clinical and mammographically unifocal breast cancers, found additional tumor foci within 2 cm of the index tumor in 56 (20%) cases and greater than 2 cm from the index cancer in 121 (43%) cases. The delivery of adjuvant radiation following lumpectomy decreases local failure rates by about 50% and increases breast cancer–specific survival.[2–4,6] The Early Breast Cancer Trialists' Collaborative Group's (EBCTCG) meta-analysis of 17 randomized trials including 10,801 women undergoing BCT demonstrated a reduction in the risk of any recurrence at 10 years from 35.0% to 19.3% and a 15-year absolute reduction in the risk of death from breast cancer of 3.8% (95% CI 1.6–6.0, $P = .00005$) with radiation. Investigators extrapolate that for every 4 recurrences that are prevented at 10 years, there is a corresponding avoidance of 1 breast cancer death at 15 years.[6]

These data specifically focused on the delivery of conventional WBI consisting of 50 Gy in 25 fractions, daily, over the course of approximately 5 to 7 weeks, followed by a boost of approximately 10 Gy to the tumor bed. Hypofractionated WBI reduces the number of treatments needed by delivering a larger fraction over a shorter period of time and allowing completion of treatment in approximately 3 weeks. Equivalent local recurrence rates at 5 and 10 years, no difference in overall survival, and improved cosmetic outcomes compared with conventional fractionation were observed in randomized trials.[32–34] Partial breast irradiation (PBI) involves radiation of a limited volume of breast tissue centered around the tumor cavity. PBI can be delivered using various techniques, including interstitial or intracavitary brachytherapy, intraoperative radiotherapy, or traditional external beam treatment. Potential advantages of PBI include shorter treatment time and irradiation of only a portion of the breast, possibly allowing repeat BCT should a new primary tumor develop. There are ongoing trials aimed at determining whether or not PBI is as effective as conventional or hypofractionated WBI in terms of local control, survival, and cosmesis.

A subgroup of BCT patients not benefitting from radiotherapy has not been identified using conventional tumor pathologic features. However, 2 prospective randomized trials demonstrated acceptable local control rates without radiation in older postmenopausal women, with small estrogen receptor–positive tumors receiving adjuvant endocrine therapy.[35,36] Women 70 years of age and older with estrogen receptor–positive stage I breast cancer who will receive endocrine therapy are considered candidates for this approach.

Several studies have shown an improvement in quality-of-life outcomes following BCT, greater cosmetic satisfaction with BCT compared with mastectomy without reconstruction, and equivalent satisfaction compared with mastectomy with immediate reconstruction.[37–40] The most important factor affecting cosmetic outcome after BCT is the volume of tissue removed, with a higher likelihood of a cosmetically significant defect when greater than 20% of the breast volume is excised.[41] Given that current guidelines do not require margins wider than no tumor on ink, a minority of patients require such large resections. In these instances, an onco-plastic procedure may be used to improve cosmetic outcomes. Oncoplastic procedures use plastic surgery tissue rearrangement and mastopexy techniques to fill in the lumpectomy defect, improving the contour of the conserved breast. The parenchymal rearrangement often results in displacement of the tumor bed and can be problematic for radiation planning. Placement of surgical clips to mark the boundaries of the lumpectomy cavity before tissue rearrangement is usually done to ensure accurate cavity localization during radiation therapy. Small retrospective series of patients undergoing large resections report greater patient satisfaction with cosmesis, and similar complication and recurrence rates as conventional BCT, with the exception of fat necrosis, which is higher in oncoplastic procedures (10% vs 25%).[42,43]

MASTECTOMY

In patients undergoing mastectomy, total mastectomy (simple mastectomy), skin-sparing mastectomy, and nipple areolar–sparing mastectomy are options for most patients. Total mastectomy removes the breast parenchyma, nipple areolar complex, and excess skin from the chest wall,

leaving only enough skin to close the incision. It is generally used when patients will not undergo immediate reconstruction. The skin-sparing mastectomy was developed to facilitate immediate reconstruction and removes the breast parenchyma and nipple areolar complex, leaving the skin as a natural envelope for placement of the tissue expander/implant or autologous flap. Multiple studies have confirmed the oncologic safety of the skin-sparing mastectomy, with local recurrence rates of approximately 6%, comparable with those observed for the traditional simple mastectomy.[44–47] The nipple areolar-sparing mastectomy preserves the nipple areolar complex in addition to the skin envelope and was initially used mainly in the prophylactic setting, and is now increasingly used in patients with invasive carcinoma. Local recurrence rates of 2% to 5% are reported, with the median follow-up ranging from 2 to 5 years.[48–51] Most of these data represent single-institution retrospective series with limited follow-up; until long-term oncologic safety has been established, patients should be carefully selected for this procedure. Although eligibility criteria vary by institution, the authors suggest limiting this procedure to patients with tumors less than 3 cm and at a distance of at least 1 cm from the nipple that do not have extensive calcifications suggesting an extensive intraductal component.

POSTMASTECTOMY RADIATION

Postmastectomy radiation (PMRT) is a well-established component of breast cancer treatment in patients with advanced disease. The role of PMRT in patients with early disease, as well as those undergoing NAC, remains in evolution. The most important predictor of LRR after mastectomy is the extent of axillary nodal disease. Patients with 4 or more positive axillary lymph nodes have a 25% or greater risk of developing an LRR.[52,53] A tumor size of 5 cm or greater is also associated with an increased risk of chest wall recurrence of greater than 20%.[52,53] For this reason, PMRT has been considered standard in these patients for many years.[13,54] PMRT in women with 1 to 3 positive lymph nodes and T1-2 breast cancers is an area of ongoing debate. A meta-analysis by the EBCTCG demonstrated a decreased risk of local recurrence and mortality after PMRT in women with 1 to 3 positive lymph nodes. However, the studies included in this meta-analysis antedated the availability of modern systemic therapies; rates of LRR in the control arms (20%) were substantially higher than expected based on more contemporary studies.[55–57] In a study at

Memorial Sloan Kettering Cancer Center examining outcomes in 1331 women with T1-2 tumors and 1 to 3 positive axillary lymph nodes treated with mastectomy between 1995 and 2006 whereby radiation was selectively administered, 15% had PMRT. At 5 years, the LRR rate was 3.2% in the PMRT group versus 4.3% in the group not receiving radiation (P = .57). Age less than 50 years and lympho-vascular invasion were identified as risk factors for recurrence.[55] These data suggest that the decision to administer PMRT in this group should be approached in a multidisciplinary setting. Factors determining the risk of recurrence in a particular patient, such as age, life expectancy, comorbidity, pathologic findings in the breast and axilla associated with a low disease burden, and biological characteristics of the tumor associated with greater effectiveness of systemic therapy, should be considered.[58]

As the use of NAC in operable breast cancer has increased, there is uncertainty as to whether the pre-NAC stage, post-NAC stage, or a combination of the two should be used to determine the need for PMRT. In general, PMRT is recommended following NAC in patients who present with clinical T3-4 tumors, N2-3 nodal involvement, or who have persistent nodal disease following NAC.[59] The benefit of PMRT in patients with clinical T1-2, N1 disease who have a pathologic complete response is an area of ongoing study.

STAGING AND MANAGEMENT OF THE AXILLA

The axillary nodes are the initial site of metastases in most patients with breast cancer, and approximately 25% of those with a normal physical examination will have nodal metastases.[60] The mainstay of axillary staging for almost 2 decades has been the sentinel lymph node biopsy. With the exception of older patients and those with severe comorbid conditions whereby information on nodal status will not change therapy, all newly diagnosed patients with invasive breast cancer who present with a clinically negative axilla should undergo axillary staging by sentinel lymph node biopsy. A sentinel node can be identified in 97% to 99% of patients using blue dye, radioactive tracers, or a combination of the two.[61–64] The sentinel node predicts the status of the remaining axillary nodes in greater than 95% of cases in the hands of experienced surgeons, and the risk of an isolated axillary recurrence after a negative sentinel node biopsy is less than 1%.[65,66] For more than a decade, completion ALND was routinely performed for any positive axillary nodes found on sentinel node biopsy, even though approximately 50% to 70% of patients

with positive sentinel nodes had no additional positive nodes on completion ALND.[67–69] The American College of Surgeons Oncology Group's (ACOSOG Z0011 trial randomized patients with T1-2 N0 invasive breast cancer with 1 or 2 positive sentinel lymph nodes to ALND versus no further axillary surgery.[7] At a median follow-up of 9.25 years, there were no differences in local recurrence, nodal recurrences,[71] or overall survival between the two groups.[72] With the implementation of the Z0011 results into clinical practice, approximately 85% of patients who would have previously undergone a completion ALND based on positive sentinel lymph nodes are now spared this procedure.[73] Completion ALND is indicated in patients with 3 or more positive sentinel lymph nodes and those found to have matted nodes intraoperatively. Importantly, Z0011 is not applicable to patients undergoing mastectomy, those receiving neoadjuvant therapy, and those treated with PBI. A completion ALND following a positive sentinel lymph node biopsy remains the standard of care for these patients. The After Mapping of the Axilla: Radiotherapy or Surgery (AMAROS) trial enrolled a similar patient population to ACOSOG Z0011 but randomized those with 1 to 2 positive sentinel nodes to ALND or no further surgery with radiation of the axillary and medial supraclavicular fields. This study reported no differences in regional recurrence or survival between groups at a follow-up of 5 years and a lower risk of lymphedema in the radiotherapy group.[74] Because AMAROS also included patients undergoing mastectomy, if the finding of metastases in 1 to 2 sentinel nodes is a sufficient indication for PMRT axillary dissection can be avoided. However, AMAROS does not indicate that all node-positive patients require axillary radiation because the results of ACOSOG Z0011, in the absence of nodal radiation, are comparable. At present, patients thought to be at higher risk for LRR based on the number of involved sentinel nodes, primary tumor size, presence of lympho-vascular invasion, microscopic extracapsular tumor extension in the nodes, and young age are selected for nodal radiation therapy.[75]

It is often assumed that preoperative imaging is useful in selecting patients undergoing BCT who require axillary dissection. However, the clinical question has shifted from the identification of any nodal metastases to identification of patients with 3 or more nodal metastases who are not candidates for sentinel node biopsy alone, and current imaging modalities (mammogram, ultrasound and MR imaging) do not reliably make this distinction. Pilewskie and colleagues[76] examined the utility of preoperative imaging in predicting the need for additional axillary surgery in 425 patients with clinical T1-2 N0 tumors and 1 or 2 positive sentinel nodes. Among patients with abnormal axillary nodes identified by mammogram, axillary ultrasound, or MR imaging, 71% did not require ALND using the Z0011 criteria.[76] Even among patients with a needle biopsy demonstrating nodal metastases, only 45% required ALND.[77] Thus, preoperative axillary imaging in patients with clinically node-negative disease should be reserved for those undergoing mastectomy whereby the finding of any nodal disease is an indication for ALND or preoperative chemotherapy to downstage the axilla.

NEOADJUVANT CHEMOTHERAPY

NAC was initially used as a way of rendering locally advanced, inoperable breast cancer resectable. More recently, NAC has been used in operable tumors to downstage disease in the breast and axilla with the intention of facilitating breast conservation and, in some instances, avoiding ALND. The oncologic safety and equivalent survival outcomes of NAC have been studied in several randomized trials.[78–80] A meta-analysis of patients treated with NAC versus surgery followed by chemotherapy has shown no differences in survival or LRR with NAC and a 17% decrease in the mastectomy rate in patients receiving NAC.[81] Seventeen percent is a minimal estimate because many of the women enrolled in these studies were candidates for BCT at presentation and, thus, could not benefit from NAC. NAC is most likely to allow BCT in the woman with a unicentric cancer, which is large relative to the size of her breast, and in those with HER2-positive or triple-negative breast cancers.

Accurate evaluation of the response to therapy and the feasibility of BCT can be problematic. MR imaging is more accurate than mammography or ultrasound in predicting the extent of residual disease, but a normal MR imaging does not exclude the presence of scattered foci of viable carcinoma, which may preclude BCT.[82] Mammography is complementary to MR imaging in evaluating suitability for BCT after NAC, as calcifications present at diagnosis infrequently resolve with NAC. Calcifications may also become apparent after neoadjuvant therapy when breast densities related to the tumor have resolved or secondary to tumor cell death. Loss of enhancement on MR imaging does not reliably indicate that calcifications are benign or due to dead cancer cells,[83] and excision of any residual palpable masses or radiographic abnormalities is standard. Of note, the entire volume originally occupied by the tumor does not need to be removed in the lumpectomy specimen and a pathologic complete response is not a requirement for successful BCT after NAC. Lumpectomy should include any residual clinical or imaging abnormalities, or, in the case of a clinical and radiographic complete response, removal of the marker at the tumor site and a generous sample of surrounding breast tissue.

Administration of NAC significantly reduces the rate of axillary metastases in clinically node-negative women,[80] and performance of sentinel lymph node biopsy after NAC is standard in this population.[84–87] More effective systemic regimens have led to increased rates of pathologic complete response in both the breast and axilla after NAC. Three prospective randomized clinical trials have examined the accuracy of sentinel node biopsy after NAC in patients presenting with nodal metastases (**Table 1**). The ACOSOG Z1071 and SENTINA (Sentinel Neoadjuvant) studies suggest that with the use of dual-tracer mapping and identification of 3 or more negative sentinel nodes, false-negative rates are less than 10%, similar to what is accepted for sentinel node biopsy in the primary surgical setting. In a prospective study from the Memorial Sloan Kettering Cancer Center, 48% of 288 patients who presented with nodal metastases and became clinically node negative after NAC had a nodal pathologic complete response and 3 or more identifiable sentinel nodes, and were able to avoid axillary dissection.[88] In patients who remain node positive, completion ALND is standard. The question of whether or not axillary radiation can be substituted for a completion ALND in the setting of a positive axillary sentinel node after NAC is currently being addressed in the Alliance A011202 trial.

Table 1
False-negative rate of sentinel lymph node biopsy following neoadjuvant chemotherapy in clinically node-positive breast cancer

| Trial | False-Negative Rate (%) | | |
	Overall	Radioactive isotope and blue dye	≥3 sentinel nodes removed
ACOSOG Z1071 (n = 649)	12.6	10.8	9.1
SENTINA (n = 642)	14.2	8.6	7.3
SN FNAC (n = 153)	13.3	5.2	4.9[a]

Abbreviation: SN FNAC, Sentinel Node Biopsy Following Neoadjuvant Chemotherapy.
[a] False-negative rate with more than 2 sentinel lymph nodes removed.

ADJUVANT MEDICAL THERAPIES FOR BREAST CANCER

Following surgical resection of the primary breast cancer, patients often receive adjuvant systemic therapy with the goal of eradicating clinically and radiographically occult micrometastatic disease that may develop into frank metastatic disease if left untreated. Selection of adjuvant systemic therapies is based on risk stratification of patients. Two factors affect risk: disease burden (number of lymph nodes, size of the primary tumor) and disease biology as determined by HR and HER2 status and genomic assays. Although patients with triple-negative and HER2-positive cancers are generally considered to be high risk, there is considerable biological diversity among those with HR-positive, HER2-negative cancers. Based on trials demonstrating a small but statistically significant benefit for the treatment of HR-positive, HER2-negative, node-negative breast cancers with chemotherapy in addition to endocrine therapy, chemotherapy has been the standard for healthy women in this group.[89] Commercially available genomic assays examine cancer-related genes in tumor-derived DNA to determine the risk of recurrence and potential chemotherapy benefit. These commercially available tests have given clinicians more clarity on which patients should receive chemotherapy.

CHEMOTHERAPY

In high-risk patients, systemic chemotherapy is generally recommended. There are several standard chemotherapy options, typically containing both an anthracycline and a taxane. In the United States, doxorubicin and cyclophosphamide for 4 cycles followed by paclitaxel for 4 cycles (AC-T) is a common regimen. Dose-dense AC-T given every 2 weeks with growth factor support after each chemotherapy cycle is superior to an older schedule of every 3 weeks.[90] Other optimal schedules of AC followed by a taxane include weekly paclitaxel for 12 weeks or every 3 weekly docetaxel for 4 cycles.[91,92] Another standard option is docetaxel with AC (DAC); however, this is not superior to the aforementioned regimens; docetaxel is associated with more toxicity than paclitaxel and higher febrile neutropenia rates in particular.[93]

Meta-analyses have demonstrated the benefit of adjuvant chemotherapy in reducing recurrence and breast cancer mortality, with a greater magnitude of benefit in those with HR-negative disease.[94] Berry and colleagues[95] analyzed trial data from Cancer and Leukemia Group B and US Breast Cancer Intergroup and demonstrated that chemotherapy provided 21% to 25% relative risk (RR) reduction in patients with HR-negative cancer, compared with 8% to 12% RR reduction in those with HR-positive disease. For patients with HR-positive, node-negative breast cancer, the Oncotype DX genomic assay provides an estimate of chemotherapy benefit; patients with high Oncotype recurrence scores ($\geq$ 31) have a large reduction in risk of recurrence with chemotherapy (RR 0.26), whereas those with low scores derive minimal, if any, benefit from chemotherapy.[96] There is insufficient evidence to provide a unanimous recommendation on the adjuvant treatment of patients with intermediate-risk Oncotype recurrence scores, pending the results of the Trial Assigning Individualized Options for Treatment (TAILORx trial) (**Fig. 2**). In this trial, patients with Oncotype recurrence scores of 11 to 25 were randomized to treatment with endocrine therapy alone or endocrine therapy plus chemotherapy. Chemotherapy for patients in this group may consist of anthracycline-containing or anthracycline-sparing regimens. In patients with low Oncotype recurrence scores, especially scores less than 11, endocrine therapy alone is sufficient. These patients have an excellent outcome, with a 5-year overall survival of 98% with endocrine therapy alone.[97]

Patients with node-positive breast cancer are generally recommended chemotherapy because of their worse prognosis relative to patients with node-negative breast cancer. This recommendation has been called into question by some retrospective analyses; Albain and colleagues[98] demonstrated the absence of a chemotherapy benefit in patients with HR-positive, lymph node-positive breast cancer with a low Oncotype recurrence score in the Southwest Oncology Group (SWOG) 8814 study. This finding led to the development of the Rx for Positive Node, Endocrine Responsive Breast Cancer (RxPONDER) trial (**Fig. 3**), which enrolled patients with HR-positive breast cancer with 1 to 3 positive nodes and Oncotype recurrence scores of 25 or less, and randomized them to chemotherapy versus none; all received standard endocrine therapy. The results of this study will determine whether some patients with node-positive disease may be spared chemotherapy.

BIOLOGICAL AND TARGETED THERAPIES

Patients with HER2-positive breast cancer are given HER2-targeted therapy in combination with a chemotherapy backbone. The availability of HER2-targeted agents has dramatically changed the prognosis of patients with HER2-positive breast cancers. Initial trials randomizing patients

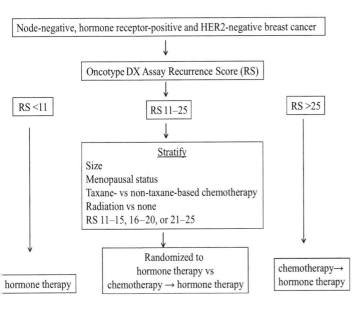

Fig. 2. TAILORx for node-negative, HR-positive and HER2-negative breast cancer. RS, recurrence score.

to chemotherapy alone or chemotherapy plus trastuzumab, a monoclonal antibody directed against the HER2 receptor, demonstrated a nearly 50% reduction in the rate of recurrence.[99–104] At present, patients with stage I HER2-positive breast cancer often receive a regimen of paclitaxel (T) with trastuzumab (H).[105] Until the U.S. Food and Drug Administration's approval of pertuzumab (P) in 2013, patients with stage II-III HER2-positive breast cancer received regimens with trastuzumab added to AC-T (AC-TH) or to docetaxel and carboplatin (DCbH). Recent data have shown an improvement in the pathologic complete response rate when pertuzumab, an HER2 dimerization inhibitor, is added to trastuzumab in the neoadjuvant setting. Administration of dual-HER2 agents (HP) in the neoadjuvant setting is now standard for patients with stage II-III HER2-positive breast cancer.[106,107] The National Comprehensive Cancer Network has also endorsed the addition of HP to chemotherapy for patients with the same burden of disease in the adjuvant setting if these therapies were not received neoadjuvantly. Recently, the APHINITY (A Study of Pertuzumab in Addition to

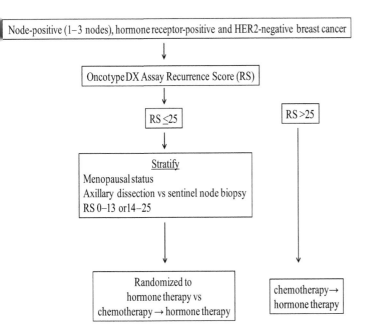

Fig. 3. RxPONDER for node-positive, HR-positive and HER2-negative breast cancer. RS, recurrence score.

Chemotherapy and Trastuzumab as Adjuvant Therapy in Participants With Human Epidermal Growth Receptor 2 (HER2)-Positive Primary Breast Cancer) trial demonstrated a small but statistically significant benefit of adjuvant HP-based over H-based therapy for 1 year.[108]

ENDOCRINE THERAPY

Endocrine therapy is recommended for most patients with HR-positive disease. Patients may be treated with endocrine therapy for 5 to 10 years, and possibly longer. Five years of adjuvant tamoxifen reduces the risk of recurrence by nearly 50% during years 0 to 4, with continued risk reduction of more than 30% in years 5 to 9. Furthermore, yearly breast cancer mortality was reduced by 30% during the first 15 years.[109] In patients who took 10 versus 5 years of tamoxifen, longer duration of therapy led to further reduction in recurrence (by about 25%) and breast cancer mortality (by almost 30%), most notably after year 10.[110] After 5 years of tamoxifen, an additional 5 years of aromatase inhibitors (AIs) provides an additional 40% RR risk reduction in recurrence as demonstrated by the MA.17 trial.[111] MA.17R randomized patients on 5 years of AI (some also had prior tamoxifen) to an additional 5 years of AI versus placebo and demonstrated a 34% risk reduction in recurrence with 10 years of AI.[112] Thus, longer duration of therapy confers additional benefit.

Tamoxifen is used in premenopausal and postmenopausal women; AIs (anastrozole, letrozole, and exemestane) are only used in postmenopausal women and are generally preferred over tamoxifen as adjuvant therapy, but may also be prescribed sequentially with tamoxifen.[113] Common side effects of these medications include hot flashes, vaginal dryness, arthralgia, and myalgia. Tamoxifen increases the risk of venous thromboembolic events and uterine cancers, and AIs may accelerate osteopenia and osteoporosis and are associated with more musculoskeletal symptoms. In premenopausal patients with high-risk HR-positive breast cancer, ovarian function suppression with AI or with tamoxifen is more effective than tamoxifen alone.[114]

SPECIAL CONSIDERATIONS

Before beginning chemotherapy, assessment of a premenopausal patient's wishes for future pregnancy is vital, as chemotherapy for breast cancer may cause premature ovarian failure. Options for fertility preservation include oocyte preservation, embryo preservation, and gonadotropin-releasing hormone (GNRH) agonist use during chemotherapy for ovarian protection. Consultation with a reproductive endocrinologist before breast cancer treatment is suggested for young women desiring future fertility, although oocyte and embryo preservation may be financially burdensome. The administration of GNRH agonists during chemotherapy is safe and inexpensive and, in one study, reduced the risk of premature ovarian failure in women less than 50 years of age from 22% to 8%.[115] Pregnancy after breast cancer does not seem to negatively impact survival.[116]

Patients with HR-positive ductal carcinoma in situ may be offered endocrine therapy to reduce the likelihood of a future breast cancer in the affected breast if conserved, and in the contralateral breast. Tamoxifen and AIs are both options.[117,118]

The management of breast cancer in elderly women is highly individualized and requires collaboration across disciplines (medical oncology, surgical oncology, and radiation oncology). A comprehensive assessment of performance status, comorbidities, and life expectancy is critical. In patients older than 65 years deemed fit for chemotherapy, standard chemotherapy regimens are superior to capecitabine monotherapy.[119]

SURVEILLANCE

Surveillance after adjuvant therapy for breast cancer is composed primarily of history, physical examination, and annual mammography. Routine computed tomography or PET imaging in the absence of symptoms has not been shown to improve survival; there is currently no proven role for surveillance imaging.[120] Serum tumor markers (cancer antigen 15–3 and carcinoembryonic antigen) are nonspecific and may prompt unnecessary imaging and procedures; they have no role in postadjuvant therapy surveillance in asymptomatic patients.[121] After a breast cancer diagnosis, patients should be encouraged to make lifestyle modifications that can decrease their likelihood of recurrence, including maintaining a normal body mass index.[122] Of note, there are emerging observational data demonstrating that physical activity may reduce the risk of breast cancer–specific recurrence and mortality, but definitive prospective studies are needed[123,124]

SUMMARY

Patients receive adjuvant systemic therapies in addition to local therapy to treat micrometastatic disease and prevent distant recurrence. Adjuvant therapy is tailored to a patient's risk of recurrence and may include chemotherapy, biological therapy, and endocrine therapy. Following adjuvant systemic treatment, there is currently no role for routine cross-sectional imaging in the absence of symptoms.

REFERENCES

1. Hortobagyi GN, Buzdar AU. Management of locally advanced breast cancer. Am J Clin Oncol 1988; 11(5):597–601.
2. Fisher B, Anderson S, Bryant J, et al. Twenty-year follow-up of a randomized trial comparing total mastectomy, lumpectomy, and lumpectomy plus irradiation for the treatment of invasive breast cancer. N Engl J Med 2002;347(16):1233–41.
3. Veronesi U, Cascinelli N, Mariani L, et al. Twenty-year follow-up of a randomized study comparing breast-conserving surgery with radical mastectomy for early breast cancer. N Engl J Med 2002; 347(16):1227–32.
4. Poggi MM, Danforth DN, Sciuto LC, et al. Eighteen-year results in the treatment of early breast carcinoma with mastectomy versus breast conservation therapy: the National Cancer Institute Randomized Trial. Cancer 2003;98(4):697–702.
5. Voogd AC, Nielsen M, Peterse JL, et al. Differences in risk factors for local and distant recurrence after breast-conserving therapy or mastectomy for stage I and II breast cancer: pooled results of two large European randomized trials. J Clin Oncol 2001;19(6):1688–97.
6. Darby S, McGale P, Correa C, et al. Effect of radiotherapy after breast-conserving surgery on 10-year recurrence and 15-year breast cancer death: meta-analysis of individual patient data for 10,801 women in 17 randomised trials. Lancet 2011; 378(9804):1707–16.
7. van Dongen JA, Voogd AC, Fentiman IS, et al. Long-term results of a randomized trial comparing breast-conserving therapy with mastectomy: European Organization for Research and Treatment of Cancer 10801 trial. J Natl Cancer Inst 2000; 92(14):1143–50.
8. Wapnir IL, Anderson SJ, Mamounas EP, et al. Prognosis after ipsilateral breast tumor recurrence and locoregional recurrences in five National Surgical Adjuvant Breast and Bowel Project node-positive adjuvant breast cancer trials. J Clin Oncol 2006; 24(13):2028–37.
9. Anderson SJ, Wapnir I, Dignam JJ, et al. Prognosis after ipsilateral breast tumor recurrence and locoregional recurrences in patients treated by breast-conserving therapy in five National Surgical Adjuvant Breast and Bowel Project protocols of node-negative breast cancer. J Clin Oncol 2009; 27(15):2466–73.
10. Clarke M, Collins R, Darby S, et al. Effects of radiotherapy and of differences in the extent of surgery for early breast cancer on local recurrence and 15-year survival: an overview of the randomised trials. Lancet 2005;366(9503):2087–106.
11. Voduc KD, Cheang MC, Tyldesley S, et al. Breast cancer subtypes and the risk of local and regional relapse. J Clin Oncol 2010;28(10):1684–91.
12. Lowery AJ, Kell MR, Glynn RW, et al. Locoregional recurrence after breast cancer surgery: a systematic review by receptor phenotype. Breast Cancer Res Treat 2012;133(3):831–41.
13. National Comprehensive Cancer Network (NCCN). Clinical practice guidelines oncology - breast cancer (Version 2.2017). 2017. Available at: https://www.nccn.org/professionals/physician_gls/pdf/breast.pdf. Accessed July 24, 2017.
14. Moran MS, Schnitt SJ, Giuliano AE, et al. Society of Surgical Oncology-American Society for Radiation Oncology consensus guideline on margins for breast-conserving surgery with whole-breast irradiation in stages I and II invasive breast cancer. J Clin Oncol 2014;32(14):1507–15.
15. Houssami N, Macaskill P, Marinovich ML, et al. The association of surgical margins and local recurrence in women with early-stage invasive breast cancer treated with breast-conserving therapy: a meta-analysis. Ann Surg Oncol 2014;21(3):717–30.
16. Kuchenbaecker KB, Hopper JL, Barnes DR, et al. Risks of breast, ovarian, and contralateral breast cancer for BRCA1 and BRCA2 mutation carriers. JAMA 2017;317(23):2402–16.
17. Morrow M, Jagsi R, Alderman AK, et al. Surgeon recommendations and receipt of mastectomy for treatment of breast cancer. JAMA 2009;302(14): 1551–6.
18. Houssami N, Ciatto S, Macaskill P, et al. Accuracy and surgical impact of magnetic resonance imaging in breast cancer staging: systematic review and meta-analysis in detection of multifocal and multicentric cancer. J Clin Oncol 2008;26(19): 3248–58.
19. Katipamula R, Degnim AC, Hoskin T, et al. Trends in mastectomy rates at the Mayo Clinic Rochester: effect of surgical year and preoperative magnetic resonance imaging. J Clin Oncol 2009;27(25): 4082–8.
20. King TA, Sakr R, Patil S, et al. Clinical management factors contribute to the decision for contralateral prophylactic mastectomy. J Clin Oncol 2011; 29(16):2158–64.
21. Sorbero ME, Dick AW, Beckjord EB, et al. Diagnostic breast magnetic resonance imaging and contralateral prophylactic mastectomy. Ann Surg Oncol 2009;16(6):1597–605.
22. Fancellu A, Soro D, Castiglia P, et al. Usefulness of magnetic resonance in patients with invasive

cancer eligible for breast conservation: a comparative study. Clin Breast Cancer 2014;14(2):114–21.

23. Pilewskie M, King TA. Magnetic resonance imaging in patients with newly diagnosed breast cancer: a review of the literature. Cancer 2014;120(14): 2080–9.

24. Houssami N, Turner R, Macaskill P, et al. An individual person data meta-analysis of preoperative magnetic resonance imaging and breast cancer recurrence. J Clin Oncol 2014;32(5):392–401.

25. Turnbull L, Brown S, Harvey I, et al. Comparative effectiveness of MRI in breast cancer (COMICE) trial: a randomised controlled trial. Lancet 2010; 375(9714):563–71.

26. Peters NH, van Esser S, van den Bosch MA, et al. Preoperative MRI and surgical management in patients with nonpalpable breast cancer: the MONET - randomised controlled trial. Eur J Cancer 2011;47(6):879–86.

27. Houssami N, Turner RM, Morrow M. Meta-analysis of pre-operative magnetic resonance imaging (MRI) and surgical treatment for breast cancer. Breast Cancer Res Treat 2017;165(2):273–83.

28. Chen AM, Obedian E, Haffty BG. Breast-conserving therapy in the setting of collagen vascular disease. Cancer J 2001;7(6):480–91.

29. Phan C, Mindrum M, Silverman C, et al. Matched-control retrospective study of the acute and late complications in patients with collagen vascular diseases treated with radiation therapy. Cancer J 2003;9(6):461–6.

30. Lin A, Abu-Isa E, Griffith KA, et al. Toxicity of radiotherapy in patients with collagen vascular disease. Cancer 2008;113(3):648–53.

31. Holland R, Veling SH, Mravunac M, et al. Histologic multifocality of Tis, T1-2 breast carcinomas. Implications for clinical trials of breast-conserving surgery. Cancer 1985;56(5):979–90.

32. Hopwood P, Haviland JS, Sumo G, et al. Comparison of patient-reported breast, arm, and shoulder symptoms and body image after radiotherapy for early breast cancer: 5-year follow-up in the randomised Standardisation of Breast Radiotherapy (START) trials. Lancet Oncol 2010; 11(3):231–40.

33. Haviland JS, Owen JR, Dewar JA, et al. The UK Standardisation of Breast Radiotherapy (START) trials of radiotherapy hypofractionation for treatment of early breast cancer: 10-year follow-up results of two randomised controlled trials. Lancet Oncol 2013;14(11):1086–94.

34. Whelan TJ, Pignol JP, Levine MN, et al. Long-term results of hypofractionated radiation therapy for breast cancer. N Engl J Med 2010;362(6):513–20.

35. Hughes KS, Schnaper LA, Bellon JR, et al. Lumpectomy plus tamoxifen with or without irradiation in women age 70 years or older with early breast cancer: long-term follow-up of CALGB 9343. J Clin Oncol 2013;31(19):2382–7.

36. Kunkler IH, Williams LJ, Jack WJ, et al. Breast-conserving surgery with or without irradiation in women aged 65 years or older with early breast cancer (PRIME II): a randomised controlled trial. Lancet Oncol 2015;16(3):266–73.

37. Engel J, Kerr J, Schlesinger-Raab A, et al. Quality of life following breast-conserving therapy or mastectomy: results of a 5-year prospective study. Breast J 2004;10(3):223–31.

38. Hartl K, Janni W, Kastner R, et al. Impact of medical and demographic factors on long-term quality of life and body image of breast cancer patients. Ann Oncol 2003;14(7):1064–71.

39. Arndt V, Stegmaier C, Ziegler H, et al. Quality of life over 5 years in women with breast cancer after breast-conserving therapy versus mastectomy: a population-based study. J Cancer Res Clin Oncol 2008;134(12):1311–8.

40. Jagsi R, Li Y, Morrow M, et al. Patient-reported quality of life and satisfaction with cosmetic outcomes after breast conservation and mastectomy with and without reconstruction: results of a survey of breast cancer survivors. Ann Surg 2015;261(6): 1198–206.

41. Bulstrode NW, Shrotria S. Prediction of cosmetic outcome following conservative breast surgery using breast volume measurements. Breast 2001; 10(2):124–6.

42. Tenofsky PL, Dowell P, Topalovski T, et al. Surgical, oncologic, and cosmetic differences between oncoplastic and nononcoplastic breast conserving surgery in breast cancer patients. Am J Surg 2014;207(3):398–402.

43. Rietjens M, Urban CA, Rey PC, et al. Long-term oncological results of breast conservative treatment with oncoplastic surgery. Breast 2007;16(4): 387–95.

44. Meretoja TJ, Rasia S, von Smitten KA, et al. Late results of skin-sparing mastectomy followed by immediate breast reconstruction. Br J Surg 2007; 94(10):1220–5.

45. Medina-Franco H, Vasconez LO, Fix RJ, et al. Factors associated with local recurrence after skin-sparing mastectomy and immediate breast reconstruction for invasive breast cancer. Ann Surg 2002;235(6):814–9.

46. Carlson GW, Styblo TM, Lyles RH, et al. The use of skin sparing mastectomy in the treatment of breast cancer: the Emory experience. Surg Oncol 2003; 12(4):265–9.

47. Lanitis S, Tekkis PP, Sgourakis G, et al. Comparison of skin-sparing mastectomy versus non-skin-sparing mastectomy for breast cancer: a meta-analysis of observational studies. Ann Surg 2010; 251(4):632–9.

48. Smith BL, Tang R, Rai U, et al. Oncologic safety of nipple-sparing mastectomy in women with breast cancer. J Am Coll Surg 2017;225(3):361–5.

49. Moo TA, Pinchinat T, Mays S, et al. Oncologic outcomes after nipple-sparing mastectomy. Ann Surg Oncol 2016;23(10):3221–5.

50. de Alcantara Filho P, Capko D, Barry JM, et al. Nipple-sparing mastectomy for breast cancer and risk-reducing surgery: the Memorial Sloan-Kettering Cancer Center experience. Ann Surg Oncol 2011;18(11):3117–22.

51. Orzalesi L, Casella D, Santi C, et al. Nipple sparing mastectomy: surgical and oncological outcomes from a national multicentric registry with 913 patients (1006 cases) over a six year period. Breast 2016;25:75–81.

52. Recht A, Gray R, Davidson NE, et al. Locoregional failure 10 years after mastectomy and adjuvant chemotherapy with or without tamoxifen without irradiation: experience of the Eastern Cooperative Oncology Group. J Clin Oncol 1999;17(6):1689–700.

53. Overgaard M, Jensen MB, Overgaard J, et al. Postoperative radiotherapy in high-risk postmenopausal breast-cancer patients given adjuvant tamoxifen: Danish Breast Cancer Cooperative Group DBCG 82c randomised trial. Lancet 1999;353(9165):1641–8.

54. Recht A, Edge SB, Solin LJ, et al. Postmastectomy radiotherapy: clinical practice guidelines of the American Society of Clinical Oncology. J Clin Oncol 2001;19(5):1539–69.

55. Moo TA, McMillan R, Lee M, et al. Selection criteria for postmastectomy radiotherapy in t1-t2 tumors with 1 to 3 positive lymph nodes. Ann Surg Oncol 2013;20(10):3169–74.

56. Sharma R, Bedrosian I, Lucci A, et al. Present-day locoregional control in patients with t1 or t2 breast cancer with 0 and 1 to 3 positive lymph nodes after mastectomy without radiotherapy. Ann Surg Oncol 2010;17(11):2899–908.

57. EBCTCG (Early Breast Cancer Trialists' Collaborative Group), McGale P, Taylor C, Correa C, et al. Effect of radiotherapy after mastectomy and axillary surgery on 10-year recurrence and 20-year breast cancer mortality: meta-analysis of individual patient data for 8135 women in 22 randomised trials. Lancet 2014;383(9935):2127–35.

58. Recht A, Comen EA, Fine RE, et al. Postmastectomy radiotherapy: an American Society of Clinical Oncology, American Society for Radiation Oncology, and Society of surgical oncology focused guideline update. J Clin Oncol 2016;34(36):4431–42.

59. Hoffman KE, Mittendorf EA, Buchholz TA. Optimising radiation treatment decisions for patients who receive neoadjuvant chemotherapy and mastectomy. Lancet Oncol 2012;13(6):e270–6.

60. McCartan D, Stempel M, Eaton A, et al. Impact of body mass index on clinical axillary nodal assessment in breast cancer patients. Ann Surg Oncol 2016;23(10):3324–9.

61. Kern KA. Concordance and validation study of sentinel lymph node biopsy for breast cancer using subareolar injection of blue dye and technetium 99m sulfur colloid. J Am Coll Surg 2002;195(4):467–75.

62. Kern KA. Sentinel lymph node mapping in breast cancer using subareolar injection of blue dye. J Am Coll Surg 1999;189(6):539–45.

63. Mertz L, Mathelin C, Marin C, et al. Subareolar injection of 99m-Tc sulfur colloid for sentinel nodes identification in multifocal invasive breast cancer. Bull Cancer 1999;86(11):939–45 [in French].

64. Boolbol SK, Fey JV, Borgen PI, et al. Intradermal isotope injection: a highly accurate method of lymphatic mapping in breast carcinoma. Ann Surg Oncol 2001;8(1):20–4.

65. Krag D, Weaver D, Ashikaga T, et al. The sentinel node in breast cancer–a multicenter validation study. N Engl J Med 1998;339(14):941–6.

66. Veronesi U, Viale G, Paganelli G, et al. Sentinel lymph node biopsy in breast cancer: ten-year results of a randomized controlled study. Ann Surg 2010;251(4):595–600.

67. Van Zee KJ, Manasseh DM, Bevilacqua JL, et al. A nomogram for predicting the likelihood of additional nodal metastases in breast cancer patients with a positive sentinel node biopsy. Ann Surg Oncol 2003;10(10):1140–51.

68. Weiser MR, Montgomery LL, Tan LK, et al. Lymphovascular invasion enhances the prediction of non-sentinel node metastases in breast cancer patients with positive sentinel nodes. Ann Surg Oncol 2001;8(2):145–9.

69. Hwang RF, Krishnamurthy S, Hunt KK, et al. Clinicopathologic factors predicting involvement of nonsentinel axillary nodes in women with breast cancer. Ann Surg Oncol 2003;10(3):248–54.

70. Giuliano AE, Hunt KK, Ballman KV, et al. Axillary dissection vs no axillary dissection in women with invasive breast cancer and sentinel node metastasis: a randomized clinical trial. JAMA 2011;305(6):569–75.

71. Giuliano AE, Ballman K, McCall L, et al. Locoregional recurrence after sentinel lymph node dissection with or without axillary dissection in patients with sentinel lymph node metastases: long-term follow-up from the American College of Surgeons Oncology Group (Alliance) ACOSOG Z0011 Randomized Trial. Ann Surg 2016;264(3):413–20.

72. Giuliano AE, Ballman KV, McCall L, et al. Effect of axillary dissection vs no axillary dissection on 10-year overall survival among women with invasive breast cancer and sentinel node metastasis: the

ACOSOG Z0011 (Alliance) Randomized Clinical Trial. JAMA 2017;318(10):918–26.

73. Dengel LT, Van Zee KJ, King TA, et al. Axillary dissection can be avoided in the majority of clinically node-negative patients undergoing breast-conserving therapy. Ann Surg Oncol 2014;21(1):22–7.

74. Donker M, Slaets L, van Tienhoven G, et al. Axillary lymph node dissection versus axillary radiotherapy in patients with a positive sentinel node: the AMAROS trial. Ned Tijdschr Geneeskd 2015;159: A9302 [in Dutch].

75. Morrow M, Van Zee KJ, Patil S, et al. Axillary dissection and nodal irradiation can be avoided for most node-positive z0011-eligible breast cancers: a prospective validation study of 793 patients. Ann Surg 2017;266(3):457–62.

76. Pilewskie M, Jochelson M, Gooch JC, et al. Is preoperative axillary imaging beneficial in identifying clinically node-negative patients requiring axillary lymph node dissection? J Am Coll Surg 2016; 222(2):138–45.

77. Pilewskie M, Mautner SK, Stempel M, et al. Does a positive axillary lymph node needle biopsy result predict the need for an axillary lymph node dissection in clinically node-negative breast cancer patients in the ACOSOG Z0011 era? Ann Surg Oncol 2016;23(4):1123–8.

78. van der Hage JA, van de Velde CJ, Julien JP, et al. Preoperative chemotherapy in primary operable breast cancer: results from the European Organization for Research and Treatment of Cancer trial 10902. J Clin Oncol 2001;19(22):4224–37.

79. Broet P, Scholl SM, de la Rochefordiere A, et al. Short and long-term effects on survival in breast cancer patients treated by primary chemotherapy: an updated analysis of a randomized trial. Breast Cancer Res Treat 1999;58(2):151–6.

80. Fisher B, Bryant J, Wolmark N, et al. Effect of preoperative chemotherapy on the outcome of women with operable breast cancer. J Clin Oncol 1998; 16(8):2672–85.

81. Mieog JS, van der Hage JA, van de Velde CJ. Neoadjuvant chemotherapy for operable breast cancer. Br J Surg 2007;94(10):1189–200.

82. Jochelson MS, Lampen-Sachar K, Gibbons G, et al. Do MRI and mammography reliably identify candidates for breast conservation after neoadjuvant chemotherapy? Ann Surg Oncol 2015;22(5): 1490–5.

83. Feliciano Y, Mamtani A, Morrow M, et al. Do calcifications seen on mammography after neoadjuvant chemotherapy for breast cancer always need to be excised? Ann Surg Oncol 2017;24(6):1492–8.

84. Classe JM, Bordes V, Campion L, et al. Sentinel lymph node biopsy after neoadjuvant chemotherapy for advanced breast cancer: results of Ganglion Sentinelle et Chimiotherapie Neoadjuvante, a French prospective multicentric study. J Clin Onc 2009;27(5):726–32.

85. Xing Y, Foy M, Cox DD, et al. Meta-analysis of sentinel lymph node biopsy after preoperative chemotherapy in patients with breast cancer. Br Surg 2006;93(5):539–46.

86. Kelly AM, Dwamena B, Cronin P, et al. Breast cancer sentinel node identification and classification after neoadjuvant chemotherapy-systematic review and meta-analysis. Acad Radiol 2009;16(5): 551–63.

87. Hunt KK, Yi M, Mittendorf EA, et al. Sentinel lymph node surgery after neoadjuvant chemotherapy is accurate and reduces the need for axillary dissection in breast cancer patients. Ann Surg 2009; 250(4):558–66.

88. Mamtani A, Barrio AV, King TA, et al. How often does neoadjuvant chemotherapy avoid axillary dissection in patients with histologically confirmed nodal metastases? Results of a prospective study. Ann Surg Oncol 2016;23(11):3467–74.

89. Early Breast Cancer Trialists' Collaborative Group (EBCTCG). Effects of chemotherapy and hormonal therapy for early breast cancer on recurrence and 15-year survival: an overview of the randomised trials. Lancet 2005;365(9472):1687–717.

90. Citron ML, Berry DA, Cirrincione C, et al. Randomized trial of dose-dense versus conventionally scheduled and sequential versus concurrent combination chemotherapy as postoperative adjuvant treatment of node-positive primary breast cancer: first report of Intergroup Trial C9741/Cancer and Leukemia Group B Trial 9741. J Clin Oncol 2003; 21(8):1431–9.

91. Sparano JA, Wang M, Martino S, et al. Weekly paclitaxel in the adjuvant treatment of breast cancer. N Engl J Med 2008;358(16):1663–71.

92. Sparano JA, Zhao F, Martino S, et al. Long-term follow-up of the E1199 phase III trial evaluating the role of taxane and schedule in operable breast cancer. J Clin Oncol 2015;33(21):2353–60.

93. Swain SM, Tang G, Geyer CE Jr, et al. Definitive results of a phase III adjuvant trial comparing three chemotherapy regimens in women with operable node-positive breast cancer: the NSABP B-38 trial. J Clin Oncol 2013;31(26):3197–204.

94. Early Breast Cancer Trialists' Collaborative Group (EBCTCG), Peto R, Davies C, Godwin J, et al. Comparisons between different polychemotherapy regimens for early breast cancer: meta-analyses of long-term outcome among 100,000 women in 123 randomised trials. Lancet 2012; 379(9814):432–44.

95. Berry DA, Cirrincione C, Henderson IC, et al. Estrogen-receptor status and outcomes of modern chemotherapy for patients with node-positive breast cancer. Jama 2006;295(14):1658–67.

96. Paik S, Tang G, Shak S, et al. Gene expression and benefit of chemotherapy in women with node-negative, estrogen receptor-positive breast cancer. J Clin Oncol 2006;24(23):3726–34.

97. Sparano JA, Gray RJ, Makower DF, et al. Prospective validation of a 21-gene expression assay in breast cancer. N Engl J Med 2015;373(21): 2005–14.

98. Albain KS, Barlow WE, Shak S, et al. Prognostic and predictive value of the 21-gene recurrence score assay in postmenopausal women with node-positive, oestrogen-receptor-positive breast cancer on chemotherapy: a retrospective analysis of a randomised trial. Lancet Oncol 2010;11(1): 55–65.

99. Cameron D, Piccart-Gebhart MJ, Gelber RD, et al. 11 years' follow-up of trastuzumab after adjuvant chemotherapy in HER2-positive early breast cancer: final analysis of the HERceptin Adjuvant (HERA) trial. Lancet 2017;389(10075):1195–205.

100. Perez EA, Romond EH, Suman VJ, et al. Trastuzumab plus adjuvant chemotherapy for human epidermal growth factor receptor 2-positive breast cancer: planned joint analysis of overall survival from NSABP B-31 and NCCTG N9831. J Clin Oncol 2014;32(33):3744–52.

101. Piccart-Gebhart MJ, Procter M, Leyland-Jones B, et al. Trastuzumab after adjuvant chemotherapy in HER2-positive breast cancer. N Engl J Med 2005;353(16):1659–72.

102. Romond EH, Perez EA, Bryant J, et al. Trastuzumab plus adjuvant chemotherapy for operable HER2-positive breast cancer. N Engl J Med 2005; 353(16):1673–84.

103. Slamon D, Eiermann W, Robert N, et al. Adjuvant trastuzumab in HER2-positive breast cancer. N Engl J Med 2011;365(14):1273–83.

104. Slamon DJ, Eiermann W, Robert NJ, et al. Ten year follow-up of the BCIRG-006 trial comparing doxorubicin plus cyclophosphamide followed by docetaxel (AC®T) with doxorubicin plus cyclophosphamide followed by docetaxel and trastuzumab (AC®TH) with docetaxel, carboplatin and trastuzumab (TCH) in HER2+ early breast cancer patients. San Antonio Breast Cancer Symposium 2015; Abstract No. S5–04. Presented December 11, 2015. Available on Page 999 at: https://www.sabcs.org/Portals/SABCS2016/Documents/SABCS-2015-Abstracts. pdf?v=5. Accessed September 29, 2017.

105. Tolaney SM, Barry WT, Dang CT, et al. Adjuvant paclitaxel and trastuzumab for node-negative, HER2-positive breast cancer. N Engl J Med 2015; 372(2):134–41.

106. Gianni L, Pienkowski T, Im YH, et al. Efficacy and safety of neoadjuvant pertuzumab and trastuzumab in women with locally advanced, inflammatory, or early HER2-positive breast cancer (NeoSphere): a randomised multicentre, open-label, phase 2 trial. Lancet Oncol 2012;13(1):25–32.

107. Schneeweiss A, Chia S, Hickish T, et al. Pertuzumab plus trastuzumab in combination with standard neoadjuvant anthracycline-containing and anthracycline-free chemotherapy regimens in patients with HER2-positive early breast cancer: a randomized phase II cardiac safety study (TRYPHAENA). Ann Oncol 2013;24(9):2278–84.

108. von Minckwitz G, Procter M, de Azambuja E, et al. Adjuvant pertuzumab and trastuzumab in early HER2-positive breast cancer. N Engl J Med 2017; 377(2):122–31.

109. Early Breast Cancer Trialists' Collaborative Group (EBCTCG), Davies C, Godwin J, Gray R, et al. Relevance of breast cancer hormone receptors and other factors to the efficacy of adjuvant tamoxifen: patient-level meta-analysis of randomised trials. Lancet 2011;378(9793):771–84.

110. Davies C, Pan H, Godwin J, et al. Long-term effects of continuing adjuvant tamoxifen to 10 years versus stopping at 5 years after diagnosis of oestrogen receptor-positive breast cancer: ATLAS, a randomised trial. Lancet 2013;381(9869):805–16.

111. Goss PE, Ingle JN, Martino S, et al. Randomized trial of letrozole following tamoxifen as extended adjuvant therapy in receptor-positive breast cancer: updated findings from NCIC CTG MA.17. J Natl Cancer Inst 2005;97(17):1262–71.

112. Goss PE, Ingle JN, Pritchard KI, et al. Extending aromatase-inhibitor adjuvant therapy to 10 years. N Engl J Med 2016;375(3):209–19.

113. Burstein HJ, Temin S, Anderson H, et al. Adjuvant endocrine therapy for women with hormone receptor-positive breast cancer: American Society of Clinical Oncology clinical practice guideline focused update. J Clin Oncol 2014;32(21):2255–69.

114. Pagani O, Regan MM, Walley BA, et al. Adjuvant exemestane with ovarian suppression in premenopausal breast cancer. N Engl J Med 2014;371(2): 107–18.

115. Moore HC, Unger JM, Phillips KA, et al. Goserelin for ovarian protection during breast-cancer adjuvant chemotherapy. N Engl J Med 2015;372(10): 923–32.

116. Azim HA Jr, Santoro L, Pavlidis N, et al. Safety of pregnancy following breast cancer diagnosis: a meta-analysis of 14 studies. Eur J Cancer 2011; 47(1):74–83.

117. Margolese RG, Cecchini RS, Julian TB, et al. Anastrozole versus tamoxifen in postmenopausal women with ductal carcinoma in situ undergoing lumpectomy plus radiotherapy (NSABP B-35): a randomised, double-blind, phase 3 clinical trial. Lancet 2016;387(10021):849–56.

118. Visvanathan K, Hurley P, Bantug E, et al. Use of pharmacologic interventions for breast cancer

risk reduction: American Society of Clinical Oncology clinical practice guideline. J Clin Oncol 2013;31(23):2942–62.

119. Muss HB, Berry DA, Cirrincione CT, et al. Adjuvant chemotherapy in older women with early-stage breast cancer. N Engl J Med 2009;360(20): 2055–65.

120. Emens LA, Davidson NE. The follow-up of breast cancer. Semin Oncol 2003;30(3):338–48.

121. Kokko R, Holli K, Hakama M. Ca 15-3 in the follow-up of localised breast cancer: a prospective study. Eur J Cancer 2002;38(9):1189–93.

122. Dal Maso L, Zucchetto A, Talamini R, et al. Effect of obesity and other lifestyle factors on mortality in women with breast cancer. Int J Cancer 2008; 123(9):2188–94.

123. Ballard-Barbash R, Friedenreich CM, Courneya KS, et al. Physical activity, biomarkers, and disease outcomes in cancer survivors: a systematic review. J Natl Cancer Inst 2012;104(11):815–40.

124. Betof AS, Dewhirst MW, Jones LW. Effects and potential mechanisms of exercise training on cancer progression: a translational perspective. Brain Behav Immun 2013;30(Suppl):S75–87.

Section 2: Current Concepts in Molecular Imaging of Breast Cancer

Section 2: Current Concepts in Mechanical Ventilation Strategies

Diagnostic Role of Fluorodeoxyglucose PET in Breast Cancer
A History to Current Application

Dhritiman Chakraborty, MD[a], Sandip Basu, MD[b],
Gary A. Ulaner, MD, PhD[c], Abass Alavi, MD[d],
Rakesh Kumar, MD, PhD[e],*

KEYWORDS

- Fluorodeoxyglucose (FDG) • Positron emission tomography (PET) • PET/CT • Breast cancer

KEY POINTS

- Histologic subtype, receptor status, and other biologic factors greatly affect the avidity of breast malignancy on fluorodeoxyglucose (FDG) PET.
- FDG PET/computed tomography (CT) has demonstrated value in the assessment of extra-axillary nodal and distant metastases.
- Patients with early-stage breast cancers do not benefit from FDG PET/CT; however, unsuspected distant metastases may be revealed by systemic staging of locally advanced breast cancers by FDG PET/CT, and this has substantial impact on patient management.
- FDG PET/CT has demonstrated value in the evaluation of treatment response and in detection of disease recurrence.

INTRODUCTION

Breast cancer is the leading cause of cancer death among women in developing countries, stands second in developed countries, and accounts for 15.3% of all cancers in the United States. Based on 2013 through 2015 Surveillance, Epidemiology, and End Results Program data, 12.4% of women will be diagnosed with breast cancer at some point during their lives.[1,2] Despite the increasing incidence of breast cancer in recent decades, survival rates have improved because of earlier diagnosis, new treatment strategies, and incorporation of molecular imaging.

Fluorodeoxyglucose (FDG) has been the molecular imaging agent of greatest impact for patients with breast cancer. Malignant tumor cells often demonstrate higher metabolism, and thus accumulate more glucose as compared with their normal counterparts. FDG, a radiolabeled glucose analogue, accumulates in cells by mechanisms similar to glucose. After intravenous administration, FDG is transported into cells by glucose transporter type 1 or 3 (GLUT-1 or GLUT-3). Subsequent

Disclosure Statement: No significant disclosures.
[a] Department of Nuclear Medicine, All India Institute of Medical Sciences, New Delhi, Delhi 110029, India;
[b] Department of Nuclear Medicine, Nuclear Medicine Academic Programme, Radiation Medicine Centre, Bhaba Atomic Research Centre, Mumbai 400012, India; [c] Department of Radiology, Memorial Sloan Kettering Cancer Center, New York, NY 10065, USA; [d] Department of Radiology, Perelman School of Medicine, University of Pennsylvania, Philadelphia, PA 19104, USA; [e] Diagnostic Nuclear Medicine Division, Department of Nuclear Medicine, All India Institute of Medical Sciences, New Delhi, Delhi 110029, India
* Corresponding author.
E-mail address: rkphulia@hotmail.com

PET Clin 13 (2018) 355–361
https://doi.org/10.1016/j.cpet.2018.02.011

intracellular phosphorylation by hexokinase leads to formation of FDG-6-phosphate. Both glucose-6-phosphate and FDG-6-phosphate are impermeable to the cell membrane, unable to be used in further glycolysis pathways, and are trapped within the cell.[3] The accumulation of FDG within highly metabolic cells allows for their visualization on FDG PET imaging. Minn and Soini[4] were the first to study the utility of FDG imaging in breast cancer in 1989. Since then, FDG PET has been used for primary breast cancer screening, detection of locoregional and distant metastases, and monitoring therapy response. Dual-modality PET/computed tomography (CT) allows simultaneous acquisition of anatomic and molecular information. The CT transmission information can be used for anatomic localization, attenuation correction, and corresponding CT assessment of lesions. PET/CT demonstrates greater specificity and accuracy for breast cancer staging than PET alone,[5] and thus, FDG PET/CT has become a standard modality for initial staging of advanced local breast cancer and evaluation of treatment response in metastatic breast cancer.[6] This article reviews the historical and current value of FDG PET and PET/CT in patients with breast malignancies.

FLUORODEOXYGLUCOSE PET AND TUMOR BIOLOGY

Breast cancer histology has an important impact on tumor visualization on FDG PET and FDG PET/CT. Invasive ductal breast carcinoma (IDC), the most common subtype of breast malignancy, has been shown to be a distinct genetic and molecular disease from invasive lobular carcinoma (ILC),[7] and these differences effect their imaging. In initial studies of primary breast malignancies, FDG uptake was significantly higher in IDC than ILC, with a mean tumor-to-background ratio of 17.3 and 6.5, respectively.[8] This phenomenon extends to metastatic disease from breast malignancies. Osseous metastases from ILC demonstrate lower FDG avidity than those from IDC, and are more likely to be overlooked on FDG PET due to avidity being no higher than background.[9] The lower avidity of ILC results in a lower rate of upstaging from FDG PET/CT as compared with IDC.[10]

Receptor status, tumor grade, and proliferation index are additional important components of tumor biology that impact FDG avidity. Currently, the most important receptors that are analyzed on breast tumors are estrogen receptor (ER), progesterone receptor (PR), and human epidermal growth factor receptor 2 (HER2). These receptors are important for patient prognosis and selection of systemic therapies. Primary breast malignancies that lack ER, PR, and HER2, often known as triple-negative breast cancer (TNBC), are significantly more FDG avid than non-TNBC.[11] Breast cancer tumor grade significantly correlates with the magnitude of FDG uptake. Primary Grade 3 carcinomas demonstrate greatest FDG avidity than grade 1 to 2 carcinomas (6.2 vs 4.9, respectively).[12] A statistically significant positive correlation between Ki-67 and FDG accumulation has been demonstrated in ductal breast cancers.[8] There is also significant correlation between proliferation index and FDG uptake, a biomarker that can be measured noninvasively and may facilitate clinical trials involving women with TNBC.[13]

Several additional biologic correlates have been proposed to effect tumor FDG avidity. Using preoperative FDG PET scans in 55 patients, Bos and colleagues[14] demonstrated that FDG accumulation in the breast tumor is a function of microvasculature density for delivering nutrients ($P = .005$), GLUT1 for transportation of the tracer into the cell ($P<.001$), hexokinase for entering the tracer into glycolysis ($P = .02$), number of viable cancerous cells per volume ($P = .009$), the proliferation rate ($P = .001$), the number of lymphocytes ($P = .03$), and the HIF-1a upregulation of GLUT1. These characteristics may help clarify why breast cancers vary in FDG uptake. MCF-7 (Michigan Cancer Foundation-7) breast cancer cells show hypoxia-induced increase in FDG accumulation in part related to an increase in GLUT activity resulting from modification of the glucose transport proteins.[15]

IMAGING OF THE PRIMARY BREAST MALIGNANCY

Early detection of breast cancer is the most effective strategy to reduce mortality. To date, mammography is the only screening method that has been shown to affect patient survival. Breast cancer often presents as a subcentimeter area of abnormality on screening mammography. An appropriate diagnostic modality must be able to demonstrate nonpalpable, small (<1.0 cm), invasive, and in situ malignancies. Conventional imaging modalities, such as mammography and ultrasonography primarily depend on changes in anatomic structure for disease detection. Whole-body FDG PET can help to detect accelerated metabolic activity that occurs before anatomic structural changes. However, it is not generally suitable for routine screening purposes because of the low sensitivity of whole-body FDG PET for primary breast cancers,[16,17] expense of the examination, and the involved radiation exposure.

As malignant lesions demonstrate greater increase in FDG avidity with increased FDG uptake time than benign lesions, dual time point (DP) imaging was proposed to improve FDG PET evaluation of breast lesions. The theoretic basis for this approach is that the dephosphorylation of FDG-6-phosphate in neoplastic cells is likely to be slower than in normal cells owing to the low glucose-6-phosphatase content.[18] The potential clinical usefulness of DP (at ~63 and ~101 minutes) FDG PET for identifying malignant lesions in the breast was evaluated in 54 patients with 57 breast lesions by Kumar and colleagues.[19] They concluded that, over time, there is an increase in the uptake of FDG in breast malignancies, whereas the uptake in inflammatory lesions and normal breast tissues decreases. A percentage change of 3.75 or more in standardized uptake value (SUV) differentiated inflammatory lesions from malignant ones. DP technique was used in a prospective study that demonstrated sensitivities of the DP imaging method in detecting invasive cancer measuring larger than 10 mm, 4 to 10 mm, and noninvasive breast cancer to be 90.1%, 82.7%, and 76.9%, respectively.[20] DP imaging may be of greater value than traditional whole-body FDG PET/CT to differentiate benign and malignant processes in the breast, although the superiority of mammography, ultrasound, and MR imaging for characterizing breast lesions has not led to the routine use of DP imaging.

Positron emission mammography (PEM) visualizes the FDG radiotracer with a small field of view, breast-specific positron imaging apparatus. In this method, 2 planar detectors are integrated into a conventional mammographic system that enables co-registration of mammographic and emission FDG images of the breast.[21] The advantages of PEM, compared with whole-body 18F-FDG PET, include higher spatial resolution, shorter imaging time, and reduced attenuation. PEM also shows higher count sensitivity and permits PEM-guided biopsy. A multicenter trial by Berg and colleagues[22] suggested that PEM may aid in the detection and characterization of both invasive and in situ breast carcinoma. The same group evaluated the effect of PEM using Flex Solo II (Naviscan PET system, SanDiego, CA) in breast cancer presurgical planning and compared it with MR imaging. This study involved 388 participants with newly diagnosed invasive or intraductal breast cancer who were candidates for breast conservation surgery, and who voluntarily underwent PEM and MR imaging within 5 days of each other. Both MR imaging and PEM led to higher sensitivity compared with mammography, whereas a combination of PEM with MR imaging led to an additional gain in sensitivity for detecting previously unknown malignant lesions. Specificity of PEM is better compared with MR imaging, although sensitivity of PEM and MR imaging is similar, with MR imaging being slightly higher.[23] Continued advances in PEM instrumentation have led to new rotating detector–based and stationary full or partial detector ring-based PEM scanners for imaging uncompressed hanging breasts in the prone position, which leads to increased sensitivity and spatial resolution. PEM systems can help in providing an accurate definition of the extent of disease in a breast, and hold great promise as further research defines their role in evaluating malignancy within the breast.

Imaging of Nodal Disease

Axillary nodes are often the first site of metastases from primary breast cancer, and are a critical prognostic feature. Thus, the evaluation of potential axillary nodal metastases is part of the workup of all patients with breast cancer. Unfortunately, FDG PET/CT has demonstrated poor sensitivity for the detection of axillary nodal metastases.[24,25] A meta-analysis[26] of 26 studies (total patients = 2591) evaluating diagnostic accuracy of PET or PET-CT for the assessment of axilla showed that mean sensitivity was only 63% (95% confidence interval [CI] 52%–74%; range 20%–100%), but the mean specificity was as high as 94% (95% CI 91%–96%; range 75%–100%). Given the low sensitivity of FDG PET/CT for detection of axillary nodal metastases, surgical sampling by sentinel lymph node biopsy or axillary dissection remains the method of choice for staging the axilla.

FDG PET/CT has demonstrated value in the detection of unsuspected extra-axillary nodal disease.[25–30] Groheux and colleagues[28] reported that PET-CT revealed additional N3 nodal disease (infra or supra clavicular and internal mammary nodes) in 32 (27.3%) of 117 patients. Identification of N3 disease upstages the disease and leads to change in therapeutic decisions related to extent of surgery or placement of radiation portals.[29]

Imaging of distant metastases

FDG PET/CT demonstrates its greatest value in patients with breast malignancies in detecting distant metastases. Almost all studies have revealed high sensitivity and specificity of PET-CT as compared with conventional imaging in diagnosing distant metastasis. PET-CT leads to upstaging, both interstage, that is, Stage III to IV due to identification of distant metastasis, and intrastage, that is, within stage III due to identification of additional regional lymph nodes.[31–36] This upstaging can result in change in management in a significant number of patients (**Fig. 1**). Patients with locally advanced breast cancer (LABC) have a high rate of distant metastases.[28] In these patients, the systemic staging with FDG PET/CT may be considered at diagnosis.[6] Osseous metastases are better detected by FDG PET/CT than by conventional CT and bone scanning.[37] Sclerotic osseous metastases may not be appreciably FDG avid, but the ability to visualize them on the corresponding CT images still allows their detection on PET/CT.[9,32] Liver metastases may be detected on FDG PET before being visualized on CT, particularly in a steatotic liver in which a low-attenuation metastasis may not be appreciated as separate from the low-attenuation steatotic liver. Smaller lung metastases may be missed on FDG PET due to respiratory motion and partial volume effects, but can be recognized on the CT component of hybrid PET/CT imaging. Overall, FDG PET/CT provides an excellent evaluation of nodes, bone, liver, and lungs, the most common sites of distant metastases from primary breast cancers. After definitive therapy, FDG PET/ CT demonstrated superior ability to detect recurrent breast cancer malignancy than conventional CT and bone scan, for both local and distant disease, in a prospective trial[38] (**Fig. 2**).

Imaging therapy response

Neoadjuvant chemotherapy has been shown to be effective in downstaging the primary tumor before surgery and is now increasingly being used in the management of patients with LABC.[39] Many studies have demonstrated that nonresponders may achieve an improved survival with the use of alternative and/or more prolonged courses of chemotherapy.[40] Therefore, it is very important to differentiate between responders and nonresponders as soon as possible so that ineffective toxic and expensive chemotherapy is avoided. In a study of 23 patients with LABC, Kumar and colleagues[41] concluded that sensitivity, specificity, and accuracy of PET/CT in detecting responders were 93%, 75%, and 87%, respectively. The investigators conducted the follow-up scan after 2 cycles of chemotherapy to assess response; they considered 50% reduction in SUV as the cutoff value to differentiate

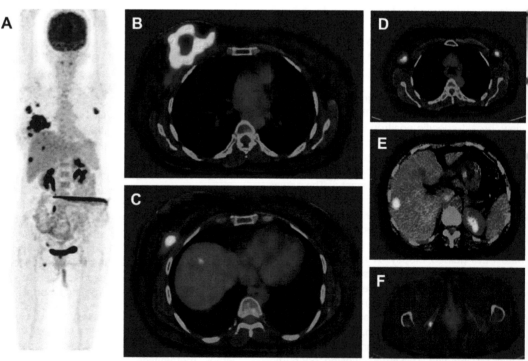

Fig. 1. A 48-year-old woman with carcinoma of right breast lump. 18F-FDG PET/CT shows FDG avid soft tissue lesion with poorly defined margins in the upper inner quadrant of the right breast measuring approximately 4.1 × 5.0 × 5.9 cm (*A, B*). The lesion is reaching toward the retro-areolar region and involving the nipple-areolar complex causing retraction of the nipple without involving underlying chest wall structures and skin (*B*). A conglomerated FDG avid rounded left axillary level I lymph nodal mass measuring 2.5 × 1.6 cm and multiple ipsilateral left level I and level II axillary lymph nodes are noted (*D*). FDG avid right internal mammary lymph node, multiple hypodense lesions in the liver, and lytic lesion in right ischium is noted (*C, E, F*).

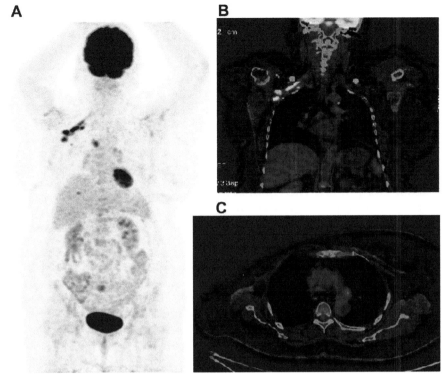

Fig. 2. A 67-year-old woman with carcinoma of the right breast, post right mastectomy, 18F-FDG PET/CT showed FDG avid ill-defined soft tissue thickening along the neurovascular bundles in right axilla exiting over right first rib laterally into axilla (likely brachial plexus involvement) (*A, B*), FDG avid right axillary lymph nodes (22 × 13 mm) (*B*). FDG avid subcentimetric right internal mammary lymph node and parasternal soft tissue mass with subtle lytic erosion of manubrium noted (*C*). Lytic lesions with increased FDG avid are also noted in right ninth rib posteriorly, manubrium, and sacrum (*A*).

between responders and nonresponders, as changes in FDG metabolism often precede morphologic changes in tumor. A separate article by Groheux, elsewhere in this issue of *PET Clinics*, provides an in-depth review of using FDG PET/CT for evaluating therapy response in patients with breast cancer.

PET/Magnetic Resonance

PET/MR is a promising emerging technology in the field of breast cancer imaging like improved differentiation of malignant from benign breast lesions.[42] Given the better evaluation of bone marrow by MR than CT, FDG PET/MR may detect more osseous metastases in patients with breast cancer than FDG PET/CT.[43] FDG PET/CT also may have an advantage in visualization of liver metastases, although PET/CT may be superior for lung metastases.[44] Work with PET/MR is still developing, and large prospective studies will be needed to fully evaluate the potential of PET/MR in patients with breast malignancies.

SUMMARY

Histologic subtype, receptor status, and other biologic factors greatly affect the avidity of breast malignancy on FDG PET. Although FDG PET/CT is outperformed by other modalities for evaluation of the primary breast malignancy and axillary nodal metastases, FDG PET/CT has demonstrated excellent value in the evaluation of extra-axillary nodal and distant metastases. Patients with early-stage breast cancers do not benefit from FDG PET/CT; however, unsuspected distant metastases may be revealed by systemic staging of LABCs by FDG PET/CT, and this has substantial impact on patient management. FDG PET/CT has demonstrated value in the evaluation of treatment response and in detection of disease recurrence. Overall, FDG PET/CT has made a substantial impact on the management of patients with breast cancer. Further work, including randomized trials on PET/CT, PET/MR, and other molecular imaging modalities is needed to optimize the use of these tools.

REFERENCES

1. Available at: https://seer.cancer.gov/statfacts/html/breast.html. Accessed May 3, 2018.
2. Siegel RL, Miller KD, Jemal A. Cancer statistics, 2017. CA Cancer J Clin 2017;67(1):7–30.
3. Pauwels EK, Ribeiro MJ, Stoot JH, et al. FDG accumulation and tumor biology. Nucl Med Biol 1998;25:317–22.
4. Minn H, Soini I. F-18 fluorodeoxyglucose scintigraphy in diagnosis and follow-up of treatment in advanced breast cancer. Eur J Nucl Med Mol Imaging 1989;15:61–6.
5. Lim HS, Yoon W, Chung TW, et al. FDG PET/CT for the detection and evaluation of breast diseases: usefulness and limitations. Radiographics 2007;27(Suppl 1):S197–213.
6. Gradishar WJ, Anderson BO, Balassanian R, et al. Invasive breast cancer version 1.2016, NCCN clinical practice guidelines in oncology. J Natl Compr Cancer Netw 2016;14(3):324–54.
7. Ciriello G, Gatza ML, Beck AH, et al. Comprehensive molecular portraits of invasive lobular breast cancer. Cell 2015;163(2):506–19.
8. Buck A, Schirrmeister H, Kuhn T, et al. FDG uptake in breast cancer: correlation with biological and clinical prognostic parameters. Eur J Nucl Med Mol Imaging 2002;29:1317–23.
9. Dashevsky BZ, Goldman DA, Parsons M, et al. Appearance of untreated bone metastases from breast cancer on FDG PET/CT: importance of histologic subtype. Eur J Nucl Med Mol Imaging 2015;42(11):1666–73.
10. Hogan MP, Goldman DA, Dashevsky B, et al. Comparison of 18F-FDG PET/CT for systemic staging of newly diagnosed invasive lobular carcinoma versus invasive ductal carcinoma. J Nucl Med 2015;56(11):1674–80.
11. Basu S, Chen W, Tchou J, et al. Comparison of triple-negative and estrogen receptor-positive/progesterone receptor-positive/HER2-negative breast carcinoma using quantitative fluorine-18 fluorodeoxyglucose/positron emission tomography imaging parameters: a potentially useful method for disease characterization. Cancer 2008;112(5):995–1000.
12. Crippa F, Seregni E, Agresti R, et al. Association between [18F]-fluorodeoxyglucose uptake and postoperative histopathology, hormone receptor status, thymidine labeling index, and p53 in primary breast cancer: a preliminary observation. Eur J Nucl Med 1998;25:1429–34.
13. Tchou J, Sonnad S, Bergey MR, et al. Degree of tumor FDG uptake correlates with proliferation index in triple-negative breast cancer. Mol Imaging Biol 2010;12(6):657–62.
14. Bos R, van Der Hoeven JJ, van Der Wall E, et al. Biologic correlates of 18fluorodeoxyglucose uptake in human breast cancer measured by positron emission tomography. J Clin Oncol 2002;20:379–87.
15. Burgman P, O'Donoghue JA, Humm JL, et al. Hypoxia-induced increase in FDG uptake in MCF7 cells. J Nucl Med 2001;42:170–5.
16. Rosen EL, Eubank WB, Mankoff DA. FDG PET, PET/CT, and breast cancer imaging. Radiographics 2007;27(Suppl 1):S215–29.
17. Avril N, Rose CA, Schelling M, et al. Breast imaging with positron emission tomography and fluorine-18 fluorodeoxyglucose: use and limitations. J Clin Oncol 2000;18:3495–502.
18. Nelson CA, Wang JQ, Leav I, et al. The interaction among glucose transport, hexokinase, and glucose-6-phosphatase with respect to 3H-2-deoxyglucose retention in murine tumor models. Nucl Med Biol 1996;23:533–41.
19. Kumar R, Loving VA, Chauhan A, et al. Potential of dual-time-point imaging to improve breast cancer diagnosis with (18)F-FDG-PET. J Nucl Med 2005;46:1819–24.
20. Mavi A, Urhan M, Yu JQ, et al. Dual time point 18F-FDG-PET imaging detects breast cancer with high sensitivity and correlates well with histologic subtypes. J Nucl Med 2006;47:1440–6.
21. Buscombe JR, Holloway B, Roche N, et al. Position of nuclear medicine modalities in the diagnostic work-up of breast cancer. Q J Nucl Med Mol Imaging 2004;48(2):109–18.
22. Berg WA, Weinberg IN, Narayanan D, et al. High-resolution fluorodeoxyglucose positron emission tomography with compression ("positron emission mammography") is highly accurate in depicting primary breast cancer. Breast J 2006;12:309–23.
23. Berg WA, Madsen KS, Schilling K, et al. Breast cancer: comparative effectiveness of positron emission mammography and MR imaging in presurgical planning for the ipsilateral breast. Radiology 2011;258:59–72.
24. Wahl RL, Siegel BA, Coleman RE, et al. Prospective multicenter study of axillary nodal staging by positron emission tomography in breast cancer: a report of the staging breast cancer with PET Study Group. J Clin Oncol 2004;22(2):277–85.
25. Pritchard KI, Julian JA, Holloway CM, et al. Prospective study of 2-[(1)(8)F]fluorodeoxyglucose positron emission tomography in the assessment of regional nodal spread of disease in patients with breast cancer: an Ontario clinical oncology group study. J Clin Oncol 2012;30(12):1274–9.
26. Cooper KL, Harnan S, Meng Y, et al. Positron emission tomography (PET) for assessment of axillary lymph node status in early breast cancer: a systematic review and meta-analysis. Eur J Surg Oncol 2011;37:187–98.
27. Jung NY, Kim SH, Kim SH, et al. Effectiveness of breast MRI and 18 F-FDG PET/CT for the preoperative staging of invasive lobular carcinoma versus ductal carcinoma. J Breast Cancer 2015;18:63–72.

28. Groheux D, Giacchetti S, Delord M, et al. 18 F-FDG PET/CT in staging patients with locally advanced or inflammatory breast cancer: comparison to conventional staging. J Nucl Med 2013;54:5–11.

29. Groheux D, Hindié E, Rubello D, et al. Should FDG PET/CT be used for the initial staging of breast cancer? Eur J Nucl Med Mol Imaging 2009;36:1539–42.

30. Robertson IJ, Hand F, Kell MR. FDG-PET/CT in the staging of local/regional metastases in breast cancer. Breast 2011;20:491–4.

31. Tran A, Pio BS, Khatibi B, et al. 18F-FDG PET for staging breast cancer in patients with inner-quadrant versus outer-quadrant tumors: comparison with long-term clinical outcome. J Nucl Med 2005; 46(9):1455–9.

32. Groheux D, Espie M, Giacchetti S, et al. Performance of FDG PET/CT in the clinical management of breast cancer. Radiology 2013;266(2):388–405.

33. Groheux D, Giacchetti S, Espie M, et al. The yield of 18F-FDG PET/CT in patients with clinical stage IIA, IIB, or IIIA breast cancer: a prospective study. J Nucl Med 2011;52(10):1526–34.

34. Groheux D, Hindie E, Delord M, et al. Prognostic impact of (18)FDG-PET-CT findings in clinical stage III and IIB breast cancer. J Natl Cancer Inst 2012; 104(24):1879–87.

35. Ulaner GA, Castillo R, Goldman DA, et al. (18) F-FDG-PET/CT for systemic staging of newly diagnosed triple-negative breast cancer. Eur J Nucl Med Mol Imaging 2016;43(11):1937–44.

36. Ulaner GA, Castillo R, Wills J, et al. 18F-FDG-PET/CT for systemic staging of patients with newly diagnosed ER-positive and HER2-positive breast cancer. Eur J Nucl Med Mol Imaging 2017;44(9):1420–7.

37. Morris PG, Lynch C, Feeney JN, et al. Integrated positron emission tomography/computed tomography may render bone scintigraphy unnecessary to investigate suspected metastatic breast cancer. J Clin Oncol 2010;28(19):3154–9.

38. Hildebrandt MG, Gerke O, Baun C, et al. [18F] Fluorodeoxyglucose (FDG)-positron emission tomography (PET)/computed tomography (CT) in suspected recurrent breast cancer: a prospective comparative study of dual-time-point FDG-PET/CT, contrast-enhanced CT, and bone scintigraphy. J Clin Oncol 2016;34(16):1889–97.

39. Wang H, Lo S. Future prospects of neoadjuvant chemotherapy in treatment of primary breast cancer. Semin Surg Oncol 1996;12:59–66.

40. Heys SD, Eremin JM, Sarkar TK, et al. Role of multimodality therapy in the management of locally advanced carcinoma of the breast. J Am Coll Surg 1994;179:493–504.

41. Kumar A, Kumar R, Seenu V, et al. The role of 18 F-FDG PET/CT in evaluation of early response to neoadjuvant chemotherapy in patients with locally advanced breast cancer. Eur Radiol 2009;19: 1347–57.

42. Pinker K, Bogner W, Baltzer P, et al. Improved differentiation of benign and malignant breast tumors with multiparametric 18fluorodeoxyglucose positron emission tomography magnetic resonance imaging: a feasibility study. Clin Cancer Res 2014;20(13): 3540–9.

43. Catalano OA, Nicolai E, Rosen BR, et al. Comparison of CE-FDG-PET/CT with CE-FDG-PET/MR in the evaluation of osseous metastases in breast cancer patients. Br J Cancer 2015;112(9):1452–60.

44. Melsaether AN, Raad RA, Pujara AC, et al. Comparison of whole-body (18)F FDG PET/MR imaging and whole-body (18)F FDG PET/CT in terms of lesion detection and radiation dose in patients with breast cancer. Radiology 2016;281(1):193–202.

Dedicated Breast Gamma Camera Imaging and Breast PET: Current Status and Future Directions

Deepa Narayanan, MS[a],*, Wendie A. Berg, MD, PhD[b]

KEYWORDS

- Molecular breast imaging • Positron emission mammography • Breast PET • Breast cancer
- Breast PET tracers

KEY POINTS

- Dedicated breast imaging using gamma and PET scanners provide high sensitivity and specificity, and can be used as an adjunct to mammography in women with breast cancer.
- Dedicated breast PET and dedicated gamma camera images must be interpreted together with mammography and other prior breast imaging, biopsy history, and patient risk factors.
- Dose reduction strategies are critical to allowing greater use of nuclear medicine modalities, especially in the screening setting.
- Newer technologies and tracers are under development to improve the performance of nuclear breast imaging.

Anatomic imaging such as mammography and ultrasound imaging are the mainstay of conventional breast imaging. Contrast-enhanced MR imaging, which is both anatomic and shows areas of increased vascularity and vascular permeability, is widely used for high-risk screening and assessing disease extent and response. Functional breast imaging techniques using dedicated gamma cameras or PET scanners can complement conventional imaging by providing specific cellular information to aid in the diagnosis, staging, and treatment of breast cancer. The 2 most common radiotracers used for breast imaging are the gamma-emitting ^{99m}Tc-sestamibi (140 keV, half-life of 6 hours) that measures mitochondrial activity and the positron emitting glucose analog $_{18}$F-fluorodeoxyglucose (FDG; 511 keV, half-life of 110 minutes) that measures metabolic activity. Conventional whole-body gamma cameras and whole-body PET systems with a large field

of view have limited spatial resolution and low sensitivity for smaller tumors.[1,2] The development of high-resolution dedicated breast scanners has resulted in improved lesion detectability, particularly for subcentimeter lesions, owing to technical improvements in detector performance, the ability to position these compact cameras closer to the breast, and the availability of projections similar to those of mammography.[3] The goal of this article is to discuss existing clinical data for nuclear medicine imaging in breast cancer and review technologies in development.

DEDICATED SINGLE PHOTON GAMMA IMAGING

Dedicated breast gamma imaging uses semiconductor-based gamma cameras in a mammographic configuration to visualize the uptake of ^{99m}Tc-sestamibi. Sestamibi, originally

---

Disclosures: None.
[a] National Cancer Institute, 9609 Medical Center Drive, Rockville, MD 20850, USA; [b] Department of Radiology, University of Pittsburgh School of Medicine, Magee-Womens Hospital of UPMC, 300 Halket Street, Pittsburgh, PA 15213
* Corresponding author.
E-mail address: mndeepa@gmail.com

PET Clin 13 (2018) 363–381
https://doi.org/10.1016/j.cpet.2018.02.008
1556-8598/18/Published by Elsevier Inc.

developed as a cardiac tracer, is approved by the US Food and Drug Administration for breast cancer imaging, accumulating selectively in breast tumors rather than the surrounding normal breast tissue.[4] There are 3 different commercially available dedicated gamma camera systems. The breast-specific gamma imaging (BSGI) detector system from Dilon Technologies (Newport News, VA) was the first dedicated breast gamma imaging system on the market. The original BSGI scanner consists of a single panel detector with NaI crystals and a field of view of 20 × 20 cm; a recent version uses cesium iodide crystals with a larger field of view of 25 × 20 cm. Lumagem (previously Gamma Medica Inc., Salem, NH; recently acquired by CMR Naviscan, Carlsbad, CA) and the Discovery NM750b (GE Healthcare, Milwaukee, WI) systems are dual panel systems that use 2 cadmium zinc telluride (CZT)

detector panels with a field of view of 20 × 16 cm and 24 × 16 cm, respectively **Table 1**. Single panel detector systems are called BSGI systems and dual-panel systems are referred to as molecular breast imaging (MBI) systems in much of the literature on this topic and are so named in this paper. Dual-panel MBI systems show improved lesion detection sensitivity compared with single-panel systems, owing to reduced lesion-to-detector distance, especially in women with large breasts and smaller lesions.[5,6] Stereotactic biopsy capability is available for the Dilon and GE systems.

In all dedicated breast gamma camera imaging systems, patients are positioned similar to mammography to obtain craniocaudal (CC) and mediolateral oblique (MLO) views with only gentle compression applied to stabilize the breast. Screening Patients are scheduled for imaging

Table 1
Gamma camera breast imaging

	Dilon Diagnostics (Newport News, VA)	Gamma Medica Inc. (Salem, NH)	GE Healthcare (Milwaukee, WI)
	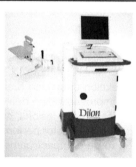	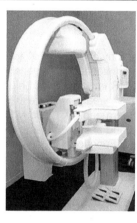	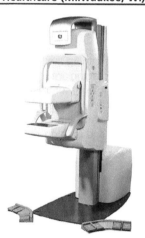
SYSTEM	Dilon Diagnostics 6800	Gamma Medica LumaGEM 3200S	GE Healthcare Discovery NM750b
Detector	NaI	CZT	CZT
Detector Geometry	Single panel detector	Dual panel detectors	Dual panel detectors
FOV (cm)	20 × 20	20 × 16	24 × 16
Biopsy	Available	In Development	Available
Spatial Resolution	4–4.2 mm	4.8–5.6 mm	4.4–4.6 mm
Injected dose	10–12 mCi	4–8 mCi	4-8 mCi
Pixel size	3 mm	1.6 mm	2.5 mm

Abbreviations: CZT, cadmium zinc telluride; FOV, field of view.
Adapted from Hsu DF, Freese DL, Levin CS. Breast-dedicated radionuclide imaging systems. J Nucl Med 2016;57 Suppl 1:40S–5S.

during days 7 to 14 of their menstrual cycle to decrease background tracer uptake. The early literature showed that patients were typically injected with 555 to 1100 MBq (15–30 mCi) of 99mTc-sestamibi, but lower doses of 370 to 444 MBq (10–12 mCi) for BSGI and 148 to 296 MBq (4–8 mCi) for MBI imaging are common in current practice. Before injection, keeping the patient in a warm and sedentary state, sitting quietly with a warming blanket is recommended to improve tracer uptake in the breast.[7] Patients are imaged beginning 5 minutes after injection. For the Dilon and Lumagem systems, a single planar image is produced for each view. The GE system displays results from each of the upper and lower detectors and also creates an "average" CC and MLO view of each breast.

DEDICATED BREAST PET

Breast-specific PET uses detectors positioned close to the breast. Because most malignancies metabolize glucose at a faster rate than normal tissue, FDG uptake provides a functional map of tumor presence and activity. There are several breast-specific PET systems being developed and broadly they fall into 2 categories: positron emission mammography (PEM), where 2 planar detectors are placed on either side of the breast with the patient positioned analogous to mammography, and dedicated breast PET (dbPET) systems, where the patient is prone and the breast imaged with a ring-shaped detector (**Table 2**). Freifelder and Karp[8] compared the designs of both ring and planar scanners, and concluded there was no significant difference in lesion detection between PEM and dbPET scanners. Although dbPET detectors had a higher image contrast, better depth resolution, and slightly better overall performance, PEM scanners had lower image noise, were more accommodating of different imaging configurations, including different breast sizes, and potentially had a lower cost.

The PEM Flex Solo II scanner from Naviscan (CMR Naviscan) is the most clinically validated breast-specific PET system available. The Solo II consists of two 6 × 16.4-cm opposing lutetium-yttrium oxyorthosilicate (LYSO) crystal-based PET detectors that move linearly within compression paddles placed on either side of a gently stabilized breast, covering a field of view 24 × 16.4 cm[9]. Patients are seated upright and positioned in either CC or MLO positions. Limited angle reconstruction is performed to display 12 tomographic slices (slice thickness is the total breast compressed thickness divided by 12) for each view (**Fig. 1**). The in-plane resolution for

PEM systems is 2.4 mm using the maximum likelihood estimation method reconstruction and 1.8 mm using the high-resolution reconstruction mode.[9,10] The z-axis resolution is lower (4–6 mm) owing to limited angle tomography (2 parallel planar detectors are unable to provide 360° coverage for the breast). In addition, a PEM-guided biopsy system that is approved by the US Food and Drug Administration is available to sample suspicious breast lesions.[11] Eo and colleagues[12] found that PEM was more sensitive for smaller invasive tumors (**Fig. 2**) than PET-computed tomography (CT): 11 of 15 T1a or T1b (73%), 42 of 44 T1c (95%), and 44 of 44 T2 tumors (100%) were seen on PEM compared with 9 of 15 T1a or T1b (60%), 37 of 44 T1c (84%), and 42 of 44 T2 tumors (95%) on PET-CT (with a P value for the overall sensitivity difference of .004).

The MAMmography with Molecular Imaging PET system (Oncovision, Valencia, Spain) is a commercially available true tomographic ring scanner using lutetium-yttrium oxyorthosilicate-based PET detectors, (**Fig. 3**) with an intrinsic spatial resolution of 1.6 mm.[13] Each breast is imaged separately, with the patient prone; the breast hangs pendulous (no compression) within a ring of detectors rotating around it. A prototype biopsy system is under development.[14] Shimadzu (Kyoto, Japan) has developed the El Mammo dbPET systems and obtained clinical data with 2 different positioning configurations. The O-scanner is a tomographic ring system using a Lutetium gadolinium oxyorthosilicate (LGSO) detector with 2.0-mm resolution in all 3 dimensions. Shimadzu's C-PEM consists of a C-shaped detector ring with the patient positioned semiprone leaning into the scanner, offering better access to image the axillary nodes.[15]

For breast-specific PET imaging, patients are injected with approximately 185 to 370 MBq (5–10 mCi) of FDG after fasting for 4 to 6 hours. Blood glucose should be within normal limits before FDG injection. Patients must wait for 60 to 90 minutes after the injection to allow for optimal tracer uptake before imaging and should be resting quietly in a warm environment during the circulation time. PEM systems require that both breasts be imaged with standard mammographic CC and MLO views with scan time typically 10 minutes per breast per view (a total of 40 minutes or more if additional views are needed). Positioning (**Fig. 4**) can be challenging for women with large breasts where tiling may be necessary, for those with very small breasts, and for lesions close to the chest wall. The most posterior tissues are difficult to fully image owing to positioning the relatively bulky detectors (especially with dual-head MBI) and the need for coincidence detection on PET. For these

Table 2
Dedicated PET breast imaging

	CMR Naviscan (Carlsbad, CA)	Oncovision (Valencia, Spain)	Shimadzu Corporation (Kyoto, Japan)	Shimadzu Corporation (Kyoto, Japan)
System	PEM Flex Solo II	MAMMI PET	ElMammo-O-Scanner	C-PEM
Detector configuration	Planar detector	Ring detector	Ring detector	C-shaped detector
Detector	LYSO	LYSO	LGSO	LGSO
Patient position	Upright, like mammography	Prone	Prone	Semiprone
FOV	24 × 16.4 cm	Transaxial FOV is 170 mm	Transaxial FOV is 183 mm	Transaxial FOV is 216 mm
Biopsy	Yes	Under development	No	No
Spatial resolution[a]	1.8–2.4 mm (Z axis = 6–8.5 mm)	1.8 × 1.9 × 1.6 (x,y,z)	<2 mm	<2 mm
Compression	Gentle compression	No	No	No
Images	Tomographic 3D	3D	3D	Tomographic 3D

Abbreviations: FOV, field of view; LGSO, Lutetium gadolinium oxyorthosilicate, LYSO, lutetium-yttrium oxyorthosilicate; MAMMI, MAMmography with Molecular Imaging.

[a] Resolution changes based on reconstruction algorithms.

Adapted from Hsu DF, Freese DL, Levin CS. Breast-dedicated radionuclide imaging systems. J Nucl Med 2016;57 Suppl 1:405–5S; and Miyake KK, Nakamoto Y, Togashi K. Current status of dedicated breast PET imaging. Curr Radiol Rep 2016;4(4):16.

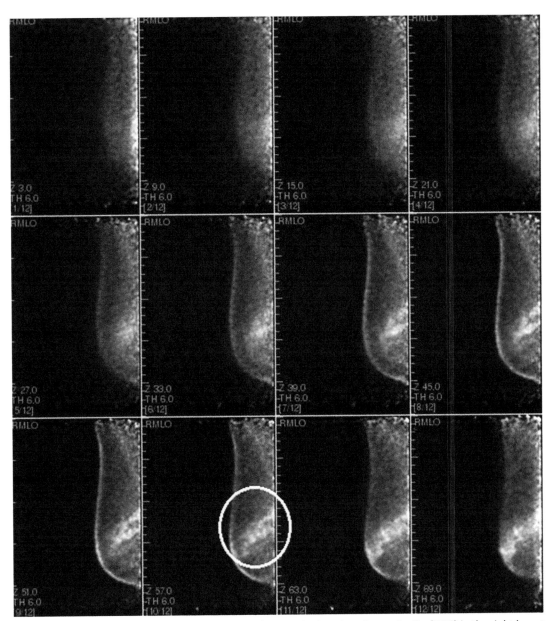

Fig. 1. A 55-year-old woman with extensive high nuclear grade ductal carcinoma in situ (DCIS) in the right breast. Twelve-slice positron emission mammography image showed increased ^{18}F-fluorodeoxyglucose uptake in the area of DCIS segmental distribution (*circle*). (*Courtesy of* Dr Wendie Berg, Magee-Womens Hospital of UPMC, Pittsburgh, PA.)

reasons, the use of trained technologists with experience in proper breast positioning as for mammography is recommended.

IMAGING TECHNIQUES AND INTERPRETATION
Interpretive Criteria

Standardized terminology to characterize and interpret findings has been developed for both MBI[16] and PEM images,[17] similar to the Breast Imaging and Reporting and Data System (BI-RADS) lexicon for MR imaging.[18] Experienced breast imagers have achieved high diagnostic accuracy and interobserver agreement after minimal training (approximately 2 hours) on either MBI or PEM. For 6 observers interpreting MBI, the median sensitivity was 100% (range, 90%–100%), specificity 88% (range, 83%–97%), and area under the receiver operating characteristic curve

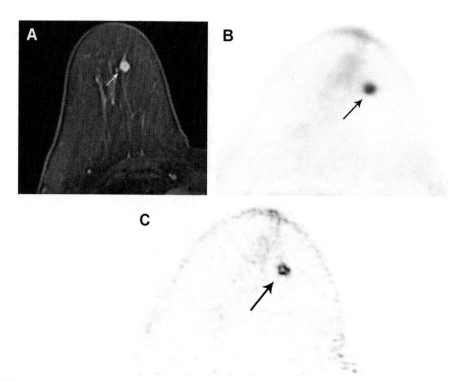

Fig. 2. A 74-year-old woman with mass in her right breast detected by screening mammography and ultrasound imaging. The tumor is well-visualized by both contrast-enhanced MR imaging (*A, arrow*) and Elmammo PET scanner (*B and C, arrows*). The patient was imaged for 5 minutes per breast and images are obtained in both standard (*B*) and enhanced resolution reconstruction mode (*C*). Pathology showed a 7-mm mucinous carcinoma with negative sentinel nodes. (*Courtesy of* Kanae K. Miyake and Yuji Nakamoto, Kyoto University Graduate School of Medicine, Kyoto, Japan.)

(AUC) 0.94 (range, 0.93–0.98).[19] Interobserver agreement was substantial for lesion type (κ = 0.79) and nonmass distribution (κ = 0.63), and excellent for final assessment (κ = 0.84).[19] Across 36 observers from 15 sites interpreting PEM images, the mean sensitivity, specificity, and AUC for PEM were 96% (range, 75%–100%), 84% (range, 66%–97%), and 0.95 (range,

0.82–1.0), respectively.[20] Interobserver agreement in the description of PEM findings was moderate to substantial with a kappa of 0.57 for lesion type (focus, mass or nonmass uptake) and 0.63 for final assessment. Because fat necrosis, fibro-adenomas, and other benign and atypical lesions can show radiotracer accumulation, both modalities must be interpreted together with mammography and other current or prior breast imaging and appropriate patient history. The use of BI-RADS final assessment category 3, probably benign, is not recommended for either PEM or MBI because lesions designated as probably benign had a malignancy rate of 9.4% (3 of 32)[17] and 8% (4 of 50)[19] respectively, greater than the expected 2% rate for lesions assessed as BI-RADS 3 and recommended for surveillance with other breast imaging modalities.[21]

Quantitative Imaging

For breast gamma imaging, quantification of uptake is not routinely available.[19] However, PEM interpretation is usually based on both visual and semiquantitative uptake.[17] Regions of interest are drawn around the lesion and around an area of

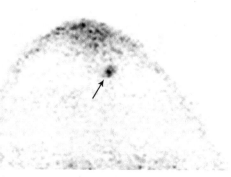

Fig. 3. MAMmography with Molecular Imaging (MAMMI)-PET image of a 60-year-old woman with a 7-mm invasive ductal carcinoma (*arrow*). (*Courtesy of* Dr R.A. Valdés Olmos, Amsterdam/Leiden, The Netherlands.)

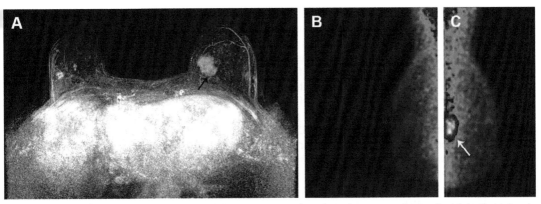

Fig. 4. A 51-year-old woman with known left breast invasive ductal carcinoma was imaged with both molecular breast imaging (MBI) and MR imaging. The maximum intensity projection of MR imaging showed enhancement at site of benign right breast stereotactic biopsy for calcifications (*A, arrow head*). On the left side, an irregular heterogeneously enhancing left breast mass in the 10 o'clock position (*A, arrow*) with predominantly washout kinetics measuring 3 cm in greatest dimension was observed, corresponding with the known cancer. MBI was performed on the GE dual head MBI system with the injection of 7.3 mCi of ^{99m}Tc-sestamibi. Mediolateral oblique views showed mild patchy background parenchymal uptake with no suspicious areas of radiotracer uptake on the right. (*B*) The known cancer was visualized on the left breast as an irregular mass measuring 2.7 cm (*C, arrow*). Because the mass is close to the chest wall, the full posterior aspect of the mass is not included in the images.

normal breast representative of mixed glandular and fatty background tissue to obtain a semiquantitative lesion-to-background (LTB) ratio, also known as a PEM uptake value (PUV). The PUV lacks attenuation and scatter correction and thereby differs from the standardized uptake value (SUV) used in whole-body PET or PET/CT, although maximum PUV (PUV_{max}) and maximum SUV (SUV_{max}) were highly correlated (r = 0.79) in a study by Wang and colleagues.[22] For dbPET detectors, the maximum uptake value for lesions on dbPET was found to be higher than whole body PET SUV for corresponding lesions.[23,24] Narayanan and colleagues[17] showed that both LTB and PUV_{max} were significantly greater (P<.001) across all malignant lesions compared with all benign lesions. In 2 separate series,[22,25] invasive ductal cancers had a higher PUV_{max} than invasive lobular cancers. PUV_{max} values for high-grade carcinomas were greater than those of lower grade cancers and were higher for triple negative breast cancers than for HER2/neu-receptor–positive or estrogen receptor–positive cancers. No specified threshold for malignancy exists, although a recent study comparing LTB and PUV_{max} recommended the use of PUV_{max} owing to its simplicity and reproducibility.[26] Another study[27] evaluated PUV_{max} and LTB using healthy tissue in the contralateral breast as background and found that both PUV_{max} and LTB were significantly higher for malignancies compared with benign lesions. In that study, Muller and colleagues[27] suggested a threshold value of PUV_{max} of greater than 1.9 and found that, among 151 pathologically proven

lesions, PEM had 100% sensitivity (26 of 26 lesions) and 96% specificity (120 of 125 lesions). This finding requires further validation; at present, it is recommended that any abnormal uptake be viewed as suspicious unless it is correlated with a known benign finding on mammography, other breast imaging, or clinical examination (eg, sebaceous cyst).

Radiation Dose

One of the biggest concerns with radionuclide breast imaging is the radiation exposure of the whole body associated with systemic radiotracer injection. All efforts must be made to reduce radiation dose while maintaining diagnostic image quality. The conventional dose of ^{99m}Tc-sestamibi for BSGI has been between 555 to 1110 MBq (15–30 mCi), with a 1110 MBq dose, resulting in an estimated whole body dose of 8.9 to 9.4 mSv. This is comparable to the effective estimated dose of 6.2 to 7.1 mSv for a 370-MBq (10 mCi) injection of FDG, and is more than 10 times greater than that from 2-view mammography (0.3–0.6 mSv).[28] The radiation dose to the breast itself from these injections is 2 mGy for ^{99m}Tc-sestamibi and 2.5 mGy for FDG, slightly less than the mean glandular dose (3.7 mGy) from digital mammography. The radiation dose and resulting estimated risks are higher to other organs such as the large intestine (40–55.5 mSv) for ^{99m}Tc-sestamibi and bladder (59 mSv) for FDG examinations.[28] For a 40-year-old woman, the estimated whole body radiation-induced cancer incidence from a single examination using conventional doses of FDG and ^{99m}Tc-sestamibi for breast imaging are 5 to 7 times higher than from mammography, whereas the radiation-induced mortality is estimated to be 20 times higher than mammography as many of the cancers potentially induced would be less treatable than breast cancer.[29] In fact, with a low dose of 300 MBq (8 mCi), the estimated benefit-to-risk ratio for dedicated breast gamma imaging for 40- to 49-year-old women (performed annually over the 10-year range) was 5 compared with 13 for mammography alone.[30] The benefit-to-risk ratio increased with screening age for both mammography and gamma imaging. To use MBI or PEM for breast cancer screening for women ages 40 to 49 with dense breasts with predicted risk-benefit ratios comparable with mammography, the administered radiotracer injections would have to be reduced to less than 150 MBq (4 mCi) for ^{99m}Tc-sestamibi and to 70 MBq (2 mCi) for FDG.

Optimization of collimators and widened energy windows coupled with improved noise reduction algorithms have allowed dose reduction of ^{99m}Tc-sestamibi to 150 to 300 MBq (4-8 mCi) in dual panel systems while maintaining equivalent image quality.[31,32] Adjustments to patient preparation by ensuring that the patient is fasting and kept warm and resting can improve ^{99m}Tc-sestamibi uptake by breast cancer and can allow further decrease in injected dose to approximately 150 MBq (4 mCi).[33] The effective whole body radiation dose from 150 MBq is 1.1 mSv, with an effective breast dose of 0.25 mGy, making it feasible to be considered for screening. Studies with low-dose BSGI (7–10 mCi) are also underway.[34] There have been similar efforts to halve the radiation dose for PEM with a corresponding increase in scan duration to maintain the total image counts[35]. Lower image counts increase noise and reduce lesion detection, but more efforts are needed to arrive at a reduced dose producing optimal images within a clinically feasible scan time.

CLINICAL EVIDENCE

The American College of Radiology recently released clinical practice parameters for the use of dedicated breast gamma imaging (both BSGI and MBI) using a gamma camera[36] and outlined potential clinical indications particularly in cases where breast MR imaging is not feasible. The clinical indications include the (a) extent of disease/preoperative staging in newly diagnosed breast cancer, (b) evaluation of response to neoadjuvant chemotherapy, (c) detection of local breast cancer recurrence, (d) evaluation for primary breast cancer in women with an unknown primary, (e) breast cancer screening for high-risk women for those who cannot undergo MR imaging, and (f) adjunct to conventional breast imaging for problem solving in indeterminate cases.

A metaanalysis of BSGI showed a pooled diagnostic sensitivity of 95% (95% confidence interval [CI]; 93%–96%) and specificity of 80% (95% CI 78%–82%) in detecting breast cancers.[37] The pooled sensitivity of BSGI in detecting subcentimeter cancers was 84% (95% CI, 80%–88%) and that of detecting ductal carcinoma in situ (DCIS) was 88% (95% CI, 81%–92%). The pooled rate of detecting additional multifocal, multicentric, or bilateral cancers in patients with known current malignancy was 6% (95% CI, 5–8). Hruska and colleagues[38] also evaluated the performance of dual-panel CZT MBI systems and showed higher sensitivity (90%; 115 of 128) compared with a single-panel CZT camera (80%; 102 of 128). In the same study, dual-panel cameras had 82% (50 of 61) sensitivity for subcentimeter lesions compared with 68% (41 of 61) for single-panel cameras. Conners and colleagues[39] retrospectively reviewed 390 invasive tumors (mean size, 1.5 cm) in 286 women injected with 8 to 33 mCi of ^{99m}Tc sestamibi who underwent MBI; invasive disease was correctly identified in 341 of 390 lesions (87.4%). MBI was better in depicting invasive ductal cancers (211 of 245; 86.1% sensitivity) than invasive lobular cancers (38 of 67 [56.7%]; P<.0001).

A recent metaanalysis of 8 prospective PEM studies in 873 women[40] with newly diagnosed breast cancer showed pooled sensitivity and specificity estimates of 85% (95% CI, 83%–88%) and 79% (95% CI, 74%–83%), respectively, and an AUC of 0.88. Cancers missed were usually small or outside the field of view.

Extent of Disease and Surgical Management

In a retrospective study[41] of 82 patients who underwent BSGI for newly diagnosed breast cancer, 18 (22%) were found to have additional suspicious findings based on BSGI including 7 of 82 (8.5%) with additional malignancy (Fig. 5). Kim[42] evaluated the adjunctive benefits of BSGI compared with MR imaging in 97 lesions in 66 patients with breast cancer with dense breasts and showed comparable sensitivity for BSGI and MR imaging at 88.8% (23 of 26; 95% CI, 69.8% to 97.6%) and 92.3% (24 of 26; 95% CI, 74.9% to 99.1%) respectively. Specificity was lower for MR imaging at 39.4% (28 of 71; 95% CI, 28.0% to 51.7%) versus 90.1% (64 of 71; 95% CI, 80.7% to 95.9%) for BSGI (P<.0001). Similar results were found in a metaanalysis comparing BSGI with MR imaging in detecting breast cancer.[43] Ten studies with 517 patients

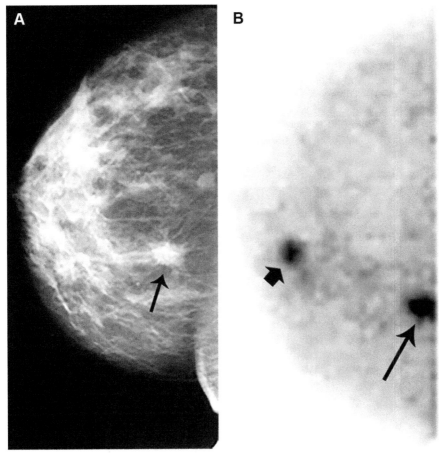

Fig. 5. Breast-specific gamma imaging showed 2 areas of focal uptake in an 82-year-old woman with dense breasts. The first (*B, arrow*) is consistent with the irregular mass noted on the mammogram (*A, arrow*). The second (*B, arrowhead*) is within an area of stable dense breast parenchyma. Pathology showed infiltrating ductal carcinoma at both sites. (*Courtesy of* Dilon, Newport News, VA; and West Valley Imaging, Las Vegas, NV.)

were included and the pooled sensitivities of BSGI and MR imaging were 84% (95% CI, 79%–88%) and 89% (95% CI, 84%–92%), respectively, and the pooled specificities of BSGI and MR imaging were 82% (95% CI, 74%–88%) and 39% (95% CI, 30%–49%), respectively. Edwards and colleagues[44] retrospectively analyzed 163 women who were candidates for breast-conserving surgery and later underwent mastectomy, 118 of whom had BSGI and 45 of whom had MR imaging. Management was changed to mastectomy in 11.9% (14 of 118) of those who had BSGI and 28.9% (13 of 45) of those who had MR imaging; in all cases, change to mastectomy was confirmed as appropriate. Percutaneous biopsy is recommended before conversion to mastectomy because some benign lesions will seem to be suspicious on BSGI. Both BSGI and MR Imaging underestimated disease extent: 15.4% of patients (16 of 104) who underwent breast-conserving therapy based on BSGI findings required a single reexcision owing

to positive surgical margins and another 15 of 104 (14.4%) required mastectomy. In the MR imaging group, 6 of 32 (18.8%) required a single reexcision, and 2 of 32 (6.3%) required mastectomy.

Berg and colleagues[45] compared the performance characteristics of PEM and MR imaging in a prospective multiinstitutional randomized study of 388 women with newly diagnosed cancer (median invasive tumor size of 1.5 cm [range, 0.4–6.9 cm]) and found that PEM and MR imaging had comparable sensitivity with PEM having greater specificity. PEM depicted 357 of 386 index malignancies (92.5%) with surgical pathology, whereas MR imaging depicted 344 of 386 (89.1%; $P = .079$). Of 388 ipsilateral breasts, 82 (21%) had additional disease (116 malignant foci) not known at study entry, with a median size of additional invasive disease of 0.7 cm; and PEM depicted cancer in 42 of 82 (51%) with MR imaging showing additional disease in 49 (60%; $P = .24$). PEM and MR imaging were complementary, with 61 of 82 breasts (74%)

with additional malignancy identified by the combination (*P*<.001 vs MR imaging alone). In another series[46] of 208 women with biopsy-proven primary breast cancer, PEM and MR imaging had equivalent sensitivity in depicting index lesions (155 of 167 [92.4%]) compared with whole body PET (117 of 173 [67.9%]; *P*<.001). There were 67 additional unsuspected ipsilateral lesions of which 40 were proven to be cancer. PEM had sensitivity of 85% (34 of 40) and specificity of 74% (20 of 27)

compared with MR imaging sensitivity of 98% (39 of 40) and specificity of 48% (13 of 27; *P* = .074, for sensitivity; *P* = .096 for specificity).

The detection sensitivity of PEM for identifying previously unsuspected DCIS was less than for invasive cancer at 41% (23 of 56)[45], similar to MRI at 22/56 in 1 multicenter series and 28 of 62 (45%) if another series by Schilling and colleagues[46] is included (**Fig. 6**). In 3 separate series,[47–49] patients with newly diagnosed DCIS were imaged with

A

B

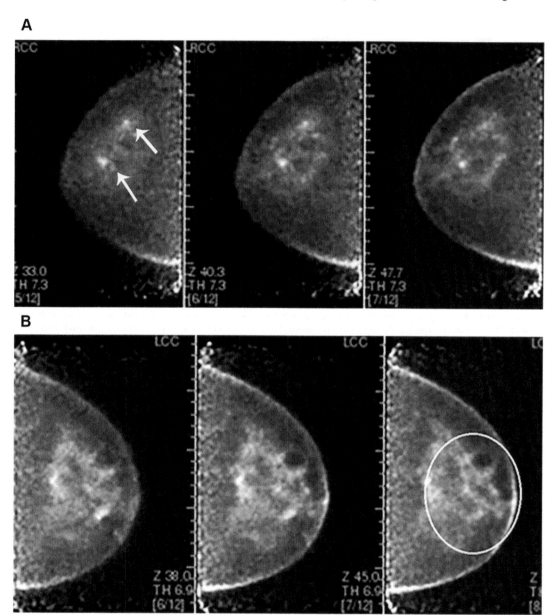

Fig. 6. A 66-year-old woman with bilateral cancer seen on positron emission mammography. The right breast has previously known high-grade ductal carcinoma in situ (DCIS). Pathology after bilateral mastectomy showed a 3.1-cm high-grade DCIS (*A, arrows*), estrogen receptor (ER)/progesterone receptor (PR) negative and node negative for the right breast and a 2.2-cm invasive ductal cancer-invasive lobular cancer with DCIS and lobular carcinoma in situ involving 3 quadrants in the left breast (*B, circle*). ER/PR positive, HER2 negative with 1 of 14 nodes positive.

BSGI and MR imaging; BSGI had a pooled sensitivity of 80% (60 of 75; range, 68.6%–91%) for DCIS, whereas the pooled MR imaging sensitivity was 91.8% (56 of 61; range, 88%–94%).

In the prospective multicenter study by Berg and colleagues[45] comparing PEM and MR imaging for surgical planning, MR imaging was better at predicting extent of disease than PEM. Eighty-nine of 388 participants (23%) required more extensive surgery: 61 of these women (69%) were identified with MR imaging, and 41 (46%) were identified with PEM (P = .003), 14 women (3.6%) had malignancies seen only on PEM. MR imaging led to more unnecessary mastectomies (n = 10) than PEM (n = 6), although this difference was not significant. In the same series, reported separately,[50] 15 women had contralateral cancer (median size, 10 mm; range, 1–22 mm) identified after study entry and only 3 (20%) were prospectively identified on PEM compared with 14 (93%) by MR imaging, although 11 of 15 (73%) were visible on PEM in a retrospective blinded independent review. One contralateral cancer was missed on both modalities.

In this same study,[50] the addition of conventional imaging (mammography and/or ultrasound imaging) improved the sensitivity of PEM imaging from 51% (42 of 82) to 65% (53 of 82; P<.001). Importantly there were 7 DCIS (7 of 82 [9%]) cases only on conventional imaging.

Similar results were observed in a retrospective study,[51] where 1024 patients who had ultrasound imaging and BSGI were retrospectively analyzed. Of the 117 cases with positive mammogram, there were 9 cases (9 of 117 [8%]) missed by BSGI, leading to the recommendation that BSGI cannot obviate biopsies recommended by mammogram. For both breast PET and breast gamma imaging, it is critical to review the images together with conventional imaging, biopsy history, and any other imaging (ie, by a radiologist trained in breast imaging). Benign findings such as fibroadenomas, fibrocystic change, fat necrosis, papillomas, atypical hyperplasia, and lobular carcinoma in situ can all show radiotracer accumulation and review of concomitant conventional imaging can improve the performance of the nuclear modalities by reducing false positives.

Monitoring Response to Treatment

Guo and colleagues[52] performed a metaanalysis to study the effectiveness of ^{99m}Tc-sestamibi in predicting the response to neoadjuvant chemotherapy in 503 patients with breast cancer. The pooled sensitivity across 14 studies was 86% (95% CI, 78%–92%), specificity was 69% (95% CI, 64%–74%), and the AUC was 0.86. Most studies used whole body single photon emission CT; only 3 used dedicated breast-specific systems. In 1 study,[53] 19 patients completed MBI imaging and neoadjuvant chemotherapy before surgery and the LTB ratio was compared with the extent of residual disease at surgery using the residual cancer burden. The decrease in the LTB ratios in MBI images performed 3 to 5 weeks after starting neoadjuvant chemotherapy was an accurate predictor of residual disease at the completion of chemotherapy. Using a threshold of a 50% decrease in the LTB ratio as a predictor for response, the sensitivity, specificity, and AUC in predicting residual disease was 92.3% (95% CI, 0.74%–0.99%), 83.3% (95% CI, 0.44%–0.99%), and 0.92, respectively. In another study,[54] 18 invasive breast cancer lesions in 17 patients undergoing neoadjuvant chemotherapy were imaged using MBI before the final surgery with a strong correlation (r = 0.681; P = .002) between measured size on MBI and residual tumor size at histopathology, although there was a decrease in LTB that was not found to be predictive of residual disease. Menes and colleagues[55] correlated the accuracy of MBI in detecting residual disease after neoadjuvant chemotherapy with molecular subtypes and found a stronger correlation with triple negative and HER2/neu positive subtypes (r = 0.92 and 0.62, respectively). The sensitivity and specificity for all 51 women (of whom 16 had pathologic complete response) was 83% (29 of 35; 95% CI, 66%–93%) and 69% (11 of 16; 95% CI, 42%–88%) compared with 88% (15 of 17; 95% CI, 62%–98%) and 75% (9 of 12; 95% CI, 43%–93%) for the subset with triple negative or HER2/neu–positive tumors. The largest of these studies was done by Lee and colleagues,[56] who compared the performance of BSGI and MR imaging in predicting residual tumor after neoadjuvant chemotherapy in a series of 122 women, of whom 104 had residual tumor at pathology. BSGI identified 77 of 104 (74.0%) with residual tumor, not statistically different from the 85 of 104 (81.7%) shown on MR imaging (P = .134). Interestingly, in this group, both MR imaging and BSGI underestimated the residual tumor size in HER2-positive tumors.

There has been only 1 study[57] to date evaluating the performance of PEM in predicting residual tumor after neoadjuvant chemotherapy. In a study comparing the performance of PEM to whole body PET in 20 patients imaged before, during, and after neoadjuvant chemotherapy, there was no difference in performance in predicting complete response between whole body PET and PEM at the completion of neoadjuvant chemotherapy. At the interim point, the SUV_{max} of whole body PET (AUC of 0.761) was superior to the PUV_{max} (AUC of 0.648) for predicting nonpathologic complete response. After neoadjuvant chemotherapy, the PUV_{max} (AUC of 0.796) was superior to the SUV_{max} of whole body PET (AUC of 0.671) in predicting residual disease. After all treatment, the PUV_{max} and LTB ratio was significantly lower in the pathologic complete response group than in the nonpathologic complete response group PUV_{max} (1.0 ± 0.2 vs 2.5 ± 2.7; $P = .0351$).

Breast Density

The BI-RADS system identifies 4 categories of breast density based on the relative amounts of fibroglandular tissue and fat present in the breast: (A) predominantly fatty, (B) scattered fibroglandular density, (C) heterogeneously dense, and (D) extremely dense. Dense breast tissue has been found to be an independent predictor of breast cancer risk.[58,59] As more and more states require that a patient's mammography results letter include information about breast density,[60] there has been an increased awareness of the masking effect of dense tissue on mammography, potentially delaying cancer diagnosis and resulting in worse outcomes. Supplemental screening using ultrasound examination, MR imaging, or other methods is being considered in women with dense breasts. Background parenchymal enhancement on MR imaging and background uptake of radiotracers may correlate with subsequent cancer risk[61,62] and may help to identify women who should undergo regular supplemental screening. Increased background uptake is correlated with an increase in breast density for BSGI and MBI,[63] although some extremely dense breasts seem to be photopenic; cancer detection is not impaired.[64]

Increased FDG uptake is seen with greater breast density and may impair cancer detection on PEM. Koo and colleagues[65] reported data from a study comparing 52 women who had both PEM and MR imaging. Increased FDG uptake correlated with increased breast density with mean $\pm$ standard deviation background ^{18}F-FDG uptake on PEM of 0.25 ± 0.13 in almost entirely fatty breasts (n = 5), 0.46 ± 0.21 in breasts with scattered fibroglandular density (n = 12), 0.62 ± 0.20 in heterogeneously dense breasts (n = 19), and 0.76 ± 0.23 in extremely dense breasts (n = 16). In the multicenter study of Berg and colleagues,[45] MR imaging was more sensitive than PEM in heterogeneously dense or extremely dense breasts: showing 34 of 60 (57%) of cancers versus 22 of 60 (37%; $P = .031$). Hormonal or menopausal status did not affect the performance of PEM.

Positioning Issues

Visualizing posterior lesions remains a challenge for dedicated breast imaging. In the multicenter series by Berg and colleagues,[45] in 6 of the 388 breasts (1.5%), the index malignancy was outside the field of view. Shimadzu tested both the O-PEM and C-PEM configurations and found that both scanners had similar sensitivity: 82% (62 of 76) and 83% (63 of 76), respectively.[66] However, 9 lesions with the O-scanner and 6 lesions with the C-scanner were outside the field of view, thereby reducing the sensitivity of dbPET. In a MAMmography with Molecular Imaging-PET study by Teixeira and colleagues,[67] 23 of 234 lesions (9.8%) were not visualized because they were too close to the pectoral muscle and out of the field of view. Similarly for an MBI study by Connors,[39,68] 8 of 360 tumor foci (2.2%) were thought to have been missed because they were outside the field of view.

Screening

Owing to proven decrease in mortality from breast cancer,[69] mammography remains the primary method for breast cancer screening. The Mayo group has studied MBI for supplemental screening in women with dense breasts, using a reduced dose of 300 MBq (8 mCi) ^{99m}Tc-sestamibi (Fig. 7).[70] In 1651 asymptomatic women with dense breasts who underwent adjunct MBI along with mammographic screening, 14 additional cancers were detected by MBI; the overall cancer detection increased from 3.2 to 12.0 per 1000 ($P<.001$; supplemental yield of MBI of 8.8 per 1000 [95% CI, 4.3–13.3]). In another supplemental screening study of 1696 women,[71] 13 mammographically occult malignancies were detected by MBI for a supplemental cancer detection rate of 7.7 per 1000 (13 of 1696; Table 3).

Yamamoto and colleagues[72] injected 265 women (165 of whom were asymptomatic and 100 with breast symptoms) with a reduced FDG dose of 4.6 mCi and imaged them using PEM. Six additional cancers were found on PEM alone with an average patient recall rate, positive predictive value, and cancer detection rate for PEM 8.3, 27.3, and 2.3% respectively. Of the 6 cancers found on PEM, 2 were found in patients with no breast symptoms, 2 were found in breasts that were previously followed for benign findings, and 2 had suspicious lesions associated with breast cancer. However, even with reduced radiation dose, it is unlikely that PEM would be used for routine screening. The requirement for fasting and study time of around 100 minutes per patient (one-hour FDG uptake time plus scan time) is not

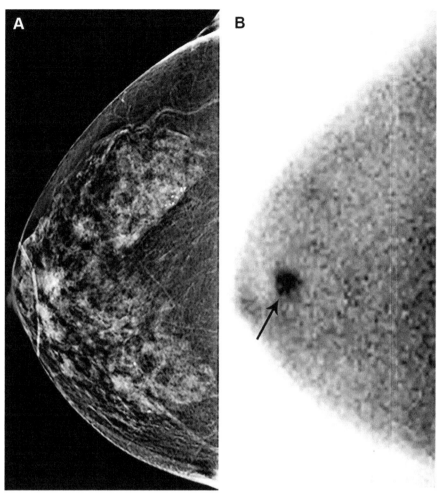

Fig. 7. An 81-year-old high-risk (based on lifetime risk assessment models) female with dense breasts had a negative mammogram (*A*) but underwent additional screening with molecular breast imaging (*B*) (MBI; 8 mCi injected dose). MBI showed intense uptake in an irregular mass (*arrow*). Biopsy showed invasive ductal carcinoma. (*Courtesy of* Robin Shermis, MD, ProMedica Toledo Hospital, Toledo, OH.)

conducive to patient throughput in a screening setting. Further, there are shielding requirements for a PEM scanner owing to the high-energy photons from FDG that make it challenging to install in most breast centers.

FUTURE DEVELOPMENTS
Instrumentation

At present, breast PET is limited to locoregional staging and monitoring response to treatment. However, there is the potential for improvement in the breast PET performance with new scanners that have optimized type of detectors, detector configurations, photomultipliers, and electronics. A dual-head PEM scanner with both detector modules rotating around a prone breast is being developed by a Portuguese Crystal Clear collaboration based at CERN.[73] In addition, there are several dbPET scanners that are still in the development phase at various academic research laboratories, including PEM/PET at West Virginia University,[74] and portable dual panel PET at Stanford University.[75] The development of integrated multimodality imaging systems combining functional imaging and anatomic imaging modalities is gaining momentum in research laboratories around the world. Several researchers are working on hybrid systems such as the dedicated simultaneous PET-MR imaging system developed at the Brookhaven National Laboratory,[76] where a PET ring detector has been integrated with a 1.5-T dedicated breast MR imaging scanner. Other multimodality systems under development include Clear PEM-Sonic, developed by CERN, that has a ring-type breast PET scanner integrated with

Table 3
BSGI/MBI screening studies

	Study Population	n	Device	Dose	No. of Cancers Detected	Cancer Detection Rate[a]	Recall Rate[b]	PPV$_1$[c]	PPV$_3$[d]	Scan Time
Rhodes et al,[70] 2010	Women with heterogeneously or extremely dense breasts + 1 additional risk factor	936	MBI	740 MBq (20 mCi)	11	7.5/1000	8% (71/936)	2% (9/73)	8% (10/36)	10 min per view
Hruska et al,[31] 2012	Women undergoing a nuclear cardiology stress	306	MBI	666–2035 MBq (18–55 mCi)	4	13.1/1000	7% (22/306)	18% (4/22)	44% (4/9)	3–5 min per view
Rhodes et al,[70] 2015	Asymptomatic women with mammographically dense breasts	1585	MBI	300 MBq (8 mCi)	21	8.8/1000	6.6% (119/1585)	14% (17/119)	33% (17/51)	10 min per view (total 40 min)
Brem et al,[34] 2016	Women with no mammographic symptoms	653	BSGI	High Dose: 781 MBq (21.1 mCi)	12	18.4/1000	25.5% (161/653)	7.4% (12/161)	15.4% (12/78)	6–10 min per view, total 40 min
Brem et al,[34] 2016[e]	Women with no mammographic symptoms	196	BSGI	Low dose: 296 MBq (8.0 mCi)	2	10.2/1000	26% (51/196)	3.9% (2/51)	10.5% (2/9)	6–10 min per view, total 40 min
Shermis et al,[71] 2017	Women with negative mammography study	1696	MBI	300 MBq (8 mCi)	13	7.7/1000	8.4 (143/1696)	9.1% (13/143)	19% (12/62)	7–10 min per view

Abbreviations: BSGI, breast-specific gamma imaging; MBI, molecular breast imaging.
[a] Detection rate: cancer detection rate of MBI or BSGI in number of women diagnosed with cancer per 1000 women screened.
[b] Recall rate: number of positive examinations per total number of patients.
[c] PPV$_1$ = number of malignancies per all abnormal BSGI examinations.
[d] PPV$_3$ = number of malignancies per all biopsies performed.
[e] Both low-dose and high-dose BSGI data are reported in the same paper. Cancer detection rate was not statistically different between the 2 groups χ^2 = 0.62, (95% confidence interval, 0.12–2.48; P = .44).
Adapted from Hruska CB. Molecular breast imaging for screening in dense breasts: state of the art and future directions. AJR Am J Roentgenol 2017;208(2):275–83.

an ultrasound system developed by Supersonic Imagine[77] (Aix-en-Provence, France). The group at University of California Davis is developing a dbPET/CT scanner consisting of a dual-head PET camera and cone-beam CT integrated into a single gantry and have performed early clinical feasibility studies.[78] A group at the University of Washington, Seattle,[79] is developing a PET/X scanner integrating dbPET with x-ray mammography to use the metabolic information from the hybrid image to assess and select effective targeted breast cancer therapies for each patient.

Dedicated multimodality gamma systems that combine CT imaging with gamma images are in development at Duke University[80] and the University of Naples,[81] and a dedicated gamma tomosynthesis system is being developed at the University of Virginia.[82] Initial evaluation of dual modality tomosynthesis in 21 lesions in 17 women injected with ^{99m}Tc-sestamibi showed a sensitivity, specificity, positive predictive value, negative predictive value, and accuracy of 86%, 100%, 100%, 93%, and 95%, respectively.[83] An integrated ultrasound, single head CZT scanner system is being developed to enable real-time registration of ultrasound imaging to MBI for the diagnostic evaluation of breast lesions detected on MBI.[84]

Radiotracers

Although FDG and ^{99m}Tc-sestamibi remain the primary radiotracers used in dedicated breast molecular imaging, new radiotracers[85] are likely to play a greater role in imaging and the clinical evaluation of breast tumors, although none are currently approved for clinical use in the United States. 3-Deoxy-3-18F-fluorothymidine (FLT) is a cell proliferative agent believed to be more specific for breast tumors than FDG PET. In several whole body PET/CT studies to monitor response to treatment,[86] FLT seemed to be a good predictor of early response to chemotherapy despite concerns regarding its surrogate proliferative status. McKinley and associates[87] reported that, because FLT PET reflects the tumor proliferative indices indirectly as a function for the thymidine salvage pathway, it creates challenges in estimating the extent of proliferation and using the magnitude of FLT uptake to quantify proliferative index.

Clinical studies evaluating ^{18}F-fluoroestradiol, an estrogen receptor expression biomarker, show benefit in patients with metastatic breast cancer and in treatment monitoring in patients undergoing endocrine therapy.[88] Building on the clinical success of HER2-targeted therapy using monoclonal antibody to the HER2 receptor (trastuzumab), there are several imaging agents being developed for both PET (eg, ^{68}Ga, [124]I, and [89]Zr) and single photon emission CT (indium-111, iodine-131, technetium-99m) imaging[89] using radiolabeled trastuzumab. Feasibility studies with [89]Zr-trastuzumab for HER2 PET imaging in 14 patients with Her2-positive metastatic breast cancer showed the ability to visualize and quantify uptake in HER-2–positive lesions.[90] Another study using [89]Zr-trastuzumab PET/CT to image patients with metastatic breast cancer with Her2-negative primary cancer showed that it could detect unsuspected HER2-positive metastases in these patients.[91] Distant metastasis may lose or gain receptor expression, leading to incorrect choice of treatment based on primary tumor characteristics alone.[92] The ability to visualize or detect receptor status by 89Zr-trastuzumab or ^{18}F-fluoroestradiol supports the idea that functional imaging of distant receptors can help to determine the appropriate treatment option for metastatic cancer.

Other PET agents that are being developed include ^{18}F-misonidazole (a hypoxia imaging agent),[93] ^{18}F-fluciclovine[94] (amino acid transport agent), and ^{18}F-FENP[95] (a progesterone receptor targeted agent). Single photon emission CT and PET radiotracers targeted to breast cancer angiogenesis makers such as vascular endothelial growth factor and integrins are also being evaluated. One such angiogenesis marker, ^{99m}Tc-NC100692[96] (Maraciclatide; GE Healthcare) was compared with ^{99m}Tc-sestamibi in 30 patients with suspected breast cancer and showed comparable diagnostic performance for both radiopharmaceuticals.[96] The AUC from receiver operating characteristic analysis was 0.83 for ^{99m}Tc-sestamibi and 0.87 for ^{99m}Tc maraciclatide ($P = .64$). Yet another technetium-based gamma imaging agent being studied is ^{99m}Tc-tetrofosmin MBI, a cardiac imaging agent that has a similar method of localization as sestamibi but with improved liver clearance. In 1 series,[97] 321 patients with suspicious breast lesions were imaged with MBI after being injected with ^{99m}Tc-tetrofosmin with sensitivity of 96.4% (267 of 277) and specificity of 86.4% (38 of 44).

SUMMARY

Nuclear medicine imaging modalities have been used for staging and additional diagnostic evaluation, and show particular promise in predicting treatment response and monitoring. Studies with PEM and BSGI/MBI have shown sensitivity comparable with breast MR imaging with better specificity. The development of a standardized interpretation lexicon, breast biopsy, and efforts to reduce radiation dose are critical to the further evolution of these new modalities. The American College of Radiology practice guideline suggests that MBI could be used for breast screening in women identified as high risk and for those with dense breasts who cannot undergo MR imaging, but the overall radiation dose must be reduced to make this a clinically reasonable alternative. Although Naviscan's PEM scanner, Dilon's BSGI systm and GE's MBI system have developed biopsy guidance, it is important for all nuclear breast imaging modalities to have similar capabilities. New breast imaging–specific radiotracers are expected to help in the molecular characterization of breast tumors to facilitate appropriate personalized treatment.

REFERENCES

1. Khalkhali I, Iraniha S, Diggles LE, et al. Scintimammography: the new role of technetium-99m Sestamibi imaging for the diagnosis of breast carcinoma. Q J Nucl Med 1997;41(3):231–8.
2. Avril N, Rose CA, Schelling M, et al. Breast imaging with positron emission tomography and fluorine-18 fluorodeoxyglucose: use and limitations. J Clin Oncol 2000;18(20):3495–502.
3. Hruska CB, O'Connor MK. Nuclear imaging of the breast: translating achievements in instrumentation into clinical use. Med Phys 2013;40(5):050901.
4. Taillefer R. The role of 99mTc-sestamibi and other conventional radiopharmaceuticals in breast cancer diagnosis. Semin Nucl Med 1999;29(1):16–40.
5. Hruska CB, Boughey JC, Phillips SW, et al. Scientific Impact Recognition Award: molecular breast imaging: a review of the Mayo Clinic experience. Am J Surg 2008;196(4):470–6.
6. Long Z, Hruska C, O'Connor M. Low dose breast imaging-comparative performance of MBI and BSGI systems. J Nucl Med 2015;56(supplement 3):1863.
7. Swanson T, Tran T, Ellingson L, et al. High-quality molecular breast imaging: a guide for technologists from the Mayo Clinic experience. J Nucl Med 2017; 58(supplement 1):1157.
8. Freifelder R, Karp JS. Dedicated PET scanners for breast imaging. Phys Med Biol 1997;42(12): 2463–80.
9. Macdonald L, Edwards J, Lewellen T, et al. Clinical imaging characteristics of the positron emission mammography PEM Flex Solo II. IEEE Nucl Sci Symp Conf Rec (1997) 2008;11(2008): 4494–501.
10. Luo WAE, Matthews CG. Performance evaluation of a PEM scanner using the NEMA NU 4–2008 small animal PET standards. IEEE Trans Nucl Sci 2010; 57:9.
11. Kalinyak JE, Schilling K, Berg WA, et al. PET-guided breast biopsy. Breast J 2011;17(2):143–51.
12. Eo JS, Chun IK, Paeng JC, et al. Imaging sensitivi of dedicated positron emission mammography relation to tumor size. Breast 2012;21(1):66–71.
13. Koolen BB, Aukema TS, Gonzalez Martinez AJ, et al First clinical experience with a dedicated PET fo hanging breast molecular imaging. Q J Nucl Me Mol Imaging 2013;57(1):92–100.
14. Collarino A, Fuoco V, Pereira Arias-Bouda LN Sánchez AM, et al. Novel frontiers of dedicated mc lecular imaging in breast cancer diagnosis. Trans Cancer Res 2017;2017.
15. Miyake KK, Nakamoto Y, Togashi K. Current status (dedicated breast PET imaging. Curr Radiol Rei 2016;4(4):16.
16. Conners AL, Maxwell RW, Tortorelli CL, et al. Gamm camera breast imaging lexicon. AJR Am J Roen genol 2012;199(6):W767–74.
17. Narayanan D, Madsen KS, Kalinyak JE, et al. Inte pretation of positron emission mammography feature analysis and rates of malignancy. AJR Ar J Roentgenol 2011;196(4):956–70.
18. Morris EA, Comstock CE, Lee C, et al. ACR BI-RADS Magnetic Resonance Imaging. ACR BI-RADS Atlas Breast Imaging Reporting and Data System. Restor VA: American College of Radiology; 2013.
19. Conners AL, Hruska CB, Tortorelli CL, et al. Lexico for standardized interpretation of gamma camera molecular breast imaging: observer agreemen and diagnostic accuracy. Eur J Nucl Med Mol Imag ing 2012;39(6):971–82.
20. Narayanan D, Madsen KS, Kalinyak JE, et al. Inte pretation of positron emission mammography and MRI by experienced breast imaging radiologists performance and observer reproducibility. AJR An J Roentgenol 2011;196(4):971–81.
21. Sickles EA, D'Orsi CJ, Bassett LW, et al. ACR BI RADS Mammography. ACR BI-RADS Atlas, Breas Imaging Reporting and Data System. Reston, VA American College of Radiology; 2013.
22. Wang CL, MacDonald LR, Rogers JV, et al. Positror emission mammography: correlation of estrogen re ceptor, progesterone receptor, and human epiderma growth factor receptor 2 status and 18F-FDG. AJF Am J Roentgenol 2011;197(2):W247–55.
23. Nakamoto R, Nakamoto Y, Ishimori T, et al. Diag nostic performance of a novel dedicated breas PET scanner with C-shaped ring detectors. Nuc Med Commun 2017;38(5):388–95.
24. Nishimatsu K, Nakamoto Y, Miyake KK, et al. Highe breast cancer conspicuity on dbPET compared to WB PET/CT. Eur J Radiol 2017;90(Supplement C):138–45.
25. Kalinyak JE, Berg WA, Schilling K, et al. Breast can cer detection using high-resolution breast PET compared to whole-body PET or PET/CT. Eur J Nucl Med Mol Imaging 2014;41(2):260–75.
26. Yamamoto Y, Tasaki Y, Kuwada Y, et al. Positron emission mammography (PEM): reviewing standardizec

semiquantitative method. Ann Nucl Med 2013;27(9): 795–801.

27. Muller FH, Farahati J, Muller AG, et al. Positron emission mammography in the diagnosis of breast cancer. Is maximum PEM uptake value a valuable threshold for malignant breast cancer detection? Nuklearmedizin 2016;55(1):15–20.

28. Hendrick RE. Radiation doses and cancer risks from breast imaging studies. Radiology 2010; 257(1):246–53.

29. O'Connor MK, Li H, Rhodes DJ, et al. Comparison of radiation exposure and associated radiation-induced cancer risks from mammography and molecular imaging of the breast. Med Phys 2010; 37(12):6187–98.

30. Hendrick RE, Tredennick T. Benefit to radiation risk of breast-specific gamma imaging compared with mammography in screening asymptomatic women with dense breasts. Radiology 2016;281(2):583–8.

31. Hruska CB, Weinmann AL, O'Connor MK. Proof of concept for low-dose molecular breast imaging with a dual-head CZT gamma camera. Part I. Evaluation in phantoms. Med Phys 2012;39(6): 3466–75.

32. Long Z, Conners AL, Hunt KN, et al. Performance characteristics of dedicated molecular breast imaging systems at low doses. Med Phys 2016;43(6): 3062–70.

33. O'Connor MK, Hruska CB, Tran TD, et al. Factors influencing the uptake of 99mTc-sestamibi in breast tissue on molecular breast imaging. J Nucl Med Technol 2015;43(1):13–20.

34. Kuhn KJ, Rapelyea JA, Torrente J, et al. Comparative diagnostic utility of low-dose breast-specific gamma imaging to current clinical standard. Breast J 2016;22(2):180–8.

35. MacDonald LR, Hippe DS, Bender LC, et al. Positron emission mammography image interpretation for reduced image count levels. J Nucl Med 2016; 57(3):348–54.

36. American College of Radiology (ACR). ACR Practice parameter for the performance of molecular breast imaging (MBI) using a dedicated gamma camera. Available at: https://www.acr.org/~/media/ACR/Documents/PGTS/guidelines/MBI.pdf. Accessed October 26, 2017.

37. Sun Y, Wei W, Yang HW, et al. Clinical usefulness of breast-specific gamma imaging as an adjunct modality to mammography for diagnosis of breast cancer: a systemic review and meta-analysis. Eur J Nucl Med Mol Imaging 2013;40(3):450–63.

38. Hruska CB, Phillips SW, Whaley DH, et al. Molecular breast imaging: use of a dual-head dedicated gamma camera to detect small breast tumors. AJR Am J Roentgenol 2008;191(6):1805–15.

39. Conners AL, Jones KN, Hruska CB, et al. Direct-conversion molecular breast imaging of invasive breast cancer: imaging features, extent of invasive disease, and comparison between invasive ductal and lobular histology. AJR Am J Roentgenol 2015; 205(3):W374–81.

40. Caldarella C, Treglia G, Giordano A. Diagnostic performance of dedicated positron emission mammography using fluorine-18-fluorodeoxyglucose in women with suspicious breast lesions: a meta-analysis. Clin Breast Cancer 2014;14(4):241–8.

41. Killelea BK, Gillego A, Kirstein LJ, et al. George Peters Award: how does breast-specific gamma imaging affect the management of patients with newly diagnosed breast cancer? Am J Surg 2009;198(4):470–4.

42. Kim BS. Usefulness of breast-specific gamma imaging as an adjunct modality in breast cancer patients with dense breast: a comparative study with MRI. Ann Nucl Med 2012;26(2):131–7.

43. Zhang A, Li P, Liu Q, et al. Breast-specific gamma camera imaging with 99mTc-MIBI has better diagnostic performance than magnetic resonance imaging in breast cancer patients: a meta-analysis. Hell J Nucl Med 2017;20(1):26–35.

44. Edwards C, Williams S, McSwain AP, et al. Breast-specific gamma imaging influences surgical management in patients with breast cancer. Breast J 2013;19(5):512–9.

45. Berg WA, Madsen KS, Schilling K, et al. Breast cancer: comparative effectiveness of positron emission mammography and MR imaging in presurgical planning for the ipsilateral breast. Radiology 2011; 258(1):59–72.

46. Schilling K, Narayanan D, Kalinyak JE, et al. Positron emission mammography in breast cancer presurgical planning: comparisons with magnetic resonance imaging. Eur J Nucl Med Mol Imaging 2011;38(1):23–36.

47. Keto JL, Kirstein L, Sanchez DP, et al. MRI versus breast-specific gamma imaging (BSGI) in newly diagnosed ductal cell carcinoma-in-situ: a prospective head-to-head trial. Ann Surg Oncol 2012;19(1): 249–52.

48. Kim JS, Lee SM, Cha ES. The diagnostic sensitivity of dynamic contrast-enhanced magnetic resonance imaging and breast-specific gamma imaging in women with calcified and non-calcified DCIS. Acta Radiol 2014;55(6):668–75.

49. Brem RF, Fishman M, Rapelyea JA. Detection of ductal carcinoma in situ with mammography, breast specific gamma imaging, and magnetic resonance imaging: a comparative study. Acad Radiol 2007; 14(8):945–50.

50. Berg WA, Madsen KS, Schilling K, et al. Comparative effectiveness of positron emission mammography and MRI in the contralateral breast of women with newly diagnosed breast cancer. AJR Am J Roentgenol 2012;198(1):219–32.

51. Weigert JM, Bertrand ML, Lanzkowsky L, et al. Results of a multicenter patient registry to determine

the clinical impact of breast-specific gamma imaging, a molecular breast imaging technique. AJR Am J Roentgenol 2012;198(1):W69–75.

52. Guo C, Zhang C, Liu J, et al. Is Tc-99m sestamibi scintimammography useful in the prediction of neoadjuvant chemotherapy responses in breast cancer? A systematic review and meta-analysis. Nucl Med Commun 2016;37(7):675–88.

53. Mitchell D, Hruska CB, Boughey JC, et al. 99mTc-sestamibi using a direct conversion molecular breast imaging system to assess tumor response to neoadjuvant chemotherapy in women with locally advanced breast cancer. Clin Nucl Med 2013; 38(12):949–56.

54. Wahner-Roedler DL, Boughey JC, Hruska CB, et al. The use of molecular breast imaging to assess response in women undergoing neoadjuvant therapy for breast cancer: a pilot study. Clin Nucl Med 2012;37(4):344–50.

55. Menes TS, Golan O, Vainer G, et al. Assessment of residual disease with molecular breast imaging in patients undergoing neoadjuvant therapy: association with molecular subtypes. Clin Breast Cancer 2016;16(5):389–95.

56. Lee HS, Ko BS, Ahn SH, et al. Diagnostic performance of breast-specific gamma imaging in the assessment of residual tumor after neoadjuvant chemotherapy in breast cancer patients. Breast Cancer Res Treat 2014;145(1):91–100.

57. Noritake M, Narui K, Kaneta T, et al. Evaluation of the response to breast cancer neoadjuvant chemotherapy using 18F-FDG positron emission mammography compared with whole-body 18F-FDG PET: a prospective observational study. Clin Nucl Med 2017;42(3):169–75.

58. Harvey JA, Bovbjerg VE. Quantitative assessment of mammographic breast density: relationship with breast cancer risk. Radiology 2004;230(1):29–41.

59. McCormack VA, dos Santos Silva I. Breast density and parenchymal patterns as markers of breast cancer risk: a meta-analysis. Cancer Epidemiol Biomarkers Prev 2006;15(6):1159–69.

60. Dense Breast Info. Legislation and regulations - what is required? Available at: http://densebreast-info.org/legislation.aspx. [Website]. Accessed March 4, 2018

61. Hruska CB, Scott CG, Conners AL, et al. Background parenchymal uptake on molecular breast imaging as a breast cancer risk factor: a case-control study. Breast Cancer Res 2016;18(1):42.

62. King V, Brooks JD, Bernstein JL, et al. Background parenchymal enhancement at breast MR imaging and breast cancer risk. Radiology 2011;260(1):50–60.

63. Hruska CB, Rhodes DJ, Conners AL, et al. Background parenchymal uptake during molecular breast imaging and associated clinical factors. AJR Am J Roentgenol 2015;204(3):W363–70.

64. Rechtman LR, Lenihan MJ, Lieberman JH, et al. Breast-specific gamma imaging for the detection of breast cancer in dense versus nondense breasts. AJR Am J Roentgenol 2014;202(2):293–8.

65. Koo HR, Moon WK, Chun IK, et al. Background (1)(8)F-FDG uptake in positron emission mammography (PEM): correlation with mammographic density and background parenchymal enhancement in breast MRI. Eur J Radiol 2013;82(10):1738–42.

66. Iima M, Nakamoto Y, Kanao S, et al. Clinical performance of 2 dedicated PET scanners for breast imaging: initial evaluation. J Nucl Med 2012; 53(10):1534–42.

67. Teixeira SC, Rebolleda JF, Koolen BB, et al. Evaluation of a hanging-breast PET system for primary tumor visualization in patients with stage I-III breast cancer: comparison with standard PET/CT. AJR Am J Roentgenol 2016;206(6):1307–14.

68. Berg WA. Nuclear breast imaging: clinical results and future directions. J Nucl Med 2016;57(Suppl 1):46S–52S.

69. Siu AL, U.S. Preventive Services Task Force. Screening for breast cancer: U.S. Preventive services task force recommendation statement. Ann Intern Med 2016;164(4):279–96.

70. Rhodes DJ, Hruska CB, Conners AL, et al. Journal club: molecular breast imaging at reduced radiation dose for supplemental screening in mammographically dense breasts. AJR Am J Roentgenol 2015; 204(2):241–51.

71. Shermis RB, Wilson KD, Doyle MT, et al. Supplemental breast cancer screening with molecular breast imaging for women with dense breast tissue. AJR Am J Roentgenol 2016;207(2):450–7.

72. Yamamoto Y, Tasaki Y, Kuwada Y, et al. A preliminary report of breast cancer screening by positron emission mammography. Ann Nucl Med 2016;30(2):130–7.

73. Abreu MC, Almeida P, Balau F, et al. Clear-PEM: a dedicated PET camera for improved breast cancer detection. Radiat Prot Dosimetry 2005;116(1–4 Pt 2):208–10.

74. Raylman RR, Abraham J, Hazard H, et al. Initial clinical test of a breast-PET scanner. J Med Imaging Radiat Oncol 2011;55(1):58–64.

75. Peng H, Levin CS. Design study of a high-resolution breast-dedicated PET system built from cadmium zinc telluride detectors. Phys Med Biol 2010;55(9): 2761–88.

76. Ravindranath B, Junnarkar S, Purschke M, et al. Results from a simultaneous PET-MRI breast scanner. J Nucl Med 2011;52(supplement 1):432.

77. Cucciati G, Auffray E, Bugalho R, et al. Development of ClearPEM-Sonic, a multimodal mammography system for PET and Ultrasound. J Instrumentation 2014;9(CD3008).

78. Bowen SL, Wu Y, Chaudhari AJ, et al. Initial characterization of a dedicated breast PET/CT scanner

during human imaging. J Nucl Med 2009;50(9):
1401–8.

79. MacDonald LR, Hunter WC, Kinahan PE, et al. Effects
of detector thickness on geometric sensitivity and
event positioning errors in the rectangular PET/X
scanner. IEEE Trans Nucl Sci 2013;60(5):3242–52.

80. Tornai MP, Shah JP, Mann SD, et al. Development of
Fully-3D CT in a Hybrid SPECT-CT Breast Imaging
System. In: Tingberg A, Lång K, Timberg P, editors.
Breast Imaging. IWDM 2016. Lecture Notes in Com-
puter Science. Switzerland: Springer, Cham; 2016.
p. 567–75.

81. Mettivier G, Bliznakova K, Sechopoulos I, et al. Evaluation of the BreastSimulator software platform for
breast tomography. Phys Med Biol 2017;62(16):
6446–66.

82. Williams MB, Judy PG, Gunn S, et al. Dual-modality breast tomosynthesis. Radiology 2010;255(1):
191–8.

83. Gong Z, Williams MB. Comparison of breast specific
gamma imaging and molecular breast tomosynthesis in breast cancer detection: evaluation in phantoms. Med Phys 2015;42(7):4250–9.

84. O'Connor MK, Morrow MM, Tran T, et al. Technical
note: development of a combined molecular
breast imaging/ultrasound system for diagnostic
evaluation of MBI-detected lesions. Med Phys
2017;44(2):451–9.

85. Meng Q, Li Z. Molecular imaging probes for diagnosis and therapy evaluation of breast cancer. Int
J Biomed Imaging 2013;2013:14.

86. Bollineni VR, Kramer GM, Jansma EP, et al.
A systematic review on [(18)F]FLT-PET uptake as a
measure of treatment response in cancer patients.
Eur J Cancer 2016;55:81–97.

87. McKinley ET, Ayers GD, Smith RA, et al. Limits of
[18F]-FLT PET as a biomarker of proliferation in
oncology. PLoS One 2013;8(3):e58938.

88. Currin E, Linden HM, Mankoff DA. Predicting
breast cancer endocrine responsiveness using
molecular imaging. Curr Breast Cancer Rep
2011;3(4):205–11.

89. Capala J, Bouchelouche K. Molecular imaging of
HER2-positive breast cancer: a step toward an individualized 'image and treat' strategy. Curr Opin Oncol 2010;22(6):559–66.

90. Dijkers EC, Oude Munnink TH, Kosterink JG, et al.
Biodistribution of 89Zr-trastuzumab and PET imaging of HER2-positive lesions in patients with metastatic breast cancer. Clin Pharmacol Ther 2010;
87(5):586–92.

91. Ulaner GA, Hyman DM, Ross DS, et al. Detection of
HER2-positive metastases in patients with HER2-
negative primary breast cancer using 89Zr-Trastuzu-
mab PET/CT. J Nucl Med 2016;57(10):1523–8.

92. Hoefnagel LD, van de Vijver MJ, van Slooten HJ,
et al. Receptor conversion in distant breast cancer
metastases. Breast Cancer Res 2010;12(5):R75.

93. Valk PE, Mathis CA, Prados MD, et al. Hypoxia in
human gliomas: demonstration by PET with fluo-
rine-18-fluoromisonidazole. J Nucl Med 1992;
33(12):2133–7.

94. Ulaner GA, Goldman DA, Gonen M, et al. Initial results of a prospective clinical trial of 18F-Fluciclovine
PET/CT in newly diagnosed invasive ductal and
invasive lobular breast cancers. J Nucl Med 2016;
57(9):1350–6.

95. Dehdashti F, McGuire AH, Van Brocklin HF, et al.
Assessment of 21-[18F]fluoro-16 alpha-ethyl-19-
norprogesterone as a positron-emitting radiopharmaceutical for the detection of progestin receptors
in human breast carcinomas. J Nucl Med 1991;
32(8):1532–7.

96. O'Connor MK, Morrow MMB, Hunt KN, et al.
Comparison of Tc-99m maraciclatide and Tc-
99m sestamibi molecular breast imaging in patients with suspected breast cancer. EJNMMI
Res 2017;7(1):5.

97. Spanu A, Chessa F, Sanna D, et al. The role of
99mTc-tetrofosmin molecular breast imaging (MBI)
in patients with breast lesions. J Nucl Med 2009;
50(supplement 2):1696.

Nuclear Medicine Imaging Techniques for Detection of Skeletal Metastases in Breast Cancer

Andrei Iagaru, MD[a],*, Ryogo Minamimoto, MD, PhD[b]

KEYWORDS

- Bone scintigraphy • SPECT • SPECT/CT • PET • PET/CT • ^{18}F-NaF • ^{18}F-FDG

KEY POINTS

- Bone is the most common site of metastases from advanced breast cancer.
- Whole-body bone scintigraphy (WBBS) has been most frequently used in the process of managing cancer patients; its advantage is that it provides rapid whole-body imaging for screening of osteoblastic or sclerotic/mixed bone metastases at reasonable cost.
- Recent advanced techniques, such as single photon emission computed tomography (SPECT)/CT, quantitative analysis, and bone scan index, contribute to better understanding of the disease state.
- More recent advances in machines and PET drugs improve the staging of the skeleton with higher sensitivity and specificity.

INTRODUCTION

In the United States, breast cancer is the most common nonskin cancer and the second leading cause of cancer-related death in women. Approximately 255,180 new cases of breast cancer and 41,070 total deaths from breast cancer are expected in 2017.[1] Breast cancer strikes women of all ages, races, ethnicities, socioeconomic strata, and geographic locales.[2]

The skeleton is the most common site of metastatic disease in advanced breast cancer. Approximately 30% to 85% of patients with metastatic breast cancer develop bone metastases, and 26% to 50% of patients with metastatic breast cancer have a bone lesion as the first site of metastasis.[3–9] The most common sites of solitary metastatic bone disease from breast cancer are the sternum (34%), pelvis (18%), thoracic spine (16%), lumbar spine (10%), ribs (7%), and pelvis, followed by skull and femur.[10,11] Over a long follow-up period, most patients presenting with a solitary bone metastasis develop metastases at other sites. Bone metastases cause skeleton-related events, including pain, fractures, hypercalcemia, and spinal cord compression; thus, the presence of bone metastases influences prognosis, quality of life, and local and systemic therapy.[12]

Imaging plays an important role in the care of patients with breast cancer. The early detection of skeletal involvement is crucial in the assessment of patients with breast cancer, because it influences clinical management.[13] This review presents data about the nuclear medicine techniques used for evaluation of the skeleton in breast cancer patients.

[a] Division of Nuclear Medicine and Molecular Imaging, Stanford University Medical Center, 300 Pasteur Drive, Room H-2200, Stanford, CA 94305, USA; [b] Division of Nuclear Medicine, National Center for Global Health and Medicine, 1-21-1, Toyama, Shinjyuku-ku, Tokyo 162-8655, Japan
* Corresponding author.
E-mail address: aiagaru@stanford.edu

PET Clin 13 (2018) 383–393
https://doi.org/10.1016/j.cpet.2018.02.002
1556-8598/18/© 2018 Elsevier Inc. All rights reserved.

BONE SCINTIGRAPHY

Whole-body bone scintigraphy (WBBS) is the most commonly used technique for detecting bone metastases.[14–17] It can identify the high osteoblastic activity and blood flow in the affected area.[16,18–20] Technetium Tc 99m (^{99m}Tc)– labeled bisphosphonates, such as methylene diphosphonate [^{99m}Tc-MDP], hydroxymethylene diphosphonate, or dicarboxypropane diphosphonate, are the most frequently used in the management of cancer patients, having the advantage of whole-body imaging at a reasonably low cost.

WBBS can accurately detect osteoblastic lesions, sclerotic/mixed bone lesions, and the reparative bone formed by osteolytic lesions; however, it is less sensitive in detecting purely osteolytic lesions, slow bone turnover, and avascular areas.[21,22] Despite the high sensitivity, the accumulation of radiotracer in sclerotic areas is not specific and reflects production of new bone in response to invasion by tumor cells.[23] WBBS identifies the metabolic reaction of bone that occurs not only in cancer but also in trauma, inflammation, and degenerative processes.[24–28]

WBBS has higher sensitivity than radiography (44% to 50%) for detecting early bone metastases[20,24,29]; for example, 30% to 75% of the normal bone mineral content has to be lost before radiographs can show the lesions in the lumbar vertebrae.[30] Limited contrast in the trabecular areas on radiographs results in difficulty identifying lesions in trabecular bone compared to cortical bone.[20] Radiographs can complement bone scintigraphy (BS), however, for the assessment of nonspecific or atypical findings or in patients with bone pain.[9]

Equivocal findings on WBBS can be further evaluated with single-photon emission CT (SPECT) and SPECT/CT, which allow 3-D imaging and can provide axial, sagittal, or coronal images.[31] Modern SPECT/CT scanners include multislice CT that provides detailed anatomic information. SPECT/CT improves both the sensitivity and the specificity for detecting bone metastases due to identification of the structural characteristics of lesions and a higher lesion to background contrast.[32] SPECT/CT improves the receiver operating characteristics (ROCs) and inter-reporter agreement for diagnosis of bone metastases compared with SPECT alone and SPECT and CT with side-by-side reading.[33] The more accurate diagnosis achieved with SPECT/CT leads to reduction in unnecessary additional studies.[34,35] Sharma and colleagues[36] reported that SPECT/CT is superior to SPECT alone for characterizing equivocal findings in patients with breast cancer.

Recent developments in SPECT/CT make possible semiquantitative measurements[37] that may play a role in characterization of a lesion as benign versus malignant as well as in assessment of response to treatment.

The detection rate of bone metastases with WBBS is 0.82% for patients with stage I disease, 2.55% for stage II disease, 16.75% for stage III, and 40.52% for those with stage IV breast cancer.[9,27,38–41] Initial detection of an abnormality or asymptomatic bone metastasis by WBBS resulted in a 14% improvement in the overall survival rate at 4 years and a 10% improvement at 5 years.[42,43] According to a large randomized study of patients with breast cancer shortly after initial treatment, semiannual screening with WBBS detected more bone metastases than clinical follow-up alone, but it did not improve 5-year survival.[44] Another randomized controlled trial showed no difference in survival between patients followed-up with physical examinations, radiographs, and BS and those followed-up with physical examinations alone.[44,45] Another study suggested that early detection of asymptomatic breast cancer recurrence at any site, including bone lesions, did not lead to improvement of overall survival.[46,47]

The American Society of Clinical Oncology guidelines do not recommend using WBBS for post-treatment surveillance of asymptomatic disease[48]; most abnormal findings are caused by benign conditions, such as trauma and inflammation. Routine WBBS screening is not recommended for patients with early (stage I or II) breast cancer.

One use of WBBS is evaluation of the response to treatment of bone lesions; WBBS can measure the associated osteoblastic response rather than tumor response. The uptake in the bone lesions is decreased when there is response to therapy, whereas increased uptake or appearance of new lesions indicates progressive disease.[9] A retrospective study of breast cancer patients with bone metastasis showed that changes in the uptake of bone lesions between baseline and post-therapy scans was related to patient survival (mean survival 5.0 ± 2.7 years compared with 3.7 ± 1.9 years for stable disease and 2.2 ± 1.3 years for progressive disease).[32,49]

One of the pitfalls of WBBS is underestimating the therapeutic response due to the so-called flare phenomenon, which makes lesions appear more intense than on previous scans due to a transient rise in osteocalcin and alkaline phosphatase bone isoenzyme.[32] The flare response occurs 3.2 months $\pm$ 1.4 months after initiation of hormone treatment or chemotherapy, and its appearance stabilizes within 6.2 months $\pm$ 3.0 months.[50]

Although response criteria have been developed, it is often difficult to apply them to osseous lesions due to complex structural changes during therapy. A recent technique is the bone scan index (BSI), which was developed as a quantitative tool to improve the interpretability and clinical relevance of bone scanning, making it possible to show the bone metastatic tumor burden.[51] The BSI has recently been reported as a response indicator in patients with metastatic breast cancer.[52,53]

An example of WBBS detection of bone metastases with CT correlate is shown in **Fig. 1**.

SODIUM FLUORIDE F 18 PET AND PET/CT

Sodium fluoride F 18 (^{18}F-NaF) is a positron-emitting radiopharmaceutical that was used briefly for skeletal scintigraphy in the 1960s.[54,55] Its clinical use was limited at that time because of the logistic difficulties in delivering a tracer with a half-life of 109.8 minutes as well as the less than ideal features of conventional gamma cameras.[54,55] ^{18}F-NaF was mainly replaced in the late 1970s by ^{99m}Tc-MDP, the characteristics of which conformed to conventional gamma cameras.[54–56]

^{18}F-NaF uptake due to bone mineralization occurs via the exchange of hydroxyl ions in the hydroxyapatite crystal. As with ^{99m}Tc-based bone agents that accumulate in bone by chemical absorption, fluorine is directly incorporated into the bone matrix, converting hydroxyapatite to fluoroapatite.[57] ^{18}F-NaF is rapidly cleared from plasma with high affinity for bone, because a smaller proportion is protein-bound in comparison with ^{99m}Tc-MDP, and it is excreted by the kidneys, with first-pass extraction of almost 100%.[58] One hour after injection, only 10% of ^{18}F-NaF remains in the plasma.[56] Its desirable characteristics of high and rapid bone uptake, accompanied by rapid blood clearance and low soft tissue uptake, result in a high bone-to-background ratio in a short time.[32]

Superior-quality and higher spatial resolution images of the bone can be obtained less than 1 hour after the intravenous administration of ^{18}F-NaF[59] (scanning started 30–45 minutes after the injection), which is shorter than of BS, at 3 hours to 4 hours after the injection.

^{18}F-NaF PET is more accurate than ^{99m}Tc-MDP planar imaging or SPECT for localizing and characterizing malignant bone lesions.[60–63] ROC

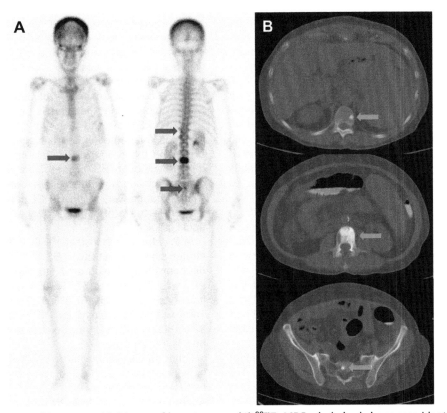

Fig. 1. A 65 year-old woman with history of breast cancer. (A) ^{99m}Tc-MDP whole-body bone scan identifies skeletal metastases (*red arrows*) correlating on (B) CT with sclerotic lesions (*green arrows*).

analysis of detection of bone lesions was higher for ^{18}F-NaF than BS (area under the curve [AUC] 0.99 vs 0.64).[62]

In a prospective study of 34 patients with breast cancer, ^{18}F-NaF PET detected more bone metastases than BS (64 bone metastases in 17 patients vs 29 bone metastases in 11 patients), and the management changed in 12% of patients.[64] Yamashita and colleagues[64] suggested that the distribution of metastatic bone lesions on the bone scan and the presence of radiographic osteosclerosis in metastatic bone lesions should be considered prognostic variables for patients with breast cancer and metastasis confined initially to bone. Petren-Mallmin and colleagues[65] investigated how the areas of pathologic uptake of ^{18}F-NaF seen on PET relate to bone structure on CT. For this purpose, both visual analysis of the radionuclide uptake and analysis of the skeletal kinetics of ^{18}F-NaF with dynamic PET imaging were performed in patients with bone metastases from breast cancer. The lytic, sclerotic, and mixed lesions found on CT all corresponded to areas with increased uptake of ^{18}F-NaF on PET. The limitation was that small lytic lesions, 2 mm to 3 mm in size, were not identified on PET. Moreover, the investigators noticed no difference in the uptake of ^{18}F-NaF between lytic and sclerotic lesions. Both lytic and sclerotic lesions had markedly higher uptake than normal bone (5–10 times higher).

In patients with metastatic breast cancer, ^{18}F-NaF improved diagnostic accuracy of bone lesions compared with BS[66–70] or CT.[71] ^{18}F-NaF PET/CT has increases diagnostic accuracy over ^{18}F-NaF PET.[68] The National Oncology PET Registry (NOPR) trial presented the impact of ^{18}F-NaF PET/CT on the management of 781 patients with breast cancer.[72] A management change occurred in 24% of those with suspected first osseous metastasis and in 60% of those with suspected progression of osseous metastases.

[18]F-NaF PET may be useful for assessing changes in bone turnover in response to therapy. Doot and colleagues[73] used dynamic ^{18}F-NaF PET to characterize the fluoride kinetics of bone metastases in patients with breast cancer, and they found that ^{18}F-NaF transport (K1) and flux (Ki) were significantly different in metastases and normal bone. The investigators also reported that these values could be estimated with reasonable precision and accuracy.

The NOPR trial also assessed the impact of ^{18}F-NaF PET/CT on treatment monitoring in 476 patients with breast cancer.[74] The incidence of a change in the management plan for patients with breast cancer was 39.3%. As with BS, a flare phenomenon can occur in ^{18}F-NaF PET after both chemotherapy and endocrine therapy in breast cancer. Therefore, an important issue that remains is the optimal time for follow-up scans.[75,76]

Despite the high performance of ^{18}F-NaF PET/CT, its clinical use remains limited because there are fewer PET/CT scanners than gamma cameras and its use is also limited by the lack of uniform reimbursement practices.

FLUDEOXYGLUCOSE F 18 PET AND PET/CT

Fludeoxyglucose F 18 (^{18}F-FDG) PET is used for evaluation of glucose metabolism in many types of cancer.[77] ^{18}F-FDG PET can be useful in distinguishing benign from malignant bone lesions.[78–81] The sensitivity of ^{18}F-FDG PET is high not only for identifying primary breast lesions and axillary lymph node involvement but also for detecting metastases in bone and other sites.[82–90] Estimates of the sensitivity of ^{18}F-FDG PET for detecting bone metastasis range from 62% to 100%, and specificity ranges from 96% to 100%.[9,84,88,91,92]

In patients with breast cancer, however, ^{18}F-FDG is sensitive for detecting osteolytic and marrow metastases, whereas it is less sensitive for detecting osteoblastic metastasis due to low accumulation of ^{18}F-FDG. ^{18}F-FDG uptake tends to reflect metabolically active tumor cells in bone, whereas BS reflects a reparative process in bone tissue close to tumor cells.[93] Cook and colleagues[77] suggested that patients with osteolytic lesions had significantly worse survival from the time of diagnosis of bone metastasis. Therefore, BS has the advantage of detecting osteoblastic type bone metastases, indicating that ^{18}F-FDG PET/CT and BS are complementary methods for detection of bone metastases and predicting the prognosis of patients with breast cancer. Although BS is one of the routine, low-cost examinations for the management of patients with breast cancer, ^{18}F-FDG PET can help clarify staging in cases of difficult or equivocal conventional staging.[93]

Many studies report that ^{18}F-FDG PET demonstrates similar sensitivity to BS.[19,88,94–98] The median sensitivity (based on 7 studies) for ^{18}F-FDG PET was 84% (range 77.7%–95.2%), and for BS it was as low as 80% (67.0%–93.3%).[19,32,88,94–98] The median specificity for ^{18}F-FDG PET was 92% (88.2%–99.0%), and for BS specificity was 85.5% (68.0%–100%).[32]

Other studies report that ^{18}F-FDG PET/CT has higher sensitivity than BS for detecting bone metastases in patients with breast cancer.[63,99] According to a study with 132 paired tests, ^{18}F-FDG PET/CT and BS were concordant in the majority (81%) of subjects, and among the discordant cases, positive cases could be confirmed in 58% of cases on ^{18}F-FDG PET/CT, in contrast to false-negative results in most cases with BS.[100] The sensitivity of ^{18}F-FDG PET/CT to detect bone metastases may depend on the histologic subtype of the breast malignancy, with greater sensitivity in ductal breast malignancies than in lobular breast malignancies.[101,102]

Identification of morphologic changes on CT and MR imaging has been the standard method for assessment of therapeutic response of bone lesions, but it does not accurately represent the metabolic alterations behind the targeted lesions, which occurred earlier than morphologic changes.[93] In patients with FDG-positive bone metastases, the change in FDG uptake (standardized uptake value [SUV]) correlated with clinical assessment of response and tumor marker changes.[103] ^{18}F-FDG PET/CT can provide information both on morphologic and metabolic aspects, which have an advantage in the accurate evaluation of the therapeutic effect on the bone lesion. During the systematic treatment of bone metastases from breast cancer, increased CT attenuation in addition to decreased FDG uptake (change of SUV) is predictive of an effective response to therapy.[104]

Fig. 2 illustrates ^{18}F-NaF PET/CT and ^{18}F-FDG PET/CT in same patient with newly diagnosed breast cancer.

FUTURE DIRECTIONS: COMBINED SODIUM FLUORIDE F 18 AND FLUDEOXYGLUCOSE F 18 PET/CT, PET/MR IMAGING

^{18}F-FDG PET/CT is not recommended for the detection of osteoblastic skeletal lesions,[95,105] whereas ^{18}F-NaF PET/CT is superior to WBBS and ^{18}F-FDG PET/CT for the detection of osteoblastic metastases.[106]

Compared with ^{18}F-FDG, ^{18}F-NaF PET/CT has the opposite pattern of uptake[19]; therefore, ^{18}F-FDG and ^{18}F-NaF PET have drawbacks and advantages for the evaluation of bone lesions, and the combination of the 2 tracers is an advantageous approach for the evaluation of cancer.[107,108] In addition, the information from the CT component of PET/CT has additional value in terms of increasing the specificity of the examination.[109]

The combined administration of ^{18}F-NaF and ^{18}F-FDG (^{18}F-NaF/^{18}F-FDG) in a single PET/CT scan for cancer detection has been advocated for detecting both extraskeletal and skeletal lesions[110,111] and a prospective international multicenter trial showed promising results.[112] The

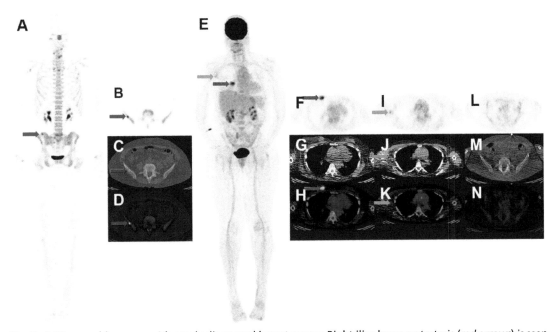

Fig. 2. A 58-year-old woman with newly diagnosed breast cancer. Right iliac bone metastasis (*red arrows*) is seen on ^{18}F-NaF maximum intensity projection image (*A*), axial PET (*B*), axial CT (*C*), and axial fused PET/CT (*D*). Right breast mass (*blue arrows*) is seen on ^{18}F-FDG maximum intensity projection image (*E*), axial PET (*F*), axial CT (*G*), and axial fused PET/CT (*H*). Right axillary lymph node metastasis (*green arrows*) is seen on ^{18}F-FDG maximum intensity projection image (*E*), axial PET (*I*), axial CT (*J*), and axial fused PET/CT (*K*). There is no ^{18}F-FDG uptake (*L–N*) in the right iliac bone lesion seen on ^{18}F-NaF.

estimated radiation dose from ^{18}F-NaF/^{18}F-FDG PET/CT (31.5 mSv) was almost equal to those of BS (4.2 mSv) and ^{18}F-FDG (26.5 mSv), which is standard for staging.[112] The recent high-sensitivity PET/CT scanners enable reduction of radiation doses from ^{18}F-NaF/^{18}F-FDG PET/CT. In the analysis of ^{18}F-NaF/^{18}F-FDG PET/CT, ^{18}F-NaF/^{18}F-FDG uptake in bony structures was mainly a reflection of ^{18}F-NaF uptake. The ^{18}F-NaF/^{18}F-FDG uptake in extraskeletal lesions showed no significant difference with the ^{18}F-FDG uptake, and a high correlation between ^{18}F-NaF/^{18}F-FDG and ^{18}F-FDG uptake was confirmed. The result indicated that the influence of ^{18}F-NaF uptake in ^{18}F-NaF/^{18}F-FDG uptake was estimated to be small in extraskeletal lesions.[113] The sensitivity of ^{18}F-NaF/^{18}F-FDG PET/CT (93.6%) is superior to that of BS (53.2%) and comparable to whole-body MR imaging (85.1%) or a combination of whole-body MR imaging and BS (93.6%) for evaluation of bone metastases in patients with breast cancer.[114] In this study, a combination of ^{18}F-NaF/^{18}F-FDG PET and whole-body MR imaging seemed much more sensitive for the detection of both skeletal and extraskeletal lesions in patients with breast cancer (93.2% vs 100.0%). The result indicates that simultaneous ^{18}F-NaF/^{18}F-FDG PET/MR imaging may provide more accurate diagnostic performance in patients with breast cancer.[114,115]

Hybrid PET/MR imaging has recently been introduced clinically. The advantage of PET/MR imaging is to be able to provide better soft tissue contrast by MR imaging than by PET/CT.[116] PET and MR imaging provide complementary information, because they evaluate different biologic processes.[117]

In the evaluation of malignant skeletal disease of 19 patients with breast cancer, ^{18}F-FDG PET/CT and PET/MR imaging showed similar lesions, but PET/MR imaging was superior to PET/CT for anatomic delineation and allocation of bone lesions.[118]

Differences in the attenuation correction (AC) methods used in PET/CT scanners versus the newly introduced whole-body simultaneous PET/MR imaging systems reportedly result in differences in uptake values in the normal skeleton.[119,120] In a recent study, MR imaging AC used in time-of-flight (TOF) PET/MR imaging provided reliable semiquantitative measurements in the normal skeleton.[121] The fast zero-echo-time AC showed more accurate AC than clinical atlas AC by improving the estimation of head-skull attenuation, which may contribute to providing accurate quantitative values on bone area when assessed with PET/MR imaging.[122] TOF PET/MR imaging has the potential to reduce metal artifact, which may help in the identification of bone lesions in patients with metallic implants in the bone.[123,124]

Fig. 3 shows findings from combined ^{18}F-NaF/^{18}F-FDG PET/MR imaging in a patient with recurrent breast cancer.

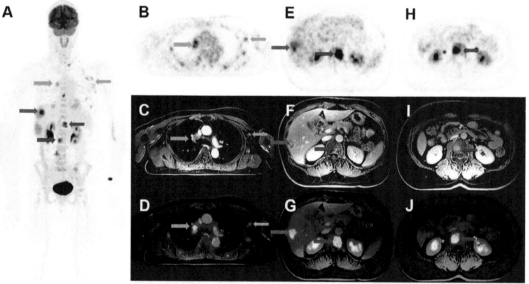

Fig. 3. A 53-year-old woman with recurrent breast cancer. Images are shown from a combined ^{18}F-NaF (1 mCi) and ^{18}F-FDG (4 mCi) PET/MR imaging study acquired using a SIGNA (GE) scanner. Selected bone metastases (*red arrows*), lymph node metastases (*green arrows*), and liver metastasis (*blue arrows*) are seen on maximum intensity projection image (*A*), axial PET (*B, E, H*), axial T1-weighted MR imaging (*C, F, I*), and axial fused PET/MR imaging (*D, G, J*).

SUMMARY

Bone is the most common site of metastases from advanced breast cancer. WBBS has been most frequently used in the process of managing cancer patients; its advantage is that it provides rapid whole-body imaging for screening of osteoblastic or sclerotic/mixed bone metastases at reasonable cost. Recent advanced techniques, such as SPECT/CT, quantitative analysis, and BSI, contribute to better understanding of the disease state.

More recent advances in machines and PET drugs improve the staging of the skeleton with higher sensitivity and specificity. Recent studies reported that ^{18}F-NaF PET is more accurate than ^{99m}Tc-MDP planar imaging or SPECT for localizing and characterizing malignant bone lesions. ^{18}F-FDG is sensitive for detecting osteolytic and marrow metastases, whereas it is less sensitive for detecting osteoblastic metastases due to low accumulation of ^{18}F-FDG. The combined administration of ^{18}F-NaF and ^{18}F-FDG in a single PET/CT scan for cancer detection has shown promising results for detecting both extraskeletal and skeletal lesions.

A greater number of osteoblastic skeletal metastases is detected with ^{18}F-NaF PET/CT. Given the high concordance between the results of the 2 scans, however, it may be possible to create a clinical workflow to evaluate patients referred for bone metastases with a ^{99m}Tc-MDP WBBS first, followed by ^{18}F-NaF PET/CT only for patients with negative or equivocal ^{99m}Tc-MDP WBBS who continue to have high clinical suspicion for bone metastases. FDG PET/CT is useful for detection of lytic bone lesions and soft tissue disease. The combination of ^{18}F-NaF and FDG in PET/CT or PET/MR imaging may become a 1-stop-shop evaluation of certain patients with advanced breast cancer. Lastly, research radiopharmaceuticals, such as those evaluating angiogenesis, estrogen receptor status,[125] and Her-2[126,127] status, may play a role in breast cancer in the future, including for evaluation of heterogeneity of bone metastases.

REFERENCES

1. Siegel RL, Miller KD, Jemal A. Cancer statistics, 2017. CA Cancer J Clin 2017;67:7–30.
2. Dumitrescu RG, Cotarla I. Understanding breast cancer risk – where do we stand in 2005? J Cell Mol Med 2005;9:208–21.
3. Solomayer EF, Diel IJ, Meyberg GC, et al. Metastatic breast cancer: clinical course, prognosis and therapy related to the first site of metastasis. Breast Cancer Res Treat 2000;59:271–8.
4. Hortobagyi GN. Unmet needs in metastatic bone disease and its complications: is progress possible? Semin Oncol 2001;28:1–3.
5. Lipton A. Bisphosphonates and metastatic breast carcinoma. Cancer 2003;97:848–53.
6. Manders K, van de Poll-Franse LV, Creemers GJ, et al. Clinical management of women with metastatic breast cancer: a descriptive study according to age group. BMC Cancer 2006;6:179.
7. Pivot X, Asmar L, Hortobagyi GN, et al. A retrospective study of first indicators of breast cancer recurrence. Oncology 2000;58:185–90.
8. Hortobagyi GN. Novel approaches to the management of bone metastases in patients with breast cancer. Semin Oncol 2002;29:134–44.
9. Hamaoka T, Madewell JE, Podoloff DA, et al. Bone imaging in metastatic breast cancer. J Clin Oncol 2004;22:2942–53.
10. Boxer DI, Todd CE, Coleman R, et al. Bone secondaries in breast cancer: the solitary metastasis. J Nucl Med 1989;30:1318–20.
11. Koizumi M, Yoshimoto M, Kasumi F, et al. Comparison between solitary and multiple skeletal metastatic lesions of breast cancer patients. Ann Oncol 2003;14:1234–40.
12. Domchek SM, Younger J, Finkelstein DM, et al. Predictors of skeletal complications in patients with metastatic breast carcinoma. Cancer 2000;89:363–8.
13. Coleman RE. Metastatic bone disease: clinical features, pathophysiology and treatment strategies. Cancer Treat Rev 2001;27:165–76.
14. Hortobagyi GN. Bone metastases in breast cancer patients. Semin Oncol 1991;18:11–5.
15. Krasnow AZ, Hellman RS, Timins ME, et al. Diagnostic bone scanning in oncology. Semin Nucl Med 1997;27:107–41.
16. Goris ML, Bretille J. Skeletal scintigraphy for the diagnosis of malignant metastatic disease to the bones. Radiother Oncol 1985;3:319–29.
17. Petren-Mallmin M, Andreasson I, Nyman R, et al. Detection of breast cancer metastases in the cervical spine. Acta Radiol 1993;34:543–8.
18. Tryciecky EW, Gottschalk A, Ludema K. Oncologic imaging: interactions of nuclear medicine with CT and MRI using the bone scan as a model. Semin Nucl Med 1997;27:142–51.
19. Cook GJ, Fogelman I. The role of positron emission tomography in the management of bone metastases. Cancer 2000;88:2927–33.
20. Rybak LD, Rosenthal DI. Radiological imaging for the diagnosis of bone metastases. Q J Nucl Med 2001;45:53–64.
21. Galasko CS, Doyle FH. The detection of skeletal metastases from mammary cancer: a regional comparison between radiology and scintigraphy. Clin Radiol 1972;23:295–7.

22. Loeffler RK, DiSimone RN, Howland WJ. Limitations of bone scanning in clinical oncology. JAMA 1975; 234:1228–32.

23. Galasko CS. The pathological basis for skeletal scintigraphy. J Bone Joint Surg Br 1975;57:353–9.

24. O'Mara RE. Skeletal scanning in neoplastic disease. Cancer 1976;37:480–6.

25. Rosenthal DI. Radiologic diagnosis of bone metastases. Cancer 1997;80:1595–607.

26. Lee YT. Bone scanning in patients with early breast carcinoma: should it be a routine staging procedure? Cancer 1981;47:486–95.

27. Coleman RE, Rubens RD, Fogelman I. Reappraisal of the baseline bone scan in breast cancer. J Nucl Med 1988;29:1045–9.

28. Dershaw DD, Osborne M. Imaging techniques in breast cancer. Semin Surg Oncol 1989;5:82–93.

29. Hortobagyi GN, Libshitz HI, Seabold JE. Osseous metastases of breast cancer. Clinical, biochemical, radiographic, and scintigraphic evaluation of response to therapy. Cancer 1984;53:577–82.

30. Vinholes J, Coleman R, Eastell R. Effects of bone metastases on bone metabolism: implications for diagnosis, imaging and assessment of response to cancer treatment. Cancer Treat Rev 1996;22: 289–331.

31. Houssami N, Costelloe CM. Imaging bone metastases in breast cancer: evidence on comparative test accuracy. Ann Oncol 2012;23:834–43.

32. Fogelman I, Gnanasegaran G, Wall HVD. Radionuclide and hybrid bone imaging. New York: Springer 2013; p. 635–89.

33. Utsunomiya D, Shiraishi S, Imuta M, et al. Added value of SPECT/CT fusion in assessing suspected bone metastasis: comparison with scintigraphy alone and nonfused scintigraphy and CT. Radiology 2006;238:264–71.

34. Strobel K, Burger C, Seifert B, et al. Characterization of focal bone lesions in the axial skeleton: performance of planar bone scintigraphy compared with SPECT and SPECT fused with CT. AJR Am J Roentgenol 2007;188:W467–74.

35. Römer W, Nömayr A, Uder M, et al. SPECT-guided CT for evaluating foci of increased bone metabolism classified as indeterminate on SPECT in cancer patients. J Nucl Med 2006;47:1102–6.

36. Sharma P, Singh H, Kumar R, et al. Bone scintigraphy in breast cancer: added value of hybrid SPECT-CT and its impact on patient management. Nucl Med Commun 2012;33:139–47.

37. Zeintl J, Vija AH, Yahil A, et al. Quantitative accuracy of clinical 99mTc SPECT/CT using ordered-subset expectation maximization with 3-dimensional resolution recovery, attenuation, and scatter correction. J Nucl Med 2010;51:921–8.

38. Brar HS, Sisley JF, Johnson RH Jr. Value of ppreoperative bone and liver scans and alkaline phosphatase in the evaluation of breast cancer patients. Am J Surg 1993;165:221–3.

39. Yeh KA, Fortunato L, Ridge JA, et al. Routine bone scanning in patients with T1 and T2 breast cancer: a waste of money. Ann Surg Oncol 1995; 2:319–24.

40. Samant R, Ganguly P. Staging investigations in patients with breast cancer: the role of bone scans and liver imaging. Arch Surg 1999;134:551–3.

41. Koizumi M, Yoshimoto M, Kasumi F, et al. What do breast cancer patients benefit from staging bone scintigraphy? Jpn J Clin Oncol 2001;31: 263–9.

42. Komaki R, Donegan W, Manoli R, et al. Prognostic value of pretreatment bone scans in breast carcinoma. AJR Am J Roentgenol 1979;132:877–81.

43. Tomin R, Donegan WL. Screening for recurrent breast cancer: its effectiveness and prognostic value. J Clin Oncol 1987;5:62–7.

44. Rosselli Del Turco M, Palli D, Cariddi A, et al. Intensive diagnostic follow-up after treatmentof primary breast cancer: a randomized trial. National Research Council Project on Breast Cancer follow-up. JAMA 1994;271:1593–7.

45. Impact of follow-up testing on survival and health-related quality of life in breast cancer patients. A multicenter randomized controlled trial. The GIVIO Investigators. JAMA 1994;271:1587–92.

46. Zwaveling A, Albers GH, Felthuis W, et al. An evaluation of routine follow-up for detectionof breast cancer recurrences. J Surg Oncol 1987;34:194–7.

47. Stierer M, Rosen HR. Influence of early diagnosis on prognosis of recurrent breast cancer. Cancer 1989;64:1128–31.

48. Smith TJ, Davidson NE, Schapira DV, et al. American Society of Clinical Oncology 1998 update of recommended breast cancer surveillance guidelines. J Clin Oncol 1999;17:1080–2.

49. Janicek MJ, Shaffer K. Scintigraphic and radiographic patterns of skeletal metastases in breast cancer: value of sequential imaging in predicting outcome. Skeletal Radiol 1995;24:597–600.

50. Janicek MJ, Hayes DF, Kaplan WD. Healing flare in skeletal metastases from breast cancer. Radiology 1994;192:201–4.

51. Erdi YE, Humm JL, Imbriaco M, et al. Quantitative bone metastases analysis based on image segmentation. J Nucl Med 1997;38:1401–6.

52. Iwase T, Yamamoto N, Ichihara H, et al. The relationship between skeletal-related events and bone scan index for the treatment of bone metastasis with breast cancer patients. Medicine (Baltimore) 2014;93:e269.

53. Idota A, Sawaki M, Yoshimura A, et al. Bone scan index predicts skeletal-related events in patients with metastatic breast cancer. Springerplus 2016; 5:1095.

54. Grant FD, Fahey FH, Packard AB, et al. Skeletal PET with 18F-fluoride: applying new technology to an old tracer. J Nucl Med 2008;49:68–78.

55. Czernin J, Satyamurthy N, Schiepers C. Molecular mechanisms of bone 18F-NaF deposition. J Nucl Med 2010;51(12):1826–9.

56. Mosci C, Iagaru A. 18F NaF PET/CT in the assessment of malignant bone disease. PET Clin 2012;7:263–74.

57. Bridges RL, Wiley CR, Christian JC, et al. An introduction to Na18F bone scintigraphy: basic principles, advanced imaging concepts, and case examples. J Nucl Med Technol 2007;35:64–76.

58. Cook GJ. PET and PET/CT imaging of skeletal metastases. Cancer Imaging 2010;10:1–8.

59. Sabbah N, Jackson T, Mosci C, et al. 18F-sodium fluoride PET/CT in oncology: an atlas of SUVs. Clin Nucl Med 2015;40:e228–31.

60. Even-Sapir E, Metser U, Mishani E, et al. The detection of bone metastases in patients with high-risk prostate cancer: 99mTc-MDP Planar bone scintigraphy, single- and multi-field-of-view SPECT, 18Ffluoride PET, and 18F-fluoride PET/CT. J Nucl Med 2006;47:287–97.

61. Krüger S, Buck AF, Mottaghy F, et al. Detection of bone metastases in patients with lung cancer: 99mTc-MDP planar bone scintigraphy, 18F-fluoride PET or 18F-FDG PET/CT. Eur J Nucl Med Mol Imaging 2009;36:1807–12.

62. Schirrmeister H, Guhlmann A, Elsner K, et al. Sensitivity in detecting osseous lesions depends on anatomic localization: planar bone scintigraphy versus 18F PET. J Nucl Med 1999;40:1623–9.

63. Iagaru A, Mittra E, Dick D, et al. Prospective evaluation of (99m)Tc MDP scintigraphy, (18)F NaF PET/CT, and (18)F FDG PET/CT for detection of skeletal metastases. Mol Imaging Biol 2012;14:252–9.

64. Yamashita K, Koyama H, Inaji H. Prognostic significance of bone metastasis from breast cancer. Clin Orthop Relat Res 1995;(312):89–94.

65. Petren-Mallmin M, Andrasson I, Ljunggren O, et al. Skeletal metastases from breast cancer: uptake of 18F-fluoride measured with positron emission tomography in correlation with CT. Skeletal Radiol 1998;27:72–6.

66. Schirrmeister H, Guhlmann A, Kotzerke J, et al. Early detection and accurate description of extent of metastatic bone disease in breast cancer with fluoride ion and positron emission tomography. J Clin Oncol 1999;17:2381–9.

67. Withofs N, Grayet B, Tancredi T, et al. 18F-fluoride PET/CT for assessing bone involvement in prostate and breast cancers. Nucl Med Commun 2011;32:168–76.

68. Even-Sapir E, Metser U, Flusser G, et al. Assessment of malignant skeletal disease: initial experience with 18F-fluoride PET/CT and comparison between 18F-fluoride PET and 18F-fluoride PET/CT. J Nucl Med 2004;45:272–8.

69. Damle NA, Bal C, Bandopadhyaya GP, et al. The role of 18F-fluoride PET-CT in the detection of bone metastases in patients with breast, lung and prostate carcinoma: a comparison with FDG PET/CT and 99mTc-MDP bone scan. Jpn J Radiol 2013;31:262–9.

70. Yoon SH, Kim KS, Kang SY, et al. Usefulness of 18F-fluoride PET/CT in breast cancer patients with osteosclerotic bone metastases. Nucl Med Mol Imaging 2013;47:27–35.

71. Piccardo A, Altrinetti V, Bacigalupo L, et al. Detection of metastatic bone lesions in breast cancer patients: fused 18F-fluoride-PET/MDCT has higher accuracy than MDCT—preliminary experience. Eur J Radiol 2012;81:2632–8.

72. Hillner BE, Siegel BA, Hanna L, et al. Impact of 18F-fluoride PET on intended management of patients with cancers other than prostate cancer: results from the National Oncologic PET Registry. J Nucl Med 2014;55:1054–61.

73. Doot RK, Muzi M, Peterson LM, et al. Kinetic analysisof 18F-Fluoride PET images of breast cancer bone metastases. J Nucl Med 2010;51:521–7.

74. Hillner BE, Siegel BA, Hanna L, et al. 18F-fluoride PET used for treatment monitoring of systemic cancer therapy: results from the National Oncologic PET Registry. J Nucl Med 2015;56:222–8.

75. Wade AA, Scott JA, Kuter I, et al. Flare response in 18F-fluoride ion PET bone scanning. AJR Am J Roentgenol 2006;186:1783–6.

76. Cook GJ, Azad GK, Goh V. Imaging bone metastases in breast cancer: staging and response assessment. J Nucl Med 2016;57(Suppl 1):27S–33S.

77. Cook GJ, Houston S, Rubens R, et al. Fogelman I. Detection of bone metastases in breast cancer by 18FDG PET: differing metabolic activity in osteoblastic and osteolytic lesions. J Clin Oncol 1998;16:3375–9.

78. Dehdashti F, Siegel BA, Griffeth LK, et al. Benign versus malignant intraosseous lesions: discrimination by means of PET with 2-[F-18]fluoro-2-deoxy-D-glucose. Radiology 1996;200:243–7.

79. Aoki J, Inoue T, Tomiyoshi K, et al. Nuclear imaging of bone tumors: FDG-PET. Semin Musculoskelet Radiol 2001;5:183–7.

80. Malhotra P, Berman CG. Evaluation of bone metastases in lung cancer: improved sensitivity and specificity of PET over bone scanning. Cancer Control 2002;9:254–60.

81. Wahl RL. Current status of PET in breast cancer imaging, staging, and therapy. Semin Roentgenol 2001;36:250–60.

82. Wahl RL, Cody RL, Hutchins GD, et al. Primary and metastatic breast carcinoma: initial clinical

evaluation with PET with the radiolabeled glucose analogue 2-[F-18]-fluoro-2-deoxy-D-glucose. Radiology 1991;179:765–70.

83. Bassa P, Kim EE, Inoue T, et al. Evaluation of preoperative chemotherapy using PET with fluorine-18-fluorodeoxyglucose in breast cancer. J Nucl Med 1996;37:931–8.

84. Moon DH, Maddahi J, Silverman DH, et al. Accuracy of whole-body fluorine-18-FDG PET for the detection of recurrent or metastatic breast carcinoma. J Nucl Med 1998;39:431–5.

85. Rostom AY, Powe J, Kandil A, et al. Positron emission tomography in breast cancer: a clinicopathological correlation of results. Br J Radiol 1999;72:1064–8.

86. Bombardieri E, Crippa F. PET imaging in breast cancer. Q J Nucl Med 2001;45:245–56.

87. Vranjesevic D, Filmont JE, Meta J, et al. Whole-body (18)F-FDG PET and conventional imaging for predicting outcome in previously treated breast cancer patients. J Nucl Med 2002;43:325–9.

88. Dose J, Bleckmann C, Bachmann S, et al. Comparison of fluorodeoxyglucose positron emission tomography and 'conventional diagnostic procedures' for the detection of distant metastases in breast cancer patients. Nucl Med Commun 2002;23:857–64.

89. Rose C, Dose J, Avril N. Positron emission tomography for the diagnosis of breast cancer. Nucl Med Commun 2002;23:613–8.

90. Shreve PD, Grossman HB, Gross MD, et al. Metastatic prostate cancer: initial findings of PET with 2-deoxy-2-[F-18]fluoro-D-glucose. Radiology 1996;199:751–6.

91. Bender H, Kirst J, Palmedo H, et al. Value of 18fluoro-deoxyglucose positron emission tomography in the staging of recurrent breast carcinoma. Anticancer Res 1997;17:1687–92.

92. Bury T, Barreto A, Daenen F, et al. Fluorine-18 deoxyglucose positron emission tomography for the detection of bone metastases in patients with non-small cell lung cancer. Eur J Nucl Med 1998;25:1244–7.

93. Eubank WB, Lee JH, Mankoff DA. Disease restaging and diagnosis of recurrent and metastatic disease following primary therapy with FDG-PET imaging. PET Clin 2009;4:299–312.

94. Abe K, Sasaki M, Kuwabara Y, et al. Comparison of 18FDG-PET with 99mTc-HMDP scintigraphy for the detection of bone metastases in patients with breast cancer. Ann Nucl Med 2005;19:573–9.

95. Nakai T, Okuyama C, Kubota T, et al. Pitfalls of FDG-PET for the diagnosis of osteoblastic bone metastases in patients with breast cancer. Eur J Nucl Med Mol Imaging 2005;32:1253–8.

96. Gallowitsch HJ, Kresnik E, Gasser J, et al. F-18 fluorodeoxyglucose positronemission tomography in the diagnosis of tumor recurrence and metastases in the follow-up of patients with breast carcinoma: a comparison to conventional imaging. Invest Radiol 2003;38:250–6.

97. Yang SN, Liang JA, Lin FJ, et al. Comparing whole body (18)F-2-deoxyglucose positron emission tomography and technetium-99m methylene diphosphonate bone scan to detect bone metastases in patients with breast cancer. J Cancer Res Clin Oncol 2002;128:325–8.

98. Ohta M, Tokuda Y, Suzuki Y, et al. Whole body PET for the evaluation of bony metastases in patients with breast cancer: comparison with 99Tcm-MDP bone scintigraphy. Nucl Med Commun 2001;22:875–9.

99. Fuster D, Duch J, Paredes P, et al. Preoperative staging of large primary breast cancer with [18F] fluorodeoxyglucose positron emission tomography/computed with conventional imaging procedures. J Clin Oncol 2008;26:4746–51.

100. Morris PG, Lynch C, Feeney JN, et al. Integrated positron emission tomography/computed tomography may render bone scintigraphy unnecessary to investigate suspected metastatic breast cancer. J Clin Oncol 2010;28:3154–9.

101. Dashevsky BZ, Goldman DA, Parsons M, et al. Appearance of untreated bone metastases from breast cancer on FDG PET/CT: importance of histologic subtype. Eur J Nucl Med Mol Imaging 2015;42:1666–73.

102. Hogan MP, Goldman DA, Dashevsky B, et al. Comparison of 18F-FDG PET/CT for systemic staging of newly diagnosed invasive lobular carcinoma versus invasive ductal carcinoma. J Nucl Med 2015;56:1674–80.

103. Stafford SE, Gralow JR, Schubert EK, et al. Use of serial FDG PET to measure the response of bone-dominant breast cancer to therapy. Acad Radiol 2002;9:913–21.

104. Tateishi U, Gamez C, Dawood S, et al. Bone metastases in patients with metastatic breast cancer: morphologic and metabolic monitoring of response to systemic therapy with integrated PET/CT. Radiology 2008;247:189–96.

105. Uematsu T, Yuen S, Yukisawa S, et al. Comparison of FDG PET and SPECT for detection of bone metastases in breast cancer. AJR Am J Roentgenol 2005;184:1266–73.

106. Hsu WK, Virk MS, Feeley BT, et al. Characterization of osteolytic, osteoblastic, and mixed lesions in a prostate cancer mouse model using 18F-FDG and 18F-fluoride PET/CT. J Nucl Med 2008;49:414–21.

107. Hoegerle S, Juengling F, Otte A, et al. Combined FDG and [F-18]fluoride whole-body PET: a feasible two-in-one approach to cancer imaging? Radiology 1998;209:253–8.

108. Cook GJ, Fogelman I. Detection of bone metasta-ses in cancer patients by 18F fluoride and 18F-flu-orodeoxyglucose positron emission tomography. Q J Nucl Med 2001;45:47–52.

109. Sampath SC, Sampath S, Mosci C, et al. Detection of osseous metastasis by 18FNaF/18F-FDG PET/CT versus CT alone. Clin Nucl Med 2015;40: e173–7.

110. Iagaru A, Mittra E, Yaghoubi SS, et al. Novel strat-egy for a cocktail 18F-fluoride and 18F-FDG PET/CT scan for evaluation of malignancy: results of the pilotphase study. J Nucl Med 2009;50:501–5.

111. Lin FI, Rao JE, Mittra ES, et al. Prospective compar-ison of combined 18F-FDG and 18F-NaF PET/CT vs. 18F-FDG PET/CT imaging for detection of ma-lignancy. Eur J Nucl Med Mol Imaging 2012;39: 262–70.

112. Iagaru A, Mittra E, Mosci C, et al. Combined 18F-fluoride and 18F-FDG PET/CT scanning for evaluation of malignancy: results of an international multicenter trial. J Nucl Med 2013;54:176–83.

113. Minamimoto R, Mosci C, Jamali M, et al. Analysis of the biodistribution of the combined 18F-NaF and 18F-FDG administration for PET/CT imaging. J Nucl Med 2015;56:688–94.

114. Minamimoto R, Loening A, Jamali M, et al. Pro-spective comparison of 99mTc-MDP scintigraphy, combined 18F-NaF and 18F-FDG PET/CT, and whole-body MRI in patients with breast and pros-tate cancer. J Nucl Med 2015;56:1862–8.

115. Ida SI, Minamimoto R, Taviani V, et al. Imaging pa-tients with breast and prostate cancers using com-bined 18F NaF/18F FDG and TOF simultaneous PET/MRI. J Nucl Med 2017;58(Suppl 1):755.

116. Iagaru A, Mittra E, Minamimoto R, et al. Simulta-neous whole-body time-of flight 18F-FDG PET/MRI: a pilot study comparing SUVmax with PET/CT and assessment of MR image quality. Clin Nucl Med 2015;40:1–8.

117. Pichler BJ, Kolb A, Nägele T, et al. PET/MRI: paving the way for the next generation of clinical multimo-dality imaging applications. J Nucl Med 2010;51: 333–6.

118. Eiber M, Takei T, Souvatzoglou M, et al. Perfor-mance of whole-body integrated 18F-FDG PET/MR in comparison to PET/CT for evaluation of malig-nant bone lesions. J Nucl Med 2014;55:191–7.

119. Samarin A, Burger C, Wollenweber SD, et al. PET/MR imaging of bone lesions: implications for PET quantification from imperfect attenuation correction. Eur J Nucl Med Mol Imaging 2010;39: 1154–60.

120. Keereman V, van Holen R, Mollet P, et al. The effect of errors in segmented attenuation maps on PET quantification. Med Phys 2011;38:6010–9.

121. Minamimoto R, Xu G, Jamali M, et al. Semi-quanti-tative assessment of 18F FDG uptake in the normal skeleton: comparison of PET/CT and time of flight simultaneous PET/MRI. AJR Am J Roentgenol 2017;209(5):1136–42.

122. Sekine T, Ter Voert EE, Warnock G, et al. Clinical evaluation of Zero-Echo-Time attenuation correc-tion for brain 18F-FDG PET/MRI: comparison with atlas attenuation correction. J Nucl Med 2016;57: 1927–32.

123. Minamimoto R, Levin C, Jamali M, et al. Improve-ments in PET image quality in time of flight (TOF) simultaneous PET/MRI. Mol Imaging Biol 2016;18: 776–81.

124. Svirydenka H, Delso G, Barbosa DG, et al. The effect of susceptibility artifacts related to metal im-plants on adjacent lesion assessment in simulta-neous TOF PET/MR. J Nucl Med 2017;58:1167–73.

125. Kurland BF, Peterson LM, Lee JH, et al. Estrogen receptor binding (18F-FES PET) and glycolytic ac-tivity (18F-FDG PET) predict progression-free sur-vival on endocrine therapy in patients with ER+ breast cancer. Clin Cancer Res 2017;23:407–15.

126. Ulaner GA, Hyman DM, Ross DS. Detection of HER2-positive metastases in patients with HER2-negative primary breast cancer using 89Zr-Trastuzumab PET/CT. J Nucl Med 2016;57(10): 1523–8.

127. Ulaner GA, Hyman DM, Lyashchenko SK, et al. 89Zr-Trastuzumab PET/CT for detection of human epidermal growth factor receptor 2-positive metas-tases in patients with human epidermal growth fac-tor receptor 2-negative primary breast cancer. Clin Nucl Med 2017;42(12):912–7.

Role of Fludeoxyglucose in Breast Cancer

Treatment Response

David Groheux, MD, PhD

KEYWORDS

- FDG-PET/CT • Breast cancer • Treatment response • Neoadjuvant chemotherapy
- Metastatic breast cancer

KEY POINTS

- Changes in metabolic activity generally occur earlier than changes in tumor size.
- The metabolic information provided by PET has been shown to be valuable for the early assessment of the response to neoadjuvant chemotherapy, but the methodology for image acquisition and analysis needs to be standardized; breast cancer subtype and treatment type need to be considered in interpreting the change in fludeoxyglucose uptake with therapy.
- In the metastatic setting, there is evidences that PET/computed tomography (CT) performed better than CT alone, especially to assess the response in bone metastases.
- In the metastatic setting, PET/CT has the ability to evaluate different sites of metastases in a single examination and to detect a heterogeneous response (coexistence of responding and nonresponding lesions within the same patient).
- The use of PET/CT in patients with metastatic breast cancer is hampered by the absence of consensus of the criteria to use to assess the response, of the number of metastatic sites to analyze, and of the optimal date to perform PET during treatment.

INTRODUCTION

The role of fludeoxyglucose (FDG) PET in the management of patients with breast cancer (BC) is evolving. Combined PET and computed tomography (CT) systems (PET/CT) have replaced PET alone in most nuclear medicine departments. The CT portion of PET/CT provides the anatomic information useful for accurate interpretation of PET signal.

Most patients with stage II-III BC are treated by neoadjuvant chemotherapy (NAC). This strategy allows more patients to undergo breast-conserving surgery and increases the chances of surgery in patients with primary inoperable disease; it also provides precious information on the efficacy of chemotherapy. Early assessment of the response to NAC should be helpful, as it might reduce the toxicity from inefficacious chemotherapy or allow a refinement of treatment. The number of studies has pointed out the efficacy of FDG PET/CT in early assessing the response to NAC.[1–12] Nevertheless, PET/CT for assessment of the response to NAC has not yet entered routine clinical practice.

Early response of treatment is also important in the metastatic setting to use the most efficient drugs and to stop early ineffective chemotherapy. Changes in metabolic activity generally occur earlier than changes in tumor size. FDG PET/CT has shown high performances to assess the response in metastatic patients with BC.[13–25]

Disclosure Statement: No conflict of interest.
Department of Nuclear Medicine, Saint-Louis Hospital, 1 Avenue Claude Vellefaux, Paris 75475 Cedex 10, France
E-mail address: dgroheux@yahoo.fr

PET Clin 13 (2018) 395–414
https://doi.org/10.1016/j.cpet.2018.02.003

When compared with conventional imaging, FDG PET/CT has shown better accuracy, especially to assess the response in bone lesions. However, PET is not currently used in the metastatic setting.

In this review, the author briefly describes the principles of PET/CT imaging in BC and the tools that could be used to assess the treatment response. Then, the author assesses the advantages and limits of FDG PET/CT to early evaluation of the response in the neoadjuvant setting and afterward in the metastatic setting.

GENERAL INFORMATION
Fludeoxyglucose PET/Computed Tomography Procedure

Imaging usually starts 60 minutes after the intravenous injection of FDG. CT and PET data are acquired sequentially before being fused. Patients are imaged from the base of the skull to the mid-thigh, except for specific situations. Imaging usually begins with CT acquisition. Questions remain as to whether the CT part of PET/CT should be performed as a contrast-enhanced full-dose diagnostic CT or as a nonenhanced, low-dose CT, with additional focused segmental examination in case of inconclusive findings. Some technical constraints imposed by the PET component, such as free breathing, might limit the full diagnostic power of CT when performed as part of PET/CT imaging.

Modern whole-body PET systems typically have a reconstructed spatial resolution of 5- to 6-mm full width at half maximum, based on phantom measurements. However, detection depends not only on tumor size but also on the degree of FDG avidity, tumor-to-background ratio, impact of motion (respiration), and so forth.

Fludeoxyglucose Uptake Depends on Breast Tumor Characteristics

Most malignant breast tumors overexpress glucose transporters (especially Glut-1 and Glut-3) and show increased hexokinase activity.[26,27] However, FDG uptake can be undetectable or weak in some tumors. In the case of low FDG uptake at baseline, PET/CT has limited value to assess the treatment response.

Invasive ductal carcinoma exhibits higher FDG uptake than invasive lobular carcinoma.[28–30] FDG uptake in carcinoma in situ is usually weak as compared with invasive tumors.[29] FDG uptake increases with the tumor proliferation index (Ki67 expression).[29] High-grade tumors exhibit higher FDG uptake than intermediate- and low-grade tumors.[29,30] FDG uptake is higher in tumors that are negative for hormone receptors.[29,30] Triple-negative breast tumors (negative for estradiol and progesterone receptors and without human epidermal growth factor receptor 2 [HER2] overexpression) are usually highly FDG avid.[30,31]

Available Fludeoxyglucose PET/Computed Tomography Parameters to Assess Treatment Response

Tumor FDG uptake can be expressed by using a so-called standardized uptake value (SUV). This index is calculated based on the amount of activity injected and the patients' body mass, as follows: SUV = measured activity in the volume of interest/[injected activity/body weight of patients]. Different methods to define the SUV are available, the most used being maximum SUV (SUV_{max}) (value of the voxel with the highest SUV), SUV_{peak} (mean of voxels intensities in a spherical region of interest of 1 cm^3 around the SUV_{max} voxel[32]), and SUV_{mean} (mean of voxels intensities within the tumor volume). The ability of SUV_{max} to assess the treatment response has been evaluated in numerous series. This robust parameter is the most used in clinical practice.

Some parameters mixing volume and FDG intensity can also be used to assess the treatment response. The metabolic active tumor volume (MATV) is determined as the tumor volume with significant FDG uptake.[33] Different methods can be used to define the MATV. The total lesion glycolysis (TLG) corresponds to the MATV multiplied by the SUV_{mean}.

Recently, some texture features, such as the entropy and the heterogeneity, were evaluated to define the breast tumor.[34–36] However, the ability of those parameters to assess the treatment response needs to be evaluated in large series.

The question remains open on whether 60 minutes after injection is the optimal timing for FDG PET/CT imaging. No optimal time has been defined in the literature. Uptake in breast tumors (and so the SUV value) continues to increase beyond 60 minutes.[37] Nevertheless, this time point, which has the advantage of simplicity, is widely used. It is a key point within a given institution to apply the same time delay after injection. The delay used at baseline imaging should be reproduced if patients are referred for response evaluation. Some investigators developed methods to make appropriate time corrections for tumor SUVs.[37,38] Also, when performing SUV measurements for response assessment, there is a risk of underestimation of SUV values when the residual tumor is small (partial volume effect). The time delay between the last chemotherapy use and FDG imaging might also influence the response assessment.

Various working groups have proposed specific PET criteria based on SUV measurements for determining the therapeutic response. The most currently used[32,39] criteria are those developed by the European Organization for Research and Treatment of Cancer (EORTC criteria)[39] and by Wahl and colleagues[32] (PET Response Criteria in Solid Tumors, PERCIST). In its last revision, the Response Evaluation Criteria in Solid Tumors (RECIST 1.1) include PET/CT findings.[40,41]

PET Procedures Standardization

The use of FDG PET and SUV to tailor treatment requires standardization of methods for PET/CT calibration, patient preparation, image acquisition, and image analysis. Preparation procedures and instrumental factors can introduce differences in the measurement of SUV. The standardization guidelines of the European Association of Nuclear Medicine (EANM)[42] and of the Society of Nuclear Medicine[43] are provided to help the physician, physicist, and technologist. The EANM's guidelines recommend that the blood glucose level should be lower than 200 mg/dL for clinical studies and lower than 150 mg/dL for research studies.[42] Patients should not consume any food for at least 4 hours before FDG injection.[42] A 60-minute interval is recommended for the uptake time (time between injection and acquisition).[42] When repeating an FDG PET/CT study in the same patient in the context of therapy response assessment, it is crucial to apply the same uptake interval to within 10 minutes. The same protocol, with identical acquisition and reconstruction settings, should be used when performing multiple examinations in the same patient.

Use of quantitative parameters, such as SUV, MATV, or TLG, in a multicenter setting requires that these parameters be comparable among patients and sites, regardless of the PET/CT system used. Harmonization programs, such as the EANM Research Ltd, aiming at using FDG PET as a quantitative imaging biomarker within multicenter studies have been developed.[44]

TREATMENT RESPONSE ASSESSMENT IN THE NEOADJUVANT SETTING
Neoadjuvant Chemotherapy in Patients with Breast Cancer

NAC is the first treatment in nonoperable locally advanced and inflammatory BC. NAC is also commonly used in case of an operable but large tumor.[45] This strategy allows more patients to undergo breast-conserving treatment and increases the chances of surgery in patients with primary inoperable disease; it provides information on the efficacy of chemotherapy.[46] Early assessment of the response to NAC should allow refinement of treatment in nonresponding patients.[47,48] Various teams have pointed out the potential of FDG PET or PET/CT in early assessment of the response to NAC.[1–12]

However, interim PET/CT in BC has not yet gained a wide audience, as opposed to other similar diseases, such as lymphomas.[49] This circumstance is in part due to a lack of consensus that early evaluation of the response can be used to direct change in therapy in the BC neoadjuvant setting, and only limited data showing that response-adaptive therapy lead to improved outcomes.[50]

Assessing Response to Neoadjuvant Treatment Using Fludeoxyglucose PET/ Computed Tomography

FDG PET/CT has shown potential for early detection of residual disease.[1–12] Four meta-analyses, encompassing 920,[12] 781,[51] 745,[52] and 1119 patients,[53] have been published. The sensitivity and specificity of PET were 84% and 66%, respectively, in the first,[12] 84% and 71% in the second,[51] 80.5% and 79.0% in the third,[52] and 81.9% and 79.3% in the last meta-analysis.[53] The sensitivity was, therefore, near 80% to 85% and the specificity a little less. A fifth meta-analysis, comparing PET with MR imaging to predict pathologic complete response (pCR), showed that PET was more sensitive and MR imaging more specific.[54] Overall, these meta-analyses highlighted large disparities between the different studies: differences in the populations studied, differences in the date of the PET evaluation (at 1, 2, or 3 cycles), differences in the site used to measure the SUV value (primary tumor only or taking axillary nodes into account), differences in the criteria used to define the pathologic response, and differences in the choice of the quantification parameter (SUV_{max}, SUV_{mean}, blood flow, TLG).

The PET image-derived parameter used in most studies was the decrease in SUV_{max} under therapy (ΔSUV_{max}), whereas a few teams also examined less common PET parameters, such as changes in tumor blood flow[3,7] or changes in TLG values.[55,56] **Table 1** shows the main studies evaluating the decrease of SUV_{max} (ΔSUV_{max}) to assess the response to NAC in patients with BC of mixed phenotypes. The CT part of the hybrid system is not decisive, and the hybrid PET/CT system performed no better than PET alone.

Most teams defined an optimal threshold value of a decrease in SUV_{max} in the primary tumor that discriminates metabolic responders from

Table 1
Studies evaluating the decrease of maximum standardized uptake value during neoadjuvant chemotherapy for breast cancer with fludeoxyglucose PET/computed tomography, without taking into account the breast cancer subtype

Study	Country	PET or PET/CT	n° Patients	Number of NAC cycles	Timing of PET Evaluation	Definition of Pathologic Responders	Is Axillary Uptake Analyzed?	Optimal Timing	Optimal SUV Threshold
Schelling et al,[2] 2000	Germany	PET	22	2–4	After 1 and 2 cycles	pCR or residual microscopic foci	No	After 2 cycles	55%
Smith et al,[1] 2000	United Kingdom	PET	30	8	After 1 and 4 cycles and before surgery	Partial response and complete response	Yes	NR	NR
Rousseau et al,[4] 2006	France	PET/CT	64	4–6	After 1, 2, and 3 cycles and before surgery	Therapeutic effect >50%	No	After 2 cycles	40%
Berriolo-Riedinger et al,[5] 2007	France	PET	47	4 or 6	After 1 cycle	Total or near total therapeutic effect	Yes	—	60%
McDermott et al,[6] 2007	United Kingdom	PET	96	6 or 8	After 1 cycle, at midpoint, at end point	pCR or malignant cells <25% of the tumor area	No	Between the end of the first cycle and the midpoint	24% after one cycle, 58% at midpoint, and 64% at end point
Duch et al,[10] 2009	Spain	PET/CT	50	4	After 2 cycles	pCR or malignant cells <25% of the tumor area	No	—	40%
Kumar et al,[9] 2009	India	PET/CT	23	6	After 2 cycles	pCR or malignant cells <25% of the tumor area	No	—	Just 50% of decrease is performed
Schwarz-Dose et al,[8] 2009[a]	Germany	PET	104	4–6	After 1 and 2 cycles	pCR or residual microscopic foci	No	PET after 1 and 2 cycles perform equally	45% after one course and 55% after 2 courses

Abbreviation: NR, not reported.
[a] Twenty-four patients with a baseline SUV less than 3 were excluded.

nonresponders and predicts the pathologic response. Unfortunately, the percentage change in FDG uptake that was considered discriminant varied dramatically across studies, which refrained translation of the technique in clinical practice. Several factors could explain these differences. First, the definition of what is a good pathologic responder varied. For example, Rousseau and colleagues[4] defined tumor regression superior to 50% as good response, whereas Berriolo-Riedinger and colleagues[5] considered no residual invasive cancer cells as a requirement to define a satisfactory pathologic response. Second, in some studies the response was analyzed only in the primary tumor, whereas in others the response was also assessed in lymph nodes. Third, the timing for interim PET varied across studies.[12] Limited studies performed interim PET/CT at multiple time points.[4,6,8,11] A meta-analysis showed that early response monitoring (after 1 or 2 cycles) was more accurate than late monitoring (after 3 or more cycles) (accuracy 76% vs 65%, $P = .001$).[12] For several teams, performing PET after the second cycle of NAC is a good compromise to evidence the effects of chemotherapy, while still allowing for a possibility of early change of treatment in case of inefficacy. Fourth, the chemotherapy regimen varied widely from one study to another. Schneider-Kolsky and colleagues[11] showed that the decrease in SUV during NAC depended on the chemotherapy drugs used; therefore, the cutoff values should take into account the type of treatment. The author and colleagues performed the same observation in the specific subgroup of triple-negative cancer.[57]

Furthermore, the pretreatment tumor SUV index must be high in order to detect a meaningful reduction during treatment.[6,8] This requirement limits the use of iterative PET in case of tumors with low SUV value.

Early Assessment of Response to Neoadjuvant Treatment According to Breast Cancer Subtype

A key, but not widely recognized, limitation of almost all early studies is that they addressed populations with mixed subtypes of BC, ignoring difference in FDG uptake across tumor subtypes and differing changes in response to therapy by subtype and type of therapy.[58] BC comprises different groups of tumors with different response rates to chemotherapy, different risks of relapse, different treatment options, and different prognoses. Also, at baseline, FDG uptake differs significantly between BC phenotypes with higher uptake in aggressive subtypes particularly in triple-negative

tumors.[30,31] The extent of the decrease in FDG uptake during NAC also varies with BC phenotype.[59–61] It has been proposed to assess the response during NAC in 3 specific BC tumors subgroups based on immunohistochemistry analysis and clinically current practice[62]: triple-negative BC (TNBC), HER2-positive BC, and estrogen receptor (ER)-positive/HER2-negative BC. Several recent works confirmed the efficiency of PET prediction based on subtype-specific criteria.[58] For the two most aggressive BC subtypes, that is, TNBC and HER2-positive BC, the probability of pCR is non-negligible (30% to 60%) and would condition patient survivals.[63–65] Thus, obtaining pCR is a main objective in these patients.[47]

Triple-negative breast cancer

Several studies evaluated the value of FDG PET to predict the response to NAC in TNBC,[57,60,61,66–72] some of them in a cohort of BC with mixed phenotype.[60,61,67–69,71] **Table 2** shows results of the main studies.

TNBC often shows high FDG uptake at baseline. **Fig. 1** shows an example of a tumor with a high SUV value at baseline and a rapid decrease after 2 cycles of NAC. Koolen and colleagues[68,69] found that ΔSUV_{max} (after 1 or 3 cycles of NAC) was predictive of pCR in patients with TNBC, whereas the prediction was limited in one other study that included only 15 patients with TNBC[67] (see **Table 2**). More recently, Humbert and colleagues[72] also observed that PET has high accuracy to predict pCR early. In a prospective series of 77 women with TNBC, the author and colleagues observed that the change in FDG tumor uptake after 2 cycles of chemotherapy was not only predictive of pCR but also of event-free survival (EFS).[57] Patients were treated with 2 different chemotherapy regimens, 23 receiving a standard-dose of epirubicin plus cyclophosphamide followed by docetaxel (EC-D) and 55 being treated with a dose-dense, dose-intense regimen of epirubicin plus cyclophosphamide (SIM) (see **Table 2**). ΔSUV_{max} was more pronounced under SIM than with EC-D (-68% vs -35%, $P = .009$).[57] During 34 months, 22 patients relapsed and 10 of them died. The ΔSUV_{max} was significantly associated with EFS in patients receiving SIM ($P = .028$) as well as in those receiving EC-D ($P = .021$). The optimal ΔSUV_{max} to predict a pathologic response and EFS was, however, specific to the treatment regimen.[57] The optimal cutoff to predict residual disease was close to -65% in the SIM group and -50% in the EC-D group.[57]

The change of SUV was not the only parameter used in the TNBC subgroup. In 46 patients with TNBC, Humbert and colleagues[73] observed that

Table 2
Main studies evaluating change of [18]fludeoxyglucose uptake (decrease in maximum standardized uptake value) during neoadjuvant chemotherapy to predict pathologic complete response in triple-negative breast cancer

Study[a]	Country	N° Patients	N° Cycles of NAC	Timing of Interim PET	pCR Rate (%)	ΔSUV$_{max}$ Threshold (%)[b]	Acc (%)[b]	Se (%)	Sp (%)	PPV (%)	NPV (%)
Zucchini et al,[67] 2013	Italy	15	4	After 2 cycles	27	50	27	100	0	27	0
Koolen et al,[69] 2014	The Netherlands	31	≥6	After 1 cycle (25 patients)	52	NR	76	NR	NR	NR	NR
				After 3 cycles (28 patients)	50	NR	87	NR	NR	NR	NR
Humbert et al,[72] 2015	France	44	6	After 1 cycle	42	50	75	74	76	70	79
Groheux et al,[57] 2016[c]	France	77	8	After 2 cycles	22	50	83	100	78	56	100
			6	After 2 cycles	44	65	78	92	68	69	91

Abbreviations: Acc, accuracy; NPV, negative predictive value; NR, not reported; PPV, positive predictive value; Se, sensitivity; Sp, specificity.
[a] When several studies of the same cohort were published, the author selected the most recent one.
[b] ΔSUV$_{max}$ cutoff measured in the primary tumor and used to differentiate metabolic responders from nonresponders.
[c] PET/CT prediction is measured according to the chemotherapy regimen. Twenty-three patients were treated with epirubicin + cyclophosphamide followed by docetaxel (EC-D) and 55 patients were treated with a dose-dense, dose-intensified regimen of epirubicin + cyclophosphamide (SIM).

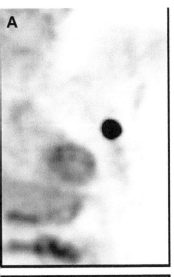
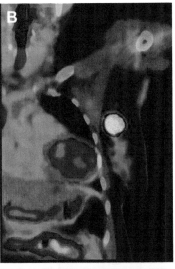
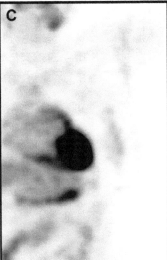
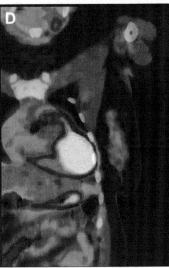

Fig. 1. FDG PET/CT to assess response early in a patient treated by NAC for a TNBC. At baseline, coronal PET (*A*) and PET/CT (*B*) fusion images show high FDG uptake in the primary tumor ($SUV_{max} = 27.3$). After 2 cycles, coronal PET (*C*) and PET/CT (*D*) fusion images show weak residual FDG uptake in the primary tumor ($SUV_{max} = 1.4$). The good metabolic response ($\Delta SUV_{max} = -95\%$) is confirmed at the completion of the NAC, surgery showing a pCR. No recurrence is observed 1 year after surgery.

tumor blood flow changes after the first cycle of chemotherapy was useful to predict patients' overall survival.

Human epidermal growth factor receptor 2–positive breast cancer

In the neoadjuvant setting, patients with HER2-positive BC receive trastuzumab plus chemotherapy.[64] Recent works have shown that dual inhibition of HER2 (trastuzumab plus lapatinib or trastuzumab plus pertuzumab)[74,75] improves the pCR rate. However, these strategies might also involve higher rates of side effects and should, therefore, be used in patients who have a low probability of achieving pCR.

Several studies evaluated the performances of PET to predict the pCR rate early in patients with HER2-positive BC.[56,60,61,67–69,76–81] Some studies were focused on patients with HER2-positive BC only,[77–80] whereas others evaluated the predictive value of PET in patients with HER2-positive BC and patients with HER2-negative BC.[60,61,67–69,76,81] PET accuracy was low in some studies,[67,68,76,81] whereas the results were promising in others.[60,77,79,80] **Table 3** shows results of the main studies.

The multicenter randomized trial AVATAXHER assessed the benefit of adding bevacizumab when patients with HER2-positive BC are predicted to be poor responders to trastuzumab plus docetaxel.[80] Of 142 patients, 69 were predicted to be responders to standard therapy according to the change in FDG uptake after one cycle. In these patients, the pCR rate was 53.6%. Of the 73 patients predicted to be poor responders, the pCR rate was 24.0% with standard

Table 3
Main studies evaluating fludeoxyglucose-PET imaging parameters during neoadjuvant chemotherapy to predict pathologic complete response in human epidermal growth factor receptor 2–positive breast cancer

Study[a]	Country	N° Patients	N° Cycles of NAC	Timing of Interim PET	pCR Rate (%)	Optimal PET Parameter	Acc (%)	Se (%)	Sp (%)	PPV (%)	NPV (%)
Martoni et al,[76] 2010	Italy	7	6–8 cycles	After 2 cycles	17	ΔSUV_{max} (cutoff of 50%) is the only criterion applied	29	17	100	100	17
Groheux et al,[56] 2013	France	30	8	After 2 cycles	53	Breast tumor and axilla SUV_{max} absolute value at interim PET ($SUV_{max}<3$)	90	94	86	88	92
Gebhart et al,[78] 2013	Belgium	77	18 wk	After 2 wk (68 patients) After 6 wk (66 patients)	35	ΔSUV_{max} (cutoff of 15% after 2 wk and of 25% after 6 wk) is only criterion applied	NR	NR	NR	NR	NR[d]
Zucchini et al,[67] 2013	Italy	14	4	After 2 cycles	29	ΔSUV_{max} (cutoff of 50%) is only criterion applied	43	100	20	33	100

Study	Country	n		Timing		Criterion	Se	Sp	PPV	NPV	Acc
Koolen et al,[69] 2014	The Netherlands	26	3	After 3 wk (21 patients)	67	ΔSUV_{max} in the site with the highest baseline SUV_{max} (either in the breast or axilla)	72	NR	NR	NR	NR
				After 8 wk (25 patients)	68		64	NR	NR	NR	NR
Humbert et al,[79] 2014[b]	France	54	6	After 1 cycle	44	SUV_{max} value at interim PET at interim PET ($SUV_{max}<2.1$)	76	NR	NR	76	76
Coudert et al,[80] 2014[c]	France	94	6	After 1 cycle	46	ΔSUV_{max}	NR	NR	NR	53	75
Cheng et al,[81] 2015	China	34	4	After 2 cycles	56	ΔSUV_{peak}	56[d]	NR	NR	NR	NR

Abbreviations: Acc, accuracy; Se, sensitivity; Sp, specificity; PPV, positive predictive value; NPV, negative predictive value; NR, not reported.

[a] In the case of several studies by the same time, only results of the most recent are given.

[b] SUV values have been corrected for body surface area and glycaemia.

[c] There were 142 patients included; 48 metabolic nonresponders after 1 cycle received bevacizumab in addition to trastuzumab plus docetaxel. PET performances are given in the 94 patients treated with trastuzumab plus docetaxel only. Optimal ΔSUV_{max} cutoff is 76%, but results are given for 70%.

[d] Fifty-six percent is the value of the area under the curve (AUC). Receiver operating chacteristic curve (ROC) analysis showed that the ΔSUV_{peak} could not effectively predict the overall pCR; the ROC-AUC was only 0.56 (95% confidence interval 0.36–0.76, $P = .53$).

treatment alone and 43.8% when bevacizumab was added.[80]

The best parameter to use to assess the response early in HER2-positive BC remains uncertain (see **Table 3**). In a limited series, the author and colleagues observed that the absolute value of residual FDG uptake (SUV_{max} in breast or axilla) after 2 cycles of chemotherapy was more predictive of pCR than ΔSUV_{max}.[77] Humbert and colleagues[79] observed similar findings. The treatment used should also be taken into account when assessing the response in patients with HER2-positive BC.[78] Targeted therapy leads to a rapid decrease in FDG uptake, which depends on the anti-HER2 regimen.[78]

Estrogen receptor–positive/human epidermal growth factor receptor 2–negative breast cancer

For this subgroup, PET seems less promising than for the triple negative and HER2-positive BC subgroups. ER-positive/HER2-negative tumors have lower FDG uptake than aggressive subtypes, such as TNBC.[30,59,60] Chemosensitivity of ER-positive tumors is variable and mostly limited; pCR is rarely achieved, especially in the luminal-A subtype. In 2 studies evaluating the role of FDG PET according to BC subtypes, only 2% of patients with ER-positive/HER2-negative BC achieved pCR.[60,69] At baseline luminal tumors have faint FDG uptake, and the decrease of SUV under chemotherapy is lower in ER-positive/HER2-negative than in other subtypes.[30,61] Because of the lesser extent of tumor regression when ER-positive/HER2 cancer is treated by NAC, the use of PET parameters taking into account metabolic volume measurements in addition to FDG uptake have been proposed in this specific subgroup.[82,83] Moreover, several studies suggested that the baseline tumor SUV value could be helpful to predict the response to NAC and patients' outcome in luminal tumors.[36,83–86] In 84 patients with ER-postive/HER2-negative BC of stage II-III (primary tumor size >2 cm), the author and colleagues observed that a high SUV_{max} or a high TLG at baseline was associated with shorter EFS ($P<.001$ and $P = .032$, respectively).[83]

Suggestions for Using Fludeoxyglucose PET/Computed Tomography to Evaluate Response to Neoadjuvant Chemotherapy in Patients with Breast Cancer

At this time, PET can be used for early evaluation of NAC in patients with BC (and possibly to change treatment) in clinical trials only. Because patients with distant metastases have specific treatments, only patients without distant foci on baseline PET study should be included in neoadjuvant trials.[48] Patients should have a pretreatment PET and an interim-PET early during NAC.

In the absence of standardized response criteria for interim PET in BC at the present time, PET-derived parameters (SUV, TLG, and so forth) and the criteria to be used to evaluate the response in clinical trials should be chosen according to results of published studies. The following factors should be taken into account: (1) value of pretreatment tumor SUV, (2) timing of interim PET, (3) type of treatment, and (4) subtype of BC.

1. Tumor FDG uptake at baseline PET: Tumors with low FDG uptake are more difficult to distinguish from background tissues and are more affected by imaging imprecision.[6,87] Tumors with low SUV_{max} are not good candidates to evaluate the response with PET.
2. Timing of interim PET: To allow treatment adaptation, interim-PET should be performed early (ideally after 1 or 2 cycles).[47] The timing of interim PET will influence the optimal ΔSUV cutoff to be used to differentiate responders from nonresponders.[4,8]
3. Type of treatment: The decrease in SUV is larger when a targeted therapy (eg, trastuzumab) is used in addition to chemotherapy.[60] The type of chemotherapy regimen can also impact the SUV decrease, the ΔSUV cutoff being higher in the case of dose-dense, dose-intense chemotherapy than in the case of a conventional dose regimen.[57]
4. Subtype of BC: PET-imaging derived parameters to apply to predict pCR depends on the BC subtype.[61] For TNBC, ΔSUV and ΔTLG offered an excellent prediction.[61] However, for HER2-positive BC, the absolute value of SUV measured at interim PET has shown better prediction.[61,77,79]

TREATMENT RESPONSE EVALUATION IN THE METASTATIC SETTING
Assessment of Response to Chemotherapy Agents ± Targeted Therapy

Several systemic agents can be used to treat patients with metastatic BC (MBC), including chemotherapy agents (anthracyclines, taxanes, gemcitabine, capecitabine, and so forth) as well as targeted therapy, such as anti-HER2 therapy.

Anatomic imaging, especially CT, is currently used to measure the diameter of the tumor lesions before, during, and after treatment response assessment and follow-up. The RECIST criteria have been defined to standardize this response evaluation.[40,41,88] However, RECIST criteria have some limitations. In particular, several cycles of treatment are needed before anatomic imaging is able to detect a change in tumor size. Moreover, modification in some tissues, such as bone metastases and pleural effusion, which are common sites of BC dissemination, are difficult to assess with CT. Changes in metabolic activity generally occur earlier than changes in tumor size.

Some teams currently used FDG PET to assess the response to systemic treatment in BC. However, only a few studies reported on the clinical use of FDG PET/CT in patients with metastatic breast disease. In most series, the number of patients was limited and sometimes PET was performed without CT (**Table 4**). In all of these series, qualitative visual analysis of FDG PET images performed early (most of times between 1 and 3 cycles) after the beginning of the systemic treatment was helpful to assess the response. Quantitative analysis based on the change of the SUV values under treatment was also useful to predict the treatment response.[13,15,16] In 2 studies,[13,15] a high SUV decrease after 1 cycle of chemotherapy was predictive of the clinical response evaluated at the end of the treatment. In the study from Couturier and colleagues,[16] the metabolic response measured as changes in SUV after the third cycle of chemotherapy predicted not only the clinical response but also the overall survival; however, early changes in SUVs (after the first cycle of chemotherapy) were not predictive of the long-term outcome.[16] The optimal date to evaluate treatment with FDG PET remains unknown. As discussed in the neoadjuvant setting, FDG PET could allow assessment of the response early after the beginning of the systemic treatment of patients with MBC. This point is especially true for targeted therapies, because these treatments can render tumors metabolically inactive without substantial modification of their size. In 87 patients treated with lapatinib and trastuzumab for HER2-positive MBC, FDG PET performed after 1 week had a high negative predictive value (91%) for identifying patients who would not achieve an objective response according to the RECIST criteria.[23] In addition, patients identified as metabolic nonresponders after 1 week had a shorter time to progression than responding patients.[23]

Another advantage to the use of PET/CT to assess the response is its ability to evaluate different sites of metastases (except brain metastases) in a single examination.[89] PET/CT is helpful to evidence a heterogeneous response (coexistence of responding and nonresponding lesions within the same patient).[20]

Although these results to assess the treatment response in MBC are promising, FDG PET/CT is not currently recommended in this setting. The use of PET/CT in this indication is hampered by the cost of this imaging, the potential for delaying care, the risk of invasive procedures stimulated by false-positive results, the exposure to ionizing radiation, and the lack of proof that changing treatment early improves patients' survival. One other important limitation for the use of PET/CT is the absence of consensus of criteria to use to assess the response. In particular, it remains unclear if semiquantitative analysis based on FDG uptake measurement is more helpful than visual analysis. In most studies, the 2 methods mostly used to assess the response are the EORTC[39] and the PERCIST[32] criteria. In a recent study, the prognostic value of PET/CT assessed with PERCIST was compared with the prognostic value of contrast-enhanced CT (CE-CT) for the prediction of outcomes in patients with stage IV BC undergoing systemic therapy.[90] Responses according to RECIST and PERCIST both correlated with progression-free survival (PFS), but PERCIST showed a significantly higher predictive accuracy (concordance index for PFS: 0.70 vs 0.60). One-year PFS for responders versus nonresponders by RECIST was 59% versus 27%, compared with 63% versus 0% by PERCIST. Four-year disease-specific survival (DSS) of responders and nonresponders by RECIST was 50% and 38%, respectively (P = .2, concordance index: 0.55), as compared with 58% versus 18% for PERCIST (P<.001, concordance index: 0.65). The response on PET/CT was also a significantly better predictor for DSS than disease control on CE-CT.[90]

In the metastatic setting, patients may show so many lesions on FDG PET/CT that it becomes quite cumbersome to measure FDG uptake for each of them.[25] The number of lesions that needs to be measured to accurately assess the response has not yet been determined. PERCIST, although recommending an analysis of the most metabolically active lesion, also encourages averaging SUV normalized by lean body mass (SUL) for up to 5 lesions.[32] In a study,[25] the exact number of analyzed lesions did not have a major influence on the prognostic value of the response by FDG PET/CT.

Bone Metastases and Their Modification Under Treatment

The skeleton is the most common organ to be affected by metastatic cancer and the site of disease that produces the greatest morbidity.[91]

Therefore, detecting bone metastases and evaluating their evolution under treatment is a major objective in patients with high-risk BC.

Although PET was more efficient than CT or bone scan for depicting lytic or mixed bone metastases, and bone marrow lesions, several teams observed that PET could lack sensitivity for detecting purely sclerotic bone metastases.[92,93] However, others found that PET/CT was more accurate than bone scan to detect bone metastases.[94,95] Although sclerotic metastases have no FDG uptake, they show osteocondensation on the CT images so that they can be detected by the hybrid PET/CT procedure.[89]

PET imaging is a powerful tool to evaluate the response of bone metastases treated with chemotherapy (see **Table 4**). Previous studies indicated that serial whole-body FDG PET can help quantitatively assess the response of BC bone metastases to therapy.[14,17] Of 405 consecutive patients with BC referred for FDG PET, 28 were treated for metastatic bone–dominant BC.[17] They were undergoing at least 2 serial PET scans. A higher SUV on the initial FDG PET predicted a shorter time to a skeletal-related event (hazard ratio [HR] = 1.30, $P<.02$). Smaller percentage decreases in SUV (or increases in SUV) were associated with a shorter time to progression ($P<.006$). A patient with no change in SUV was twice as likely to progress compared with a patient with a 42% median decrease in SUV.[17]

More recently, studies performed with hybrid PET/CT showed the complementarity of the PET and the CT information to characterize bone metastases and to evaluate their modification under treatment. Du and colleagues[18] observed bone metastases in 67 of 408 consecutive patients with recurrent BC. Twenty-five of them (146 bone lesions) had sequential FDG PET/CT examinations (86 studies) over an average follow-up period of 23 months. At baseline, the 146 lesions were classified as osteolytic (N = 77), osteoblastic (N = 41), mixed-pattern (N = 11), or no change/negative (N = 17) on CT. Most osteolytic and mixed-pattern lesions, but fewer of the osteoblastic lesions, showed increased FDG uptake. After treatment, 58 osteolytic lesions (80.5%) became FDG negative and osteoblastic on CT and only 14 lesions (19.5%) remained FDG avid. Of the 25 FDG-avid osteoblastic lesions, 13 (52%) became FDG negative, but 12 (48%) remained FDG avid and increased in size on CT. All 17 CT-negative lesions became FDG negative; however, 9 of them became osteoblastic.[18] The study from Tateishi and colleagues[19] also brings some evidence that hybrid FDG PET/CT (when both CT information and tumor metabolic activity are considered) provides additional and useful information to assess the evaluation of systemic chemotherapy. This team retrospectively compared morphologic and metabolic changes in bone metastases in response to systemic therapy in 102 patients with MBC.[19] They observed that an increase in attenuation in bone metastases (measured in Hounsfield units) and a decrease in SUV were altogether associated with response duration.[19] In multivariate analysis, a decrease in SUV of 8.5% or more was the only significant predictor of a long response duration. The studies from Du and colleagues[18] and from Tateishi and colleagues[19] suggest that FDG PET/CT is more accurate than CT alone for early monitoring of the response to therapy, with a good prognostic stratification. In a recent retrospective study, hybrid FDG PET/CT was also found to be a powerful tool in treatment response assessment of bone metastases in BC and consistent with the clinical status of the patients, as it reflects tumor activity.[24] Bone scan was found to be insufficient for response assessment of bone metastases, as it reflects osteoblastic reaction of the bone against metastatic disease, which increases as the disease responds to treatment.[24]

Assessment of Response to Hormonal Therapy: the Paradoxal Metabolic Flare

As describe in patients treated with chemotherapy, FDG PET can be used to assess the response to endocrine therapy. Twenty-two patients scheduled to receive endocrine therapy for MBC had a PET/CT at baseline and after a mean of 10 ± 4 weeks for evaluation of the response after induction.[21] The metabolic response was assessed according to the EORTC's criteria and based on the mean difference in SUV_{max} between the two PET/CT scans. Metastatic sites were localized in bone (N = 15), lymph nodes (N = 11), chest wall (N = 3), breast (N = 5), lung (N = 3), soft tissue (N = 1), and liver (N = 1). Partial metabolic response (PMR) was observed in 11 patients (50%), stable metabolic disease (SMD) in 5 (23%) and progressive metabolic disease (PMD) in 6 (27%). The median PFS times were 20, 27, and 6 months in the PMR, SMD, and PMD groups, respectively. PFS in the PMD group differed from that in the PMR and SMD groups ($P<.0001$).[21] This study shows that the metabolic response assessed by FDG PET/CT imaging in patients with MBC treated with endocrine therapy is predictive of the patients' PFS. In another study, 17 evaluable patients with ER-positive/HER2-negative MBC were treated with the combination of an endocrine therapy, letrozole, with a

Table 4
Main studies evaluating fludeoxyglucose PET or PET/computed tomography to assess response in metastatic breast cancer

Reference	Type	PET or PET/CT	No. of Patients	Site of Metastases	Date of PET to Assess Response	Main Objective	Main Results
Gennari et al,[13] 2000	P	PET	13	No specific site	After the first cycle and at the end of TTT	To investigate the role FDG PET in the early evaluation of response to chemotherapy in patients with MBC	SUV of MBC sites shows a rapid and significant decrease in tumor glucose metabolism soon after the first cycle of TTT in responding patients.
Stafford et al,[14] 2002	R	PET	24	Bone dominant	Serial time points during the therapy	To determine the feasibility of using quantitative FDG-PET with SUV_{max} to monitor the response of BC bone metastases to therapy	Changes in FDG SUV with TTT showed correlation with the clinical response and with the change in tumor marker value.
Dose Schwarz et al,[15] 2005	P	PET	11	No specific site	After the first and second cycles	To evaluate the use of FDG PET to predict response after the first and second cycles of chemotherapy for MBC	In patients with MBC, sequential FDG PET allowed prediction of response to TTT after the first cycle of chemotherapy.
Couturier et al,[16] 2006	P	PET	20	Bone, lung, pleural, LN, and liver	After the first and third cycle	To evaluate the clinical value of PET for monitoring chemotherapy in MBC	Change in the SUV value after 3 cycles of chemotherapy is useful for monitoring the response to chemotherapy in MBC.
Specht et al,[17] 2007	R	PET	28	Bone dominant	At least 2 PET during TTT	To evaluate the prognostic power of serial FDG PET in patients with bone-dominant MBC	Changes in serial FDG PET may predict time to progression in patients with bone-dominant MBC.
Du et al,[18] 2007	R	PET/CT	25	Bone metastases	Sequential PET/CT examinations	To investigate the clinical relevance of FDG uptake features of bone metastases with various radiographic appearances	FDG uptake reflects the immediate tumor activity of bone metastases, whereas the radiographic morphology changes vary greatly with time.
Tateishi et al,[19] 2008	R	PET/CT	102	Bone metastases	After treatment	To retrospectively compare morphologic and metabolic changes in bone metastases in response to systemic therapy in patients with MBC	A decrease in SUV after treatment was an independent predictor of response duration in patients with MBC who had bone metastases.

(continued on next page)

Table 4
(continued)

Reference	Type	PET or PET/CT	No. of Patients	Site of Metastases	Date of PET to Assess Response	Main Objective	Main Results
Huyge et al,[20] 2010	R	PET/CT	25	Bone dominant	<12 mo after TTT initiation	To describe the intraindividual heterogeneity of the FDG PET/CT response among lesions in patients with bone-dominant MBC	Whole-body PET/CT allows frequent heterogeneous responses after systemic therapy to be identified in patients with bone-dominant MBC.
Mortazavi-Jehanno et al,[21] 2012	P	PET/CT	22	Bone, LN, CW, lung, ST, liver	10 ± 4 wk after TTT induction	To assess whether outcomes in patients with MBC is related to metabolic response to endocrine therapy determined by FDG PET/CT	Metabolic response assessed by FDG PET/CT imaging in patients with MBC treated with ET is predictive of the patients' PFS.
Mayer et al,[22] 2014	P	PET/CT	51	Bone, LN, lung, pleural, liver	2 wk after TTT induction	To evaluate buparlisib + letrozole in patients with ER + MBC refractory to ET	No metabolic response at 2 wk was associated with rapid disease progression.
Lin et al,[23] 2015	P	PET/CT	87	Bone, lung, liver pleural, CW, LN	Weeks 1 and 8	To evaluate the combination lapatinib + trastuzumab in HER2+ MBC	Week-1 PET/CT may allow selection of patients who can be treated with targeted regimens.
Al-Muqbel et al,[24] 2016	R	PET/CT	32 (Gr-2)	Bone metastases	No predefined date	To examine the effectiveness of BS (Gr-1) and FDG PET/CT (Gr-2) in treatment response assessment of patients with bone metastases in MBC patients	PET/CT is powerful to assess the response of bone metastases, as it reflects tumor activity; BS is insufficient, as it reflects osteoblastic reaction.
Pinker et al,[25] 2016	R	PET/CT	60	No specific site	No predefined date	To compare analysis of 1 lesion (PERCIST 1) vs analysis of up to 5 lesions (PERCIST 5) for predicting the outcome of patients with MBC	The exact number of analyzed lesions did not have a major influence on the prognostic value of the response by FDG PET/CT.
Riedl et al,[90] 2017	R	PET/CT	65	No specific site	Within 90 d after initiation of therapy	To compare FDG PET/CT and CE-CT for the prediction of outcome in patients with MBC undergoing systemic therapy	In patients with MBC, tumor response on PET/CT seems to be a superior predictor of PFS and DSS than response on CE-CT.

Abbreviations: BS, bone scintigraphy; CE-CT, contrast-enhanced CT; CW, chest wall; DSS, disease-specific survival; ET, endocrine therapy; Gr, group; LN, lymph nodes; P, prospective study; PFS, progression-free survival; R, retrospective study; ST, soft tissue; TTT, treatment.

therapy-targeted phosphoinositide-3-kinase, the buparlisib.[22] No metabolic responses measured by FDG PET/CT scan at 2 weeks was associated with rapid disease progression. Phase III trials of buparlisib and endocrine therapy in patients with ER-positive BC are ongoing.[22]

A paradoxical increase in FDG uptake during the first days after initiation of endocrine therapy has been observed in patients with good therapeutic response. This phenomenon has been described under the term "metabolic flare."[96] This effect typically occurs during the 10 days after initiation of hormone therapy.[96] An explanation for this phenomenon is that endocrine therapy has initial agonist effects before antagonist effects dominate. Therefore, an increase in the SUV value by tumors during a PET scan performed early after the initiation of hormone therapy is predictive of a good therapeutic response.[97,98] This effect was observed not only with tamoxifen[97] but also with antiaromatase and with fulvestrant.[98] However, these results have been reported on small numbers of patients; further works are needed to better analyze this phenomenon.

Prognostic Value of Fludeoxyglucose PET/Computed Tomography Findings in Patients with Metastatic Breast Cancer

As previously described, the change of SUV_{max} in metastases of BC can predict patients' survival, a high SUV_{max} decrease being associated with better outcomes.[16] Several studies also suggested that PET/CT performed at a single time point before[99,100] or after[101] completion of chemotherapy can be predictive of survival in patients with metastatic BC. Of 253 patients with MBC, pretreatment SUV_{max} was strongly associated with overall survival in patients who had bone metastases (N = 141, HR = 3.13, $P<.001$).[99] This effect was maintained on multivariate analysis (HR = 3.19, $P = .002$) after correcting for known prognostic variables. A greater risk of death was also associated with the SUV_{max} value in patients who had metastases to the liver (N = 46, HR = 2.07), lymph nodes (N = 149, HR = 1.1), and lung (N = 62, HR = 2.2), although these results were not significant ($P = .18$, $P = .31$, and $P = .095$, respectively). In another study from the same team, SUV_{max} and TLG were both predictors of survival in patients with BC with bone metastases.[100] TLG was a more informative biomarker of overall survival than SUV_{max} for patients with lymph nodes (HR = 2.3, $P<.01$) and liver metastases (HR = 4.9, $P<.01$).[100]

In a group of 47 patients, Cachin and colleagues[101] showed that patients with a negative FDG PET (complete metabolic response) following high-dose chemotherapy (HDC) had a significantly longer survival than patients with a positive FDG PET (median survival time: 24 months vs 10 months, respectively; $P<.001$). In a multivariate analysis, the FDG PET result was the most powerful and an independent predictive factor of survival.[101] A positive PET, 1 month after HDC, increases the relative risk of death by 5-fold.[101]

SUMMARY

Changes in metabolic activity generally occur earlier than changes in tumor size. The metabolic information provided by PET has been shown to be valuable for the early assessment of the response to NAC, but methodology for image acquisition and analysis needs to be standardized; BC subtype and treatment type need to be considered in interpreting the change in FDG uptake with therapy. Future studies should consider these factors and provide further validation of FDG PET/CT as an early response indicator to support its use as an integral marker in therapeutic trials and as a clinical tool to direct therapy in patients. Moreover, the place of PET in comparison with MR imaging, which is also useful in the early evaluation of NAC, remains to be better determined.[102]

PET/CT is also a powerful method for early assessment of response to treatment in the metastatic setting. An advantage to the use of PET/CT is its ability to evaluate different sites of metastases (except brain metastases) in a single examination. PET/CT is helpful to detect a heterogeneous response (coexistence of responding and nonresponding lesions within the same patient). The use of PET/CT in this indication is hampered by the cost of this imaging, the potential for delaying care, the risk of invasive procedures stimulated by false-positive results, the exposure to ionizing radiation, and the lack of proof that changing treatment early improves patients' survival. Other important limitations for the use of PET/CT are the absence of consensus of the criteria to use to assess the response, of the number of metastatic sites to analyze, and of the optimal date to perform PET during treatment. However, there is evidence that PET/CT performed better than CT alone, especially to assess the response in bone metastases.

REFERENCES

1. Smith IC, Welch AE, Hutcheon AW, et al. Positron emission tomography using [(18)F]-fluorodeoxy-D-glucose to predict the pathologic response of

breast cancer to primary chemotherapy. J Clin Oncol 2000;18:1676–88.

2. Schelling M, Avril N, Nährig J, et al. Positron emission tomography using [(18)F]fluorodeoxyglucose for monitoring primary chemotherapy in breast cancer. J Clin Oncol 2000;18:1689–95.

3. Mankoff DA, Dunnwald LK, Gralow JR, et al. Changes in blood flow and metabolism in locally advanced breast cancer treated with neoadjuvant chemotherapy. J Nucl Med 2003;44:1806–14.

4. Rousseau C, Devillers A, Sagan C, et al. Monitoring of early response to neoadjuvant chemotherapy in stage II and III breast cancer by [18F]fluorodeoxyglucose positron emission tomography. J Clin Oncol 2006;24:5366–72.

5. Berriolo-Riedinger A, Touzery C, Riedinger J-M, et al. [18F]FDG-PET predicts complete pathological response of breast cancer to neoadjuvant chemotherapy. Eur J Nucl Med Mol Imaging 2007;34:1915–24.

6. McDermott GM, Welch A, Staff RT, et al. Monitoring primary breast cancer throughout chemotherapy using FDG-PET. Breast Cancer Res Treat 2007; 102:75–84.

7. Dunnwald LK, Gralow JR, Ellis GK, et al. Tumor metabolism and blood flow changes by positron emission tomography: relation to survival in patients treated with neoadjuvant chemotherapy for locally advanced breast cancer. J Clin Oncol 2008;26:4449–57.

8. Schwarz-Dose J, Untch M, Tiling R, et al. Monitoring primary systemic therapy of large and locally advanced breast cancer by using sequential positron emission tomography imaging with [18F]fluorodeoxyglucose. J Clin Oncol 2009;27:535–41.

9. Kumar A, Kumar R, Seenu V, et al. The role of 18F-FDG PET/CT in evaluation of early response to neoadjuvant chemotherapy in patients with locally advanced breast cancer. Eur Radiol 2009;19:1347–57.

10. Duch J, Fuster D, Muñoz M, et al. 18F-FDG PET/CT for early prediction of response to neoadjuvant chemotherapy in breast cancer. Eur J Nucl Med Mol Imaging 2009;36:1551–7.

11. Schneider-Kolsky ME, Hart S, Fox J, et al. The role of chemotherapeutic drugs in the evaluation of breast tumour response to chemotherapy using serial FDG-PET. Breast Cancer Res 2010;12:R37.

12. Wang Y, Zhang C, Liu J, et al. Is 18F-FDG PET accurate to predict neoadjuvant therapy response in breast cancer? A meta-analysis. Breast Cancer Res Treat 2012;131:357–69.

13. Gennari A, Donati S, Salvadori B, et al. Role of 2-[18F]-fluorodeoxyglucose (FDG) positron emission tomography (PET) in the early assessment of response to chemotherapy in metastatic breast cancer patients. Clin Breast Cancer 2000;1: 156–61 [discussion: 162–3].

14. Stafford SE, Gralow JR, Schubert EK, et al. Use of serial FDG PET to measure the response of bone-dominant breast cancer to therapy. Acad Radiol 2002;9:913–21.

15. Dose Schwarz J, Bader M, Jenicke L, et al. Early prediction of response to chemotherapy in metastatic breast cancer using sequential 18F-FDG PET. J Nucl Med 2005;46:1144–50.

16. Couturier O, Jerusalem G, N'Guyen J-M, et al. Sequential positron emission tomography using [18F]fluorodeoxyglucose for monitoring response to chemotherapy in metastatic breast cancer. Clin Cancer Res 2006;12:6437–43.

17. Specht JM, Tam SL, Kurland BF, et al. Serial 2-[18F] fluoro-2-deoxy-D-glucose positron emission tomography (FDG-PET) to monitor treatment of bone-dominant metastatic breast cancer predicts time to progression (TTP). Breast Cancer Res Treat 2007;105:87–94.

18. Du Y, Cullum I, Illidge TM, et al. Fusion of metabolic function and morphology: sequential [18F]fluorodeoxyglucose positron-emission tomography/computed tomography studies yield new insights into the natural history of bone metastases in breast cancer. J Clin Oncol 2007;25:3440–7.

19. Tateishi U, Gamez C, Dawood S, et al. Bone metastases in patients with metastatic breast cancer: morphologic and metabolic monitoring of response to systemic therapy with integrated PET/CT. Radiology 2008;247:189–96.

20. Huyge V, Garcia C, Alexiou J, et al. Heterogeneity of metabolic response to systemic therapy in metastatic breast cancer patients. Clin Oncol (R Coll Radiol) 2010;22:818–27.

21. Mortazavi-Jehanno N, Giraudet A-L, Champion L, et al. Assessment of response to endocrine therapy using FDG PET/CT in metastatic breast cancer: a pilot study. Eur J Nucl Med Mol Imaging 2012;39:450–60.

22. Mayer IA, Abramson VG, Isakoff SJ, et al. Stand up to cancer phase Ib study of pan-phosphoinositide-3-kinase inhibitor buparlisib with letrozole in estrogen receptor-positive/human epidermal growth factor receptor 2-negative metastatic breast cancer. J Clin Oncol 2014;32:1202–9.

23. Lin NU, Guo H, Yap JT, et al. Phase II study of lapatinib in combination with trastuzumab in patients with human epidermal growth factor receptor 2-positive metastatic breast cancer: clinical outcomes and predictive value of early [18F]fluorodeoxyglucose positron emission tomography imaging (TBCRC 003). J Clin Oncol 2015;33:2623–31.

24. Al-Muqbel KM, Yaghan RJ. Effectiveness of 18F-FDG-PET/CT vs bone scintigraphy in treatment response assessment of bone metastases in breast cancer. Medicine (Baltimore) 2016;95: e3753.

25. Pinker K, Riedl CC, Ong L, et al. The impact that number of analyzed metastatic breast cancer lesions has on response assessment by 18F-FDG PET/CT using PERCIST. J Nucl Med 2016;57: 1102–4.

26. Brown RS, Wahl RL. Overexpression of Glut-1 glucose transporter in human breast cancer. An immunohistochemical study. Cancer 1993;72: 2979–85.

27. Bos R, van Der Hoeven JJM, van Der Wall E, et al. Biologic correlates of (18)fluorodeoxyglucose uptake in human breast cancer measured by positron emission tomography. J Clin Oncol 2002;20: 379–87.

28. Avril N, Rosé CA, Schelling M, et al. Breast imaging with positron emission tomography and fluorine-18 fluorodeoxyglucose: use and limitations. J Clin Oncol 2000;18:3495–502.

29. Gil-Rendo A, Martínez-Regueira F, Zornoza G, et al. Association between [18F]fluorodeoxyglucose uptake and prognostic parameters in breast cancer. Br J Surg 2009;96:166–70.

30. Groheux D, Giacchetti S, Moretti J-L, et al. Correlation of high (18)F-FDG uptake to clinical, pathological and biological prognostic factors in breast cancer. Eur. J Nucl Med Mol Imaging 2011;38: 426–35.

31. Basu S, Chen W, Tchou J, et al. Comparison of triple-negative and estrogen receptor-positive/progesterone receptor-positive/HER2-negative breast carcinoma using quantitative fluorine-18 fluorodeoxyglucose/positron emission tomography imaging parameters: a potentially useful method for disease characterization. Cancer 2008;112: 995–1000.

32. Wahl RL, Jacene H, Kasamon Y, et al. From RECIST to PERCIST: evolving considerations for PET response criteria in solid tumors. J Nucl Med 2009;50(Suppl 1):122S–50S.

33. Daisne J-F, Sibomana M, Bol A, et al. Tri-dimensional automatic segmentation of PET volumes based on measured source-to-background ratios: influence of reconstruction algorithms. Radiother Oncol 2003;69:247–50.

34. Soussan M, Orlhac F, Boubaya M, et al. Relationship between tumor heterogeneity measured on FDG-PET/CT and pathological prognostic factors in invasive breast cancer. PLoS One 2014;9: e94017.

35. Groheux D, Majdoub M, Tixier F, et al. Do clinical, histological or immunohistochemical primary tumour characteristics translate into different (18) F-FDG PET/CT volumetric and heterogeneity features in stage II/III breast cancer? Eur. J Nucl Med Mol Imaging 2015;42:1682–91.

36. Groheux D, Martineau A, Teixeira L, et al. (18)FDG-PET/CT for predicting the outcome in ER+/HER2-

breast cancer patients: comparison of clinicopathological parameters and PET image-derived indices including tumor texture analysis. Breast Cancer Res 2017;19:3.

37. Stahl AR, Heusner TA, Hartung V, et al. Time course of tumor SUV in 18F-FDG PET of breast cancer: presentation of a simple model using a single reference point for time corrections of tumor SUVs. J Nucl Med 2011;52:18–23.

38. Beaulieu S, Kinahan P, Tseng J, et al. SUV varies with time after injection in (18)F-FDG PET of breast cancer: characterization and method to adjust for time differences. J Nucl Med 2003;44: 1044–50.

39. Young H, Baum R, Cremerius U, et al. Measurement of clinical and subclinical tumour response using [18F]-fluorodeoxyglucose and positron emission tomography: review and 1999 EORTC recommendations. European Organization for Research and Treatment of Cancer (EORTC) PET Study Group. Eur J Cancer 1999;35:1773–82.

40. Eisenhauer EA, Therasse P, Bogaerts J, et al. New response evaluation criteria in solid tumours: revised RECIST guideline (version 1.1). Eur J Cancer 2009;45:228–47.

41. Schwartz LH, Litière S, de Vries E, et al. RECIST 1.1-update and clarification: from the RECIST committee. Eur J Cancer 2016;62:132–7.

42. Boellaard R, Delgado-Bolton R, Oyen WJG, et al. FDG PET/CT: EANM procedure guidelines for tumour imaging: version 2.0. Eur J Nucl Med Mol Imaging 2015;42:328–54.

43. Delbeke D, Coleman RE, Guiberteau MJ, et al. Procedure guideline for tumor imaging with 18F-FDG PET/CT 1.0. J Nucl Med 2006;47:885–95.

44. Aide N, Lasnon C, Veit-Haibach P, et al. EANM/EARL harmonization strategies in PET quantification: from daily practice to multicentre oncological studies. Eur J Nucl Med Mol Imaging 2017;44: 17–31.

45. NCCN clinical practice guidelines in oncology. Breast cancer. Version 4. 2017. Available at: http://www.nccn.org/professionals/physician_gls/f_guidelines.asp. Accessed March 03, 2018.

46. Gralow JR, Burstein HJ, Wood W, et al. Preoperative therapy in invasive breast cancer: pathologic assessment and systemic therapy issues in operable disease. J Clin Oncol 2008;26:814–9.

47. Groheux D. Predicting pathological complete response in breast cancer early. Lancet Oncol 2014;15:1415–6.

48. Hindié E, Groheux D. Pathological complete response in breast cancer. Lancet 2015;385:114.

49. Barrington SF, Mikhaeel NG, Kostakoglu L, et al. Role of imaging in the staging and response assessment of lymphoma: consensus of the International Conference on Malignant Lymphomas

Imaging Working Group. J Clin Oncol 2014;32: 3048–58.

50. Bardia A, Baselga J. Neoadjuvant therapy as a platform for drug development and approval in breast cancer. Clin Cancer Res 2013;19:6360–70.

51. Cheng X, Li Y, Liu B, et al. 18F-FDG PET/CT and PET for evaluation of pathological response to neoadjuvant chemotherapy in breast cancer: a meta-analysis. Acta Radiol 2012;53:615–27.

52. Mghanga FP, Lan X, Bakari KH, et al. Fluorine-18 fluorodeoxyglucose positron emission tomography-computed tomography in monitoring the response of breast cancer to neoadjuvant chemotherapy: a meta-analysis. Clin Breast Cancer 2013;13:271–9.

53. Tian F, Shen G, Deng Y, et al. The accuracy of (18)F-FDG PET/CT in predicting the pathological response to neoadjuvant chemotherapy in patients with breast cancer: a meta-analysis and systematic review. Eur Radiol 2017;27(11):4786–96.

54. Liu Q, Wang C, Li P, et al. The role of (18)F-FDG PET/CT and MRI in assessing pathological complete response to neoadjuvant chemotherapy in patients with breast cancer: a systematic review and meta-analysis. Biomed Res Int 2016;2016: 3746232.

55. Tateishi U, Miyake M, Nagaoka T, et al. Neoadjuvant chemotherapy in breast cancer: prediction of pathologic response with PET/CT and dynamic contrast-enhanced MR Imaging–prospective assessment. Radiology 2012;263:53–63.

56. Hatt M, Groheux D, Martineau A, et al. Comparison between 18F-FDG PET image-derived indices for early prediction of response to neoadjuvant chemotherapy in breast cancer. J Nucl Med 2013;54:341–9.

57. Groheux D, Biard L, Giacchetti S, et al. 18F-FDG PET/CT for the early evaluation of response to neoadjuvant treatment in triple-negative breast cancer: influence of the chemotherapy regimen. J Nucl Med 2016;57:536–43.

58. Groheux D, Mankoff D, Espié M, et al. (18)F-FDG PET/CT in the early prediction of pathological response in aggressive subtypes of breast cancer: review of the literature and recommendations for use in clinical trials. Eur J Nucl Med Mol Imaging 2016;43:983–93.

59. Specht JM, Kurland BF, Montgomery SK, et al. Tumor metabolism and blood flow as assessed by positron emission tomography varies by tumor subtype in locally advanced breast cancer. Clin Cancer Res 2010;16:2803–10.

60. Humbert O, Berriolo-Riedinger A, Riedinger JM, et al. Changes in 18F-FDG tumor metabolism after a first course of neoadjuvant chemotherapy in breast cancer: influence of tumor subtypes. Ann Oncol 2012;23:2572–7.

61. Groheux D, Majdoub M, Sanna A, et al. Early metabolic response to neoadjuvant treatment: FDG PET/CT criteria according to breast cancer subtype. Radiology 2015;277:358–71.

62. Groheux D, Giacchetti S, Espié M, et al. Early monitoring of response to neoadjuvant chemotherapy in breast cancer with (18)F-FDG PET/CT: defining a clinical aim. Eur. J Nucl Med Mol Imaging 2011; 38:419–25.

63. Carey LA, Dees EC, Sawyer L, et al. The triple negative paradox: primary tumor chemosensitivity of breast cancer subtypes. Clin Cancer Res 2007;13:2329–34.

64. Untch M, Fasching PA, Konecny GE, et al. Pathologic complete response after neoadjuvant chemotherapy plus trastuzumab predicts favorable survival in human epidermal growth factor receptor 2-overexpressing breast cancer: results from the TECHNO trial of the AGO and GBG study groups. J Clin Oncol 2011;29:3351–7.

65. Cortazar P, Zhang L, Untch M, et al. Pathological complete response and long-term clinical benefit in breast cancer: the CTNeoBC pooled analysis. Lancet 2014;384:164–72.

66. Groheux D, Hindié E, Giacchetti S, et al. Triple-negative breast cancer: early assessment with 18F-FDG PET/CT during neoadjuvant chemotherapy identifies patients who are unlikely to achieve a pathologic complete response and are at a high risk of early relapse. J Nucl Med 2012; 53:249–54.

67. Zucchini G, Quercia S, Zamagni C, et al. Potential utility of early metabolic response by 18F-2-fluoro-2-deoxy-D-glucose-positron emission tomography/computed tomography in a selected group of breast cancer patients receiving preoperative chemotherapy. Eur J Cancer 2013;49:1539–45.

68. Koolen BB, Pengel KE, Wesseling J, et al. FDG PET/CT during neoadjuvant chemotherapy may predict response in ER-positive/HER2-negative and triple negative, but not in HER2-positive breast cancer. Breast 2013;22:691–7.

69. Koolen BB, Pengel KE, Wesseling J, et al. Sequential (18)F-FDG PET/CT for early prediction of complete pathological response in breast and axilla during neoadjuvant chemotherapy. Eur J Nucl Med Mol Imaging 2014;41:32–40.

70. Groheux D, Hindié E, Giacchetti S, et al. Early assessment with 18F-fluorodeoxyglucose positron emission tomography/computed tomography can help predict the outcome of neoadjuvant chemotherapy in triple negative breast cancer. Eur J Cancer 2014;50:1864–71.

71. Connolly RM, Leal JP, Goetz MP, et al. TBCRC 008: early change in 18F-FDG uptake on PET predicts response to preoperative systemic therapy in human epidermal growth factor receptor 2-negative

primary operable breast cancer. J Nucl Med 2015; 56:31–7.

72. Humbert O, Riedinger J-M, Charon-Barra C, et al. Identification of biomarkers including 18FDG-PET/CT for early prediction of response to neoadjuvant chemotherapy in triple negative breast cancer. Clin Cancer Res 2015;21:5460–8.

73. Humbert O, Riedinger J-M, Vrigneaud J-M, et al. 18F-FDG PET-derived tumor blood flow changes after 1 cycle of neoadjuvant chemotherapy predicts outcome in triple-negative breast cancer. J Nucl Med 2016;57:1707–12.

74. Baselga J, Bradbury I, Eidtmann H, et al. Lapatinib with trastuzumab for HER2-positive early breast cancer (NeoALTTO): a randomised, open-label, multicentre, phase 3 trial. Lancet 2012;379:633–40.

75. Gianni L, Pienkowski T, Im Y-H, et al. Efficacy and safety of neoadjuvant pertuzumab and trastuzumab in women with locally advanced, inflammatory, or early HER2-positive breast cancer (NeoSphere): a randomised multicentre, open-label, phase 2 trial. Lancet Oncol 2012;13:25–32.

76. Martoni AA, Zamagni C, Quercia S, et al. Early (18) F-2-fluoro-2-deoxy-d-glucose positron emission tomography may identify a subset of patients with estrogen receptor-positive breast cancer who will not respond optimally to preoperative chemotherapy. Cancer 2010;116:805–13.

77. Groheux D, Giacchetti S, Hatt M, et al. HER2-over-expressing breast cancer: FDG uptake after two cycles of chemotherapy predicts the outcome of neoadjuvant treatment. Br J Cancer 2013;109: 1157–64.

78. Gebhart G, Gámez C, Holmes E, et al. 18F-FDG PET/CT for early prediction of response to neoadjuvant lapatinib, trastuzumab, and their combination in HER2-positive breast cancer: results from NeoALTTO. J Nucl Med 2013;54:1862–8.

79. Humbert O, Cochet A, Riedinger J-M, et al. HER2-positive breast cancer: ^{18}F-FDG PET for early prediction of response to trastuzumab plus taxane-based neoadjuvant chemotherapy. Eur J Nucl Med Mol Imaging 2014;41:1525–33.

80. Coudert B, Pierga J-Y, Mouret-Reynier M-A, et al. Use of [(18)F]-FDG PET to predict response to neoadjuvant trastuzumab and docetaxel in patients with HER2-positive breast cancer, and addition of bevacizumab to neoadjuvant trastuzumab and docetaxel in [(18)F]-FDG PET-predicted non-responders (AVATAXHER): an open-label, randomised phase 2 trial. Lancet Oncol 2014;15: 1493–502.

81. Cheng J, Wang Y, Mo M, et al. 18F-fluorodeoxyglucose (FDG) PET/CT after two cycles of neoadjuvant therapy may predict response in HER2-negative, but not in HER2-positive breast cancer. Oncotarget 2015;6(30):29388–95.

82. Groheux D, Hatt M, Hindié E, et al. Estrogen receptor-positive/human epidermal growth factor receptor 2-negative breast tumors: early prediction of chemosensitivity with (18) F-fluorodeoxyglucose positron emission tomography/computed tomography during neoadjuvant chemotherapy. Cancer 2013;119:1960–8.

83. Groheux D, Sanna A, Majdoub M, et al. Baseline tumor 18F-FDG uptake and modifications after 2 cycles of neoadjuvant chemotherapy are prognostic of outcome in ER+/HER2- breast cancer. J Nucl Med 2015;56:824–31.

84. Ahn SG, Lee M, Jeon TJ, et al. [18F]-fluorodeoxyglucose positron emission tomography can contribute to discriminate patients with poor prognosis in hormone receptor-positive breast cancer. PLoS One 2014;9:e105905.

85. Aogi K, Kadoya T, Sugawara Y, et al. Utility of (18)F FDG-PET/CT for predicting prognosis of luminal-type breast cancer. Breast Cancer Res Treat 2015;150:209–17.

86. Humbert O, Berriolo-Riedinger A, Cochet A, et al. Prognostic relevance at 5 years of the early monitoring of neoadjuvant chemotherapy using (18)F-FDG PET in luminal HER2-negative breast cancer. Eur J Nucl Med Mol Imaging 2014;41:416–27.

87. Doot RK, Dunnwald LK, Schubert EK, et al. Dynamic and static approaches to quantifying 18F-FDG uptake for measuring cancer response to therapy, including the effect of granulocyte CSF. J Nucl Med 2007;48:920–5.

88. Therasse P, Arbuck SG, Eisenhauer EA, et al. New guidelines to evaluate the response to treatment in solid tumors. European Organization for Research and Treatment of Cancer, National Cancer Institute of the United States, National Cancer Institute of Canada. J Natl Cancer Inst 2000;92: 205–16.

89. Groheux D, Espié M, Giacchetti S, et al. Performance of FDG PET/CT in the clinical management of breast cancer. Radiology 2013;266: 388–405.

90. Riedl CC, Pinker K, Ulaner GA, et al. Comparison of FDG-PET/CT and contrast-enhanced CT for monitoring therapy response in patients with metastatic breast cancer. Eur J Nucl Med Mol Imaging 2017; 44(9):1428–37.

91. Coleman RE. Clinical features of metastatic bone disease and risk of skeletal morbidity. Clin Cancer Res 2006;12:6243s–9s.

92. Nakai T, Okuyama C, Kubota T, et al. Pitfalls of FDG-PET for the diagnosis of osteoblastic bone metastases in patients with breast cancer. Eur J Nucl Med Mol Imaging 2005;32:1253–8.

93. Schirrmeister H. Detection of bone metastases in breast cancer by positron emission tomography. Radiol Clin North Am 2007;45:669–76, vi.

94. Morris PG, Lynch C, Feeney JN, et al. Integrated positron emission tomography/computed tomography may render bone scintigraphy unnecessary to investigate suspected metastatic breast cancer. J Clin Oncol 2010;28:3154–9.

95. Groheux D, Hindié E, Delord M, et al. Prognostic impact of 18FDG-PET-CT findings in clinical stage III and IIB breast cancer. J Natl Cancer Inst 2012; 104:1879–87.

96. Quon A, Gambhir SS. FDG-PET and beyond: molecular breast cancer imaging. J Clin Oncol 2005; 23:1664–73.

97. Mortimer JE, Dehdashti F, Siegel BA, et al. Metabolic flare: indicator of hormone responsiveness in advanced breast cancer. J Clin Oncol 2001;19: 2797–803.

98. Dehdashti F, Mortimer JE, Trinkaus K, et al. PET-based estradiol challenge as a predictive biomarker of response to endocrine therapy in women with estrogen-receptor-positive breast cancer. Breast Cancer Res Treat 2009;113:509–17.

99. Morris PG, Ulaner GA, Eaton A, et al. Standardized uptake value by positron emission tomography/computed tomography as a prognostic variable in metastatic breast cancer. Cancer 2012;118:5454–62.

100. Ulaner GA, Eaton A, Morris PG, et al. Prognostic value of quantitative fluorodeoxyglucose measurements in newly diagnosed metastatic breast cancer. Cancer Med 2013;2:725–33.

101. Cachin F, Prince HM, Hogg A, et al. Powerful prognostic stratification by [18F]fluorodeoxyglucose positron emission tomography in patients with metastatic breast cancer treated with high-dose chemotherapy. J Clin Oncol 2006;24:3026–31.

102. Loo CE, Straver ME, Rodenhuis S, et al. Magnetic resonance imaging response monitoring of breast cancer during neoadjuvant chemotherapy: relevance of breast cancer subtype. J Clin Oncol 2011;29:660–6.

Section 3: Innovative Radiotracers for Molecular Imaging of Breast Cancer

Clinical Potential of Estrogen and Progesterone Receptor Imaging

Hannah M. Linden, MD[a], Lanell M. Peterson, BA[a],*,
Amy M. Fowler, MD, PhD[b]

KEYWORDS

- FES-PET • FFNP-PET • Estrogen receptor imaging • Progesterone receptor imaging
- Breast cancer

KEY POINTS

- 16α-[^{18}F]fluoro-17β-estradiol (FES)–PET is likely to become clinically available to predict the clinical benefit from endocrine therapy given alone or in combination with new cyclin-dependent kinase 4/6 inhibitors.
- FES-PET could help predict the therapy response at multiple points in time along the course of treatment when endocrine resistance may arise.
- FES-PET could be used for pharmacodynamic imaging to help develop new ER antagonist drug therapies.
- FES-PET can identify tumor heterogeneity and may facilitate selection of the optimal biopsy site or confirm metastatic diagnosis if biopsy is not possible.
- Progesterone receptor imaging is being investigated as a method to measure the response to therapy after endocrine therapy or early response to antiestrogen therapy.

INTRODUCTION

Most breast cancers diagnosed are estrogen receptor (ER) and progesterone receptor (PR) positive, and early outcomes are better across all stages compared with ER-, PR- disease.[1] Advances in endocrine therapy show improved outcomes for patients with ER+ tumors.[2–7] Interestingly, despite the promise of molecularly targeted therapies, ER expression is the only established biomarker of the response to cyclin-dependent kinase 4/6 inhibitors.[8] It is not uncommon for patients with ER+ tumors to have late recurrences or indolent disease several years after diagnosis or present with de novo metastatic disease.[9,10] The most common site of metastases is the bone, where biopsies may be challenging to obtain and the response is difficult to measure by current clinical imaging.[11–13]

PET with ^{18}F-radiolabeled steroid hormones can be used to image tumoral expression of ER and PR in patients with primary and metastatic breast cancer. These radiotracers include 16α-[^{18}F]fluoro-17β-estradiol (FES) for ER imaging and ^{18}F-fluoro-furanyl-norprogesterone (FFNP) for PR imaging.

Disclosure statement: The authors have nothing to disclose.
This work was supported, in part, by NCI/NIH (P01CA42045, R01CA72064, R01CA148131, P30CA015704, P30CA047904, KL2TR000428), NIH/CIP N01CM-37008, Susan G Komen SAC140060, DOD W81XWH-04010675, and the Mary Kay Ash Foundation 053-08 NIH KL2TR000428.
[a] Department of Medical Oncology, Seattle Cancer Care Alliance, UWMC, 825 Eastlake Avenue East, Valley Building LV-200, Seattle, WA 98109-1023, USA; [b] Department of Radiology, University of Wisconsin, School of Medicine and Public Health, E3/366 Clinical Science Center, 600 Highland Avenue, Madison, WI 53792-3252, USA
* Corresponding author.
E-mail address: lanell@uw.edu

Tumor uptake from FES-PET imaging has been proven to correlate with ER protein[14,15] demonstrating the functional presence of ER. Likewise, FFNP uptake as measured by tumor-to-normal breast tissue ratios has been shown to be greater in PR+ breast cancers compared with PR− cancers.[16] FES- and FFNP-PET can be used to both qualitatively and quantitatively measure uptake from all metastatic sites at the same time through whole-body scanning. These molecular imaging agents may also be used in conjunction with dedicated high-resolution PET systems for breast imaging or simultaneous breast PET/MR imaging to better depict primary ER+ tumor biology and assess changes in receptor expression through preoperative window-of-opportunity drug trials.

As new endocrine therapies and novel biologics are introduced into clinic practices, better strategies are needed to individualize therapy. In this article, the authors review the research of the most commonly used PET tracer for ER, FES, and FFNP for PR imaging and their potential use in a clinical setting. For FES, the past studies include use to predict the response to endocrine therapy as a biomarker in pharmacodynamics imaging, as means to help develop ER antagonist therapy, and to identify tumor heterogeneity. Several current and upcoming trials are discussed for their potential to contribute to the promising future of using ER and PR imaging in the clinical setting.

16α-[¹⁸F]FLUORO-17β-ESTRADIOL PREDICTS RESPONSE TO ENDOCRINE THERAPY

Perhaps the most impactful use of FES-PET imaging in the clinic will be the ability to predict the effectiveness of endocrine therapy. Approximately 30% of patients with breast cancer develop tumor regression with initial endocrine therapy, and only 20% have stable disease.[17] Second- and third-line therapies are available; however, the ability to measure ER expression in all tumor sites can ultimately influence treatment decisions, especially if there is substantial heterogeneity between tumor sites. Several groups have shown that FES predicts whether patients will experience a clinical benefit with ER-directed therapies in first-line and later-line treatment.[18–21] Clinical benefit, defined as stable disease, partial response, or complete response, is clinically meaningful and a logical end point in ER+ breast cancer, whereby indolent disease does not usually show measurable tumor shrinkage. Although these data, from single centers, are convincing and clinically relevant, a multicenter trial is ongoing to confirm these single-center results.

Another study tested the ability of FES-PET to predict the response to salvage aromatase inhibitor treatment in 47 patients with heavily pretreated metastatic breast cancer with ER+ primary tumors. Treatment selection based on quantitative FES-PET and a maximum standardized uptake value (SUV$_{max}$) cutoff of 1.5 would have increased the rate of response from 23% to 34% overall and from 29% to 46% in the subset of patients with HER2− disease.[20] This study found that quantitative FES-PET provides additional information over conventional clinical criteria to predict the response to hormonal therapy in the challenging situation of patients who have received multiple prior lines of therapy.

16α-[¹⁸F]FLUORO-17β-ESTRADIOL AND FLUORODEOXYGLUCOSE PET PROVIDE PROGNOSTIC INFORMATION

Like ER expression measured using immunohistochemistry, FES-PET imaging has the potential to provide prognostic information. Kurland and colleagues[7] evaluated progression-free survival (PFS) in 84 patients with ER+/HER2− breast cancer receiving endocrine therapy and lesion uptake from fluorodeoxyglucose (FDG) and FES-PET. Patients were stratified into 3 response groups: patients with low FDG uptake (suggesting indolent disease) (29%; 24 of 84), FDG-avid tumors with high FES uptake (59%; 50 of 84), and FDG-avid tumors with low FES uptake (12%; 10 of 84). The median PFS in these groups was 26.1 months (95% confidence interval [CI]: 11.2–49.7 months), 7.9 months (95% CI: 5.6–11.8), and 3.3 months (95% CI: 1.4–not evaluable), respectively. **Fig. 1** shows images of representative cases from 3 classification groups: (**Fig. 1**A) low FDG lean body mass corrected standardized uptake value (SUL) SUL-max3, (**Fig. 1**B) high FDG SULmax3 and low FES SULmean3, and (**Fig. 1**C) high FDG SULmax3 and high FES SULmean3. This study suggested that FDG PET and FES-PET may help provide important prognostic information by identifying patients with indolent disease and aid in deciding when to select targeted and/or cytotoxic chemotherapy.[7]

ESTROGEN RECEPTOR AS A BIOMARKER IN PHARMACODYNAMIC IMAGING

PET imaging also has a unique role in pharmacodynamics, the study of biochemical and physiologic effects of a drug on the body. Serial imaging of ER can provide a noninvasive assessment of the effective dosing and delivery of a drug at early time points. In recent studies, FES-PET imaging has been shown to be a

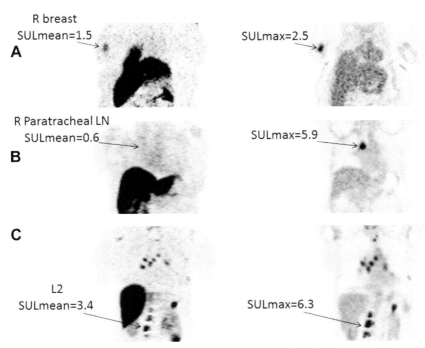

R breast
SULmean=1.5

A

SULmax=2.5

R Paratracheal LN
SULmean=0.6

B

SULmax=5.9

C

L2
SULmean=3.4

SULmax=6.3

Fig. 1. Representative cases for the 3 classification groups. Coronal view from FES-PET and FDG PET scans. Ordered subset expectation maximization (OSEM) reconstruction was used for improved presentation but not for quantitation. (*A*) Low FDG SULmax3. This 56-year-old woman had 4 lesions in her breast and lymph nodes. Geometric mean FDG SULmax for the 3 hottest lesions was 1.5 (geometric mean FES SULmean was 1.1). She was treated with an aromatase inhibitor for 5 months until progression. (*B*) High FDG SULmax3 and low FES SULmean3. This 59-year-old woman had 5 lesions in lymph nodes and spine. Geometric mean FDG SULmax for the 3 hottest lesions was 4.4. Geometric mean FES SULmean3 was 0.3. She was on tamoxifen for 3 months until progression. (*C*) High FDG SULmax3 and high FES SULmean3. This 59-year-old woman had lesions in the breast, chest wall, and hilar nodes as well as multiple bony lesions, including lumbar spine (L2). Geometric mean FDG SULmax for the 3 hottest lesions was 12.7. Geometric mean FES SULmean was 6.6. She was on exemestane for 9.5 months until progression. LN, lymph node; R, right. (*From* Kurland BF, Peterson LM, Lee JH, et al. Estrogen receptor binding [18F-FES PET] and glycolytic activity [18F-FDG PET] predict progression-free survival on endocrine therapy in patients with ER + breast cancer. Clin Cancer Res 2017;23:413; with permission.)

pharmacodynamic biomarker for ER-directed therapy. In a study by Lin and colleagues,[22] 15 patients with refractory ER+ metastatic disease were imaged with FES-PET at baseline; 8 of those patients were imaged again 1 to 5 days after administration of Z-endoxifen (a metabolite of tamoxifen). Decreases in SUV_{max} were observed (*P* = .0078) as early as 1 day after the drug was administered. Earlier studies, such as the study of metabolic flare as an indicator of hormone responsiveness,[18] concluded that the functional status of tumor ER could be predictive of tamoxifen therapy 7 to 10 days after the start of treatment in patients with advanced ER+ breast cancer. In a study by Linden and colleagues,[23] imaging revealed significant differences between agents, including differences in the efficacy of blockade by different ER antagonists. **Fig. 2** shows images from that study. In the clinical setting, the use of FES-PET could be used to test ER blockade, both quantitatively

and qualitatively, as an indicator that the drug is reaching the correct target. In addition, pharmacodynamic imaging of ER can be used to optimize drug dose and timing and whether or not complete blockade is necessary for drug effectiveness.

16α-[¹⁸F]FLUORO-17β-ESTRADIOL CAN BE USED TO HELP DEVELOP NOVEL ESTROGEN RECEPTOR ANTAGONIST THERAPY

In a recent phase I dose-escalation trial, Wang and colleagues[24] showed that FES-PET/computed tomography (CT) was a useful biomarker of ER occupancy and/or downregulation and helped optimize the dosage of the novel ER antagonist/degrader (GDC-0810) for future phase II trials. In that study, 30 patients with ER+ metastatic breast cancer underwent 2 FES-PET/CT scans, one before therapy and one at cycle 2 (day 3) of the GDC-0810 therapy. Up to 5 lesions were evaluated, and complete ER suppression was defined as a 90% or greater

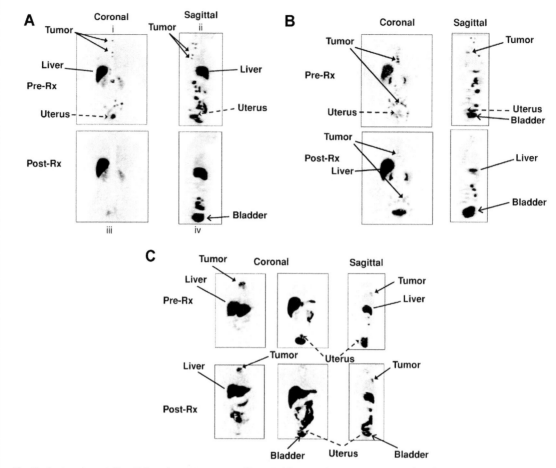

Fig. 2. Pretreatment (Pre-Rx) and posttreatment (Post-Rx) images in patients treated with ER blocking (*A,* tamoxifen; *B,* fulvestrant) and estrogen-lowering therapies (*C,* aromatase inhibitor). Top, coronal (*i*) and sagittal (*ii*) views pretreatment, and bottom panels show the same patient following treatment with coronal (*iii*) and sagittal views (*iv*). Tumor is shown with a solid arrow, uterus is shown with a dashed arrow. Liver (with diffuse uptake because of metabolism of FES) is shown with a (*thin line*), and the bladder is denoted by a (*thin arrow*). Tumor in the upper spine shows complete ER blockade. Tumor in mediastinal nodes shows incomplete ER blockade. Sternal tumor shows no blockade. (*From* Linden HM, Kurland BF, Peterson LM, et al. Fluoroestradiol positron emission tomography reveals differences in pharmacodynamics of aromatase inhibitors, tamoxifen, and fulvestrant in patients with metastatic breast cancer. Clin Cancer Res 2011;17:4802; with permission.)

decrease in the aggregate background-corrected FES SUV$_{max}$. Twenty-four patients (80%) achieved complete ER suppression. Thus, FES-PET imaging seems useful in evaluating novel ER antagonist therapies by determining the optimal dose needed to suppress ER while reducing dose-related drug toxicities.

16α-[^{18}F]FLUORO-17β-ESTRADIOL CAN BE USED TO IDENTIFY TUMOR HETEROGENEITY

Biopsy of a single metastatic site is indicated to confirm the diagnosis at the time of metastatic presentation, but the heterogeneity of ER/PR expression across all metastatic tumor sites may indicate a need for change in therapy. However, it is not feasible to biopsy all metastatic tumor sites. Furthermore, many clinical trials require biopsy before treatment to study relevant biomarkers. The authors recently reviewed ER and HER2 expression from prior evaluations of site-to-site tumor heterogeneity within patients imaged with FES-PET from 3 different studies. Of 46 patients, 6 (13%) had at least one ER-metastatic biopsy. One (2%) biopsy changed from ER+/HER2− to ER−/HER2+, and one (2%) biopsy changed from ER+/HER2+ to ER+/HER2−. Although the FDG PET or CT scan helped guide the selection of the biopsy site, the FES results correlated with each biopsy finding. Biopsy findings resulted in changes in clinical management due to change in ER/HER2 status; 3 patients were given another type of endocrine therapy, 1 patient was treated with

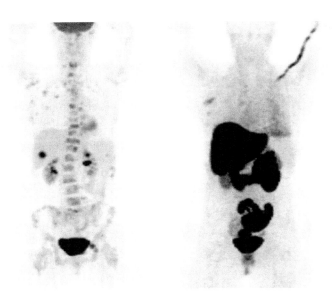

Fig. 3. A 57-year-old woman with documented de novo metastatic invasive ductal carcinoma. The primary breast tumor was ER+. FDG PET scan showed multiple lesions with intense uptake. FES-PET showed uptake in the right axilla but not in the bone lesions. Based on an ER biopsy of the liver, the patient was switched from fulvestrant to pertuzumab, trastuzumab, and paclitaxel.

surgery, and 2 patients were switched to chemotherapy plus biologics.[25] **Fig. 3** is an example of one of the patients who switched from endocrine therapy to chemotherapy after a liver biopsy. These results are consistent with pathology studies whereby receptor discordance was found in approximately 15% of metastatic lesions compared with primary lesions.[26,27] In another case report study, temporal heterogeneity was seen in serial FES scans in a patient who was imaged at 4 time points: before initiation of endocrine therapy, after response to endocrine therapy, at subsequent disease progression on endocrine therapy, and at disease progression on chemotherapy (**Fig. 4**). This study indicated an increase in the tumor's capability to bind estradiol at the time of disease progression on chemotherapy, signifying increased ER expression.[28]

PROGESTERONE IMAGING WITH 18F-FLUORO-FURANYL-NORPROGESTERONE MAY MEASURE RESPONSE TO THERAPY AFTER ENDOCRINE THERAPY OR EARLY RESPONSE TO ANTIESTROGEN THERAPY

As discussed earlier, measuring decreases in FES uptake after initiation of ER antagonist therapy (eg, tamoxifen, fulvestrant) can confirm that the drug hit the target appropriately because this reflects preferential occupancy of the receptor ligand binding pocket by the antagonist rather than FES. Antagonist binding to the receptor, however, does not guarantee that ER transcriptional function will be completely inhibited, particularly in situations of *ESR1* gene mutations.[29] This fact has prompted investigations into imaging estrogen-regulated target genes downstream of ER binding

as a method for functionally monitoring the therapy response. PR is a classic estrogen-regulated ER target gene. There are few clinical studies using progestin-based radioligands for PR imaging.[16,30] FFNP is the most commonly used PET agent for PR imaging, notably used in a first-in-human study to identify PR+ breast cancer[16] and in preclinical studies to predict the response to both fulvestrant therapy[31] and estrogen-deprivation therapy.[32] The clinical potential of PR PET imaging is likely to focus on the response to therapy after endocrine therapy or early response to antiestrogen therapy.

CURRENT AND UPCOMING CLINICAL TRIALS

Eighteen studies using FES-PET are currently listed in clinicaltrials.gov as of September 2017. Seven studies are currently enrolling patients. All of the studies currently enrolling patients include using FES-PET to measure ER status in patients with metastatic breast cancer, and one of the studies also allows patients with ER+ primary breast cancer. The outcomes include determining ER status, predicting the response to therapy, and using FES-PET to guide fulvestrant therapy. There is only one multicenter study (NCT02398773) currently recruiting patients. The primary objective of the study is to determine the negative predictive value (NPV) of FES uptake for clinical benefit of endocrine therapy at 6 months. Secondary study aims are to determine the test-retest reproducibility of quantitative assessment of tumor FES uptake by SUVs; evaluate the accuracy of FES PET for predicting the response in patients treated with first-line endocrine therapy for metastatic breast cancer;

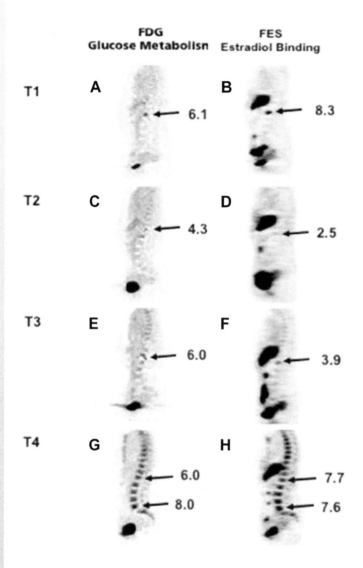

FDG
Glucose Metabolism

FES
Estradiol Binding

T1 — A ← 6.1   B ← 8.3

T2 — C ← 4.3   D ← 2.5

T3 — E ← 6.0   F ← 3.9

T4 — G ← 6.0   H ← 7.7
         ← 8.0   ← 7.6

Fig. 4. (*A, C, E*) FDG and FES-PET images at 4 time points. T1 (*A, B*): before initiation of endocrine therapy; T2 (*C, D*) after response to endocrine therapy; T3 (*E, F*): at subsequent disease progression on endocrine therapy; and T4 (*G, H*): at disease progression on chemotherapy. These quantitative changes in FES SUV suggested an increase in the tumor's capability to bind estradiol at the time of disease progression on chemotherapy, suggesting increased ER expression. (*From* Currin E, Peterson LM, Schubert EK, et al. Temporal heterogeneity of estrogen receptor expression in bone-dominant breast cancer: 18F-fluoroestradiol PET imaging shows return of ER expression. J Natl Compr Canc Netw 2016;14:145; with permission.)

evaluate the accuracy of FES-PET for predicting PFS in patients treated with first-line endocrine therapy for metastatic breast cancer; and evaluate FES SUV$_{max}$ less than 1.5 as the optimal cut point for predicting PFS to first-line endocrine therapy for metastatic breast cancer.

For FFNP-PET imaging, there are 2 studies listed in clinicaltrials.gov that are currently recruiting patients. One study (NCT02455453) aims to determine if changes in FFNP uptake measured using PET/CT in postmenopausal patients with metastatic ER+ breast cancer after 1 day of estradiol administration (estrogen challenge) predicts the response to endocrine therapy. The other study (NCT03212170) aims to compare FFNP uptake measured using PET/MR imaging in patients with newly diagnosed primary breast cancer with PR immunohistochemistry to determine the accuracy of this approach for subsequent studies investigating its predictive value for neoadjuvant endocrine therapy response.

SUMMARY

Steroid hormone receptor imaging provides a virtual assessment of receptor binding at multiple tumor sites and can identify tumor heterogeneity. There are encouraging data from many centers to suggest clinical utility of imaging to help clinicians select treatment and aid in drug development. Studies are underway to bring these tracers closer to clinical use, in a field of endocrine therapy that remains an area of growth and improvement in patient outcomes. One impactful goal of imaging is to guide patients toward the most effective and least toxic therapies in this era of precision medicine.

REFERENCES

1. Jemal A, Ward EM, Johnson CJ, et al. Annual report to the nation on the status of cancer, 1975-2014, featuring survival. J Natl Cancer Inst 2017;109(9):1–22.
2. Ellis MJ, Llombart-Cussac A, Feltl D, et al. Fulvestrant 500 mg versus anastrozole 1 mg for the first-line treatment of advanced breast cancer: overall survival analysis from the phase II FIRST study. J Clin Oncol 2015;33:3781–7.
3. Mehta RS, Barlow WE, Albain KS, et al. Combination anastrozole and fulvestrant in metastatic breast cancer. N Engl J Med 2012;367:435–44.
4. Baselga J, Campone M, Piccart M, et al. Everolimus in postmenopausal hormone-receptor-positive advanced breast cancer. N Engl J Med 2012;366:520–9.
5. Jordan VC. Endoxifen: the end, or are we at the beginning? J Clin Oncol 2017;35(30):3378–9.
6. Finn RS, Crown JP, Lang I, et al. The cyclin-dependent kinase 4/6 inhibitor palbociclib in combination with letrozole versus letrozole alone as first-line treatment of oestrogen receptor-positive, HER2-negative, advanced breast cancer (PALOMA-1/TRIO-18): a randomised phase 2 study. Lancet Oncol 2015;16:25–35.
7. Kurland BF, Peterson LM, Lee JH, et al. Estrogen receptor binding (18F-FES PET) and glycolytic activity (18F-FDG PET) predict progression-free survival on endocrine therapy in patients with ER+ breast cancer. Clin Cancer Res 2017;23:407–15.
8. Ingham M, Schwartz GK. Cell-cycle therapeutics come of age. J Clin Oncol 2017;35:2949–59.
9. Jatoi I, Anderson WF, Jeong JH, et al. Breast cancer adjuvant therapy: time to consider its time-dependent effects. J Clin Oncol 2011;29:2301–4.
10. Lim E, Metzger-Filho O, Winer EP. The natural history of hormone receptor-positive breast cancer. Oncology (Williston Park) 2012;26:688–94, 696.
11. Collignon J, Gennigens C, Jerusalem G. Assessment of response to therapy for bone metastases: is it still a challenge in oncology? PET Clin 2010;5: 311–26.
12. Cook GJ, Azad GK, Goh V. Imaging bone metastases in breast cancer: staging and response assessment. J Nucl Med 2016;57(Suppl 1):27S–33S.
13. Woolf DK, Padhani AR, Makris A. Assessing response to treatment of bone metastases from breast cancer: what should be the standard of care? Ann Oncol 2015;26:1048–57.
14. Mintun MA, Welch MJ, Siegel BA, et al. Breast cancer: PET imaging of estrogen receptors. Radiology 1988;169:45–8.
15. Peterson LM, Mankoff DA, Lawton T, et al. Quantitative imaging of estrogen receptor expression in breast cancer with PET and 18F-fluoroestradiol. J Nucl Med 2008;49:367–74.

16. Dehdashti F, Laforest R, Gao F, et al. Assessment of progesterone receptors in breast carcinoma by PET with 21-18F-fluoro-16alpha,17alpha-[(R)-(1'-alpha-furylmethylidene)dioxy]-19-norpregn- 4-ene-3,20-dione. J Nucl Med 2012;53:363–70.
17. Osborne CK, Schiff R. Mechanisms of endocrine resistance in breast cancer. Annu Rev Med 2011; 62:233–47.
18. Mortimer JE, Dehdashti F, Siegel BA, et al. Metabolic flare: indicator of hormone responsiveness in advanced breast cancer. J Clin Oncol 2001;19: 2797–803.
19. Peterson LM, Kurland BF, Schubert EK, et al. A phase 2 study of 16alpha-[18F]-fluoro-17beta-estradiol positron emission tomography (FES-PET) as a marker of hormone sensitivity in metastatic breast cancer (MBC). Mol Imaging Biol 2014;16:431–40.
20. Linden HM, Stekhova SA, Link JM, et al. Quantitative fluoroestradiol positron emission tomography imaging predicts response to endocrine treatment in breast cancer. J Clin Oncol 2006;24:2793–9.
21. van Kruchten M, Glaudemans AW, de Vries EF, et al. Positron emission tomography of tumour [(18)F]fluoroestradiol uptake in patients with acquired hormone-resistant metastatic breast cancer prior to oestradiol therapy. Eur J Nucl Med Mol Imaging 2015;42:1674–81.
22. Lin FI, Gonzalez EM, Kummar S, et al. Utility of 18F-fluoroestradiol (18F-FES) PET/CT imaging as a pharmacodynamic marker in patients with refractory estrogen receptor-positive solid tumors receiving Z-endoxifen therapy. Eur J Nucl Med Mol Imaging 2017;44:500–8.
23. Linden HM, Kurland BF, Peterson LM, et al. Fluoroestradiol positron emission tomography reveals differences in pharmacodynamics of aromatase inhibitors, tamoxifen, and fulvestrant in patients with metastatic breast cancer. Clin Cancer Res 2011; 17:4799–805.
24. Wang Y, Ayres KL, Goldman DA, et al. 18F-fluoroestradiol PET/CT measurement of estrogen receptor suppression during a phase I trial of the novel estrogen receptor-targeted therapeutic GDC-0810: using an imaging biomarker to guide drug dosage in subsequent trials. Clin Cancer Res 2017;23:3053–60.
25. Peterson LM, Kurland BF, Romine P, et al. The uses of 18F-fluoroestradial (FES) PET with and without 18F-fluorodeoxyglucose (FDG) PET in breast cancer evaluation. Chicago: ASCO; 2017.
26. Karagoz Ozen DS, Ozturk MA, Aydin O, et al. Receptor expression discrepancy between primary and metastatic breast cancer lesions. Oncol Res Treat 2014;37:622–6.
27. Qu Q, Zong Y, Fei XC, et al. The importance of biopsy in clinically diagnosed metastatic lesions in patients with breast cancer. World J Surg Oncol 2014; 12:93.

28. Currin E, Peterson LM, Schubert EK, et al. Temporal heterogeneity of estrogen receptor expression in bone-dominant breast cancer: 18F-fluoroestradiol PET imaging shows return of ER expression. J Natl Compr Canc Netw 2016;14:144–7.

29. Jeselsohn R, Yelensky R, Buchwalter G, et al. Emergence of constitutively active estrogen receptor-alpha mutations in pretreated advanced estrogen receptor-positive breast cancer. Clin Cancer Res 2014;20:1757–67.

30. Dehdashti F, McGuire AH, Van Brocklin HF, et al. Assessment of 21-[18F]fluoro-16 alpha-ethyl-19-norprogesterone as a positron-emitting radiopharmaceutical for the detection of progestin receptors in human breast carcinomas. J Nucl Med 1991;32:1532–7.

31. Fowler AM, Chan SR, Sharp TL, et al. Small-animal PET of steroid hormone receptors predicts tumor response to endocrine therapy using a preclinical model of breast cancer. J Nucl Med. 2012;53:1119–26.

32. Chan SR, Fowler AM, Allen JA, et al. Longitudinal noninvasive imaging of progesterone receptor as a predictive biomarker of tumor responsiveness to estrogen deprivation therapy. Clin Cancer Res 2015;21:1063–70.

Clinical Potential of Human Epidermal Growth Factor Receptor 2 and Human Epidermal Growth Factor Receptor 3 Imaging in Breast Cancer

Kelly E. Henry, PhD[a],*, Gary A. Ulaner, MD, PhD[a,b], Jason S. Lewis, PhD[a,b,c,d,e]

KEYWORDS

• PET • SPECT • CT • Radiotracers • HER2 • HER3 • Metastasis • Breast cancer

KEY POINTS

- The human epidermal growth factor receptor (HER) family members are of increasing interest to target by small molecules, affibody moieties, and monoclonal antibodies.
- Imaging can simultaneously assess HER expression of primary and metastatic sites, which may vary across lesions within any given patient.
- PET and SPECT imaging allows noninvasive diagnosis in breast cancer, has the ability to detect metastatic disease, and addresses the issue of tumor heterogeneity.
- Resistance against the epidermal growth factor receptor and HER2-targeting agents is a clinically relevant problem that requires optimization of targeting other members of the HER family.
- HER3 is strongly involved in the development and maintenance of many tumor types and is emerging to play a significant role in breast cancer.

INTRODUCTION

Breast cancer is the most common cancer in women worldwide, with approximately 12% of women in the United States developing invasive breast cancer in their lifetime.[1] Although breast cancer has come a long way with regard to treatment options and overall survival, there remain challenges that occur mostly from intratumoral heterogeneity[2] and metastatic disease.[3] Although significant research has emerged to identify biological processes leading to breast cancer,[4] selecting patients who would benefit from targeted therapies remains a major hurdle. Noninvasive tools to stratify patients and facilitate precision medicine are needed to address this issue.[5–7]

Disclosure Statement: The authors have nothing to disclose.
a Department of Radiology, Memorial Sloan Kettering Cancer Center, 1275 York Avenue, New York, NY 10065, USA; b Department of Radiology, Weill Cornell Medical College, 1275 York Avenue, New York, NY 10065, USA; c Program in Molecular Pharmacology and Chemistry, Memorial Sloan Kettering Cancer Center, 1275 York Avenue, New York, NY 10065, USA; d Department of Pharmacology, Weill Cornell Medical College, 1300 York Avenue, New York, NY 10065, USA; e Radiochemistry and Molecular Imaging Probes Core, Memorial Sloan Kettering Cancer Center, 1275 York Avenue, New York, NY 10065, USA
* Corresponding author.
E-mail address: henryk1@mskcc.org

PET Clin 13 (2018) 423–435
https://doi.org/10.1016/j.cpet.2018.02.010
1556-8598/18/© 2018 Elsevier Inc. All rights reserved.

Although breast cancer is typically diagnosed and staged via 3 main biomarkers, estrogen receptor, progesterone receptor, and human epidermal growth factor receptor 2 (HER2),[8] there are other biomarkers of interest that are relevant and may be beneficial to the clinical outcome of breast cancer. Reports of clinical benefit from HER2-targeted therapy in patients with a primary HER2[-] tumor have facilitated to spearhead the concept behind HER2-targeted molecular imaging for unsuspected metastases in breast cancer.[9,10] An additional biomarker of interest includes HER3.[11] HER3 overexpression has been linked with poor prognosis in multiple cancer subtypes, including breast, which has driven interest in HER3 as potential target for both imaging and therapy. Additionally, emerging resistance to HER2-targeted therapy has driven the need to explore additional targets for both imaging and therapy.[11] The HER family in general has been extensively studied in breast cancer,[12] and there are many HER2-targeted agents for therapy and molecular imaging,[13–15] and strategies to target HER3 are also increasing in clinical trials.[16,17]

Molecular imaging, particularly with tracers used in PET and single photon emission computed tomography (SPECT) have the ability to noninvasively detect heterogeneity between primary tumors and metastases in breast cancer.[6,18] PET- and SPECT-based measurement of the HER2 and HER3 expression in breast cancer offers several advantages over repeated biopsies in patient cohorts. Several groups have developed antibody, affibody, and nanoparticle-based radioligands for PET imaging preclinically and clinically,[19–22] many of which include radiotracers used to image HER2 and HER3 in breast cancer.[13,23] Pairing these targeting moieties with longer lived radioisotopes such as zirconium-89 (^{89}Zr; half-life ($t_{1/2}$) = 78 hours) for PET, along with lutetium-177 (^{177}Lu; $t_{1/2}$ = 6.7 days) and indium-111 (^{111}In; $t_{1/2}$ = 67 hours) for SPECT can be used to match the biological half-life of antibodies in vivo ($t_{1/2}$ ~72 hours for typical full-length antibodies).[24] Isotopes like copper-64 (^{64}Cu; $t_{1/2}$ = 12 hours) or technium-99m (^{99m}Tc; $t_{1/2}$ = 6 hours) can be used in PET and SPECT, respectively, for both full-length and antibody fragments, as well as affibodies.[25–27] Antibody fragments and affibody molecules are often labeled with shorter-lived isotopes such as gallium-68 (^{68}Ga; $t_{1/2}$ = 68 minutes) or fluorine-18 (^{18}F, $t_{1/2}$ = 110 minutes) to pair appropriately with shorter biological half-lives in vivo.[28–31]

Many of the PET and SPECT imaging tracers that have made it to the clinic (in phase I/II trials) to detect HER2[+] breast cancer and metastases, are summarized in our previous review.[15] This review seeks to communicate an update about the current clinical trials for both HER2- and HER3 targeted imaging, which are outlined in **Table 1** The current clinical radiotracers used to image HER3[+] and HER2[+] breast cancers are reviewed herein.

PET AND SINGLE PHOTON EMISSION COMPUTED TOMOGRAPHY IMAGING WITH MONOCLONAL ANTIBODIES IN HUMAN EPIDERMAL GROWTH FACTOR RECEPTOR 2[+] BREAST CANCER

An extensively studied target for imaging in breast cancer is HER2, because clinical trials using this target are being undertaken at cancer centers all over the world.[9,32,33] HER2 imaging can address the issue of tumor heterogeneity and reliably determine both the quantity and the functional status of tumor HER2 in individual lesions in a noninvasive manner. This technique is of critical importance to identify patients who would truly benefit from HER2-targeted therapy, and to monitor the change in HER2 status during immunotherapy.[34,35] We have previously reviewed HER2 targeted imaging,[15] and provide an update of more recent work here.

^{89}Zr-Trastuzumab

^{89}Zr-trastuzumab has been vastly studied across patient cohorts and clinical trials for both primary and metastatic breast cancer.[9,36–40] Ulaner and coworkers[9,41] have expanded the field with ^{89}Zr-trasuzumab to detect unsuspecting metastases in both HER2[+] and HER2[-] primary breast tumors. Multiple studies are being carried out at Memorial Sloan Kettering Cancer Center to image this HER2 expression discordance and guide biopsies.[41,42] Another current clinical trial using ^{89}Zr-trastuzumab is led by Laforest and coworkers[43] at Washington University in St. Louis. Twelve women were enrolled in the study, 6 with primary breast cancer and 6 with metastatic breast cancer. Eleven of these patients underwent ^{89}Zr-trastuzumab PET/CT during neoadjuvant or adjuvant therapy, and the remaining patient was imaged before neoadjuvant therapy. Laforest and colleagues found that increasing the dose to 62 ± 2 MBq (vs the average dose of 37 MBq, which was used in previous studies done by Dijkers and colleagues[38,44] in the ZEPHIR [HER2 Imaging Study to Identify HER2 Positive Metastatic Breast Cancer Patient Unlikely to Benefit From T-DM1] trial)[33] allowed for optimal images at later time points (**Figs. 1** and **2**). The dose-limiting organ was found to be the liver, with a

Table 1
Current clinical trials with PET and SPECT radiotracers targeting HER2- and HER3$^+$ breast cancer in 2017

Radiotracer	Description of Trial	Clinical Trial/Reference	Sponsor	Status
^{64}Cu-DOTA-patritumab	RO, PK, and treatment response	NCT01479023	Washington University School of Medicine	Terminated
^{89}Zr-DFO-lumretuzumab	Treatment response	NCT01482377	Hoffmann-La Roche	Completed
^{89}Zr-DFO-trastuzumab	HER2$^+$ BC	NCT02065609	Washington University School of Medicine	Recruiting
	HER2$^+$ MBC	NCT02286843	Memorial Sloan Kettering Cancer Center	Recruiting
	IMPACT-MBC	NCT01957332	University Medical Center Groningen	Recruiting
^{89}Zr-DFO-pertuzumab	HER2$^+$ MBC	NCT03109977	Memorial Sloan Kettering Cancer Center	Completed
	HER2$^+$ MBC	NCT02286843	Memorial Sloan Kettering Cancer Center	Recruiting
^{64}Cu-DOTA-trastuzumab	Treatment Response in HER2$^+$ BC	NCT02827877	City of Hope Medical Center	Recruiting
	HER2$^+$ BC	UMIN000017446	P-DIRECT	Completed
^{177}Lu-DOTA-trastuzumab	HER2$^+$ BC	Bhusari et al,[52] 2017	PGIMER	Completed
[^{131}I]-SGMIB anti-HER2 VHH1	Healthy patients and HER2$^+$ BC	NCT02683083	Camel-IDS NV	Recruiting
^{64}Cu-MM-302	HER2$^+$ MBC	NCT01304797	Merrimack Pharmaceuticals	Ongoing, Not Recruiting

Abbreviations: BC, breast cancer; IMPACT, IMaging PAtients for Cancer Drug selection; MBC, metastatic breast cancer; PK, pharmacokinetics; RO, receptor occupancy.

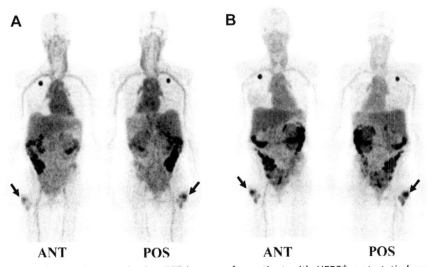

Fig. 1. Anterior and posterior reprojection PET images of a patient with HER2$^+$ metastatic breast cancer on (*A*) day 3 and (*B*) day 6 after ^{89}Zr-trastuzumab administration demonstrate greater tracer uptake in the right femoral metastatic lesion without other significant change in tracer biodistribution on day 6 compared with day 3 (*Arrows* indicate lesions at all time points). The area of intense activity in the right chest is related to administration of ^{89}Zr-trastuzumab via a port catheter. ANT, anterior; POS, posterior. (*From* Laforest R, Lapi SE, Oyama R, et al. [89Zr]Trastuzumab: evaluation of radiation dosimetry, safety, and optimal imaging parameters in women with HER2-positive breast cancer. Mol Imaging Biol 2016;18(6):955; with permission.)

A   **B**

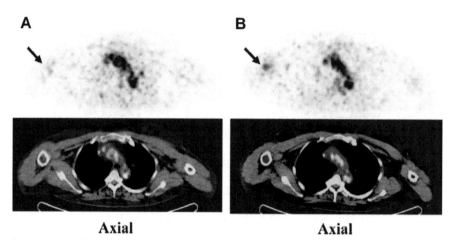

Axial   Axial

Fig. 2. Axial PET (*top*) and fused PET/computed tomography (*bottom*) images of a patient with HER2$^+$ metastatic breast cancer at the chest level on (*A*) day 2 and (*B*) day 4 after ^{89}Zr-trastuzumab administration demonstrate greater tracer uptake in the right humeral metastatic lesion on day 4 compared with day 2 (*Arrows* indicate lesions of interest). (*From* Laforest R, Lapi SE, Oyama R, et al. [89Zr]Trastuzumab: evaluation of radiation dosimetry, safety, and optimal imaging parameters in women with HER2-positive breast cancer. Mol Imaging Biol 2016;18(6):955; with permission.)

dose of 1.63 mSv/MBq. The biodistribution of ^{89}Zr-trastuzumab did not significantly change during the 7 days of imaging. Slow blood clearance was observed with a biological half-life of 113 hours and an initial level of 58% injected dose. Overall, this study showed that imaging ^{89}Zr-trastuzumab imaging is safe, has acceptable dosimetry, and provides a noninvasive means of assessing HER2 status of individual lesions in patients with breast cancer.

^{89}Zr-Pertuzumab

Because ^{89}Zr-trastuzumab has been associated with avidity on PET/CT that does not allow a correlation with HER2 positivity on pathology, additional HER2 targeted tracers have been investigated. For example, pertuzumab is a newer humanized monoclonal antibody that binds to the HER2 receptor at a site distinct from trastuzumab and seems to be more efficient than trastuzumab.[45] A first-in-human trial of ^{89}Zr-pertuzumab imaging in patients with HER2$^+$ breast cancer has demonstrated safety and dosimetry.[46] A potential clinical application of ^{89}Zr-pertuzumab and other HER2-targeting agents was demonstrated in patients with 2 primary breast malignancies, one HER2$^+$ and the other HER2$^-$, who developed brain metastases. HER2-targeted imaging allowed determination of the HER2$^-$ status of the brain metastases, and could assist in the choice of HER2-targeted therapy. In 1 patient, resection of a symptomatic brain metastasis confirmed a HER2$^+$ metastasis, as imaged on ^{89}Zr-pertuzumab PET/CT (**Fig. 3**).

^{64}Cu-Trastuzumab

^{64}Cu-DOTA-trastuzumab has also been used in multiple clinical trials to date.[25–27] The first study to use this radiotracer was to determine the safety, distribution, internal dosimetry, and initial HER2$^+$ tumor images of ^{64}Cu-DOTA-trastuzumab in humans by Tamura and colleagues.[26] Since this study, this tracer has been used for a number of studies to detect both HER2$^+$ primary and metastatic disease and assess therapy response. Tamura and coworkers[47] have expanded on this work to assess intratumoral heterogeneity in HER2$^+$ breast cancer. In a separate study, maximum standardized uptake values were correlated with HER2 immunohistochemistry (IHC) scores and assessment for HER2 status by HER2 PET imaging strongly correlated with histologic HER2 expression status. Tamura and coworkers[25] have also previously demonstrated HER2-specific ^{64}Cu-trastuzumab accumulation in a specimen of removed brain metastasis using IHC and autoradiography. An image of the month study highlighted the first report describing the visualization of HER2-specific intratumoral heterogeneity (IHC 1$^+$ and 2$^+$) using HER2 PET imaging (**Fig. 4**).[47] This interesting finding suggests that HER2 PET imaging could facilitate decision making for clinical treatment strategies. The relationship between HER2 PET imaging and the effects of anti-HER2 therapy, as well as the use of a high-resolution dedicated breast PET scanner, remain to be evaluated.

Mortimer and coworkers[48] are also using the ^{64}Cu-trastuzumab to assess metastatic breast

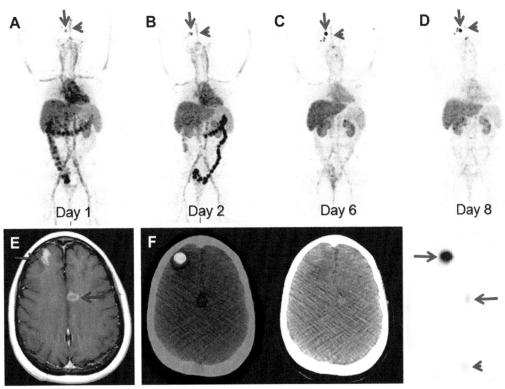

Fig. 3. A 46-year-old woman with both HER2⁺ and HER2-negative primary breast malignancies and recently diag-nosed brain metastases. Sequential maximum-intensity projection images at (*A*) 1 day, (*B*) 2 days, (*C*) 6 days, and (*D*) 8 days after the administration of ^{89}Zr-pertuzumab. Blood pool and liver background clears on sequential im-ages. Excreted bowel activity is seen on days 1 and 2. Bilateral kidney activity is visualized on all days. Increasing activity in foci overlying the skull is seen as time progresses (*arrows*). Decreasing activity is seen in the blood pool of the superior sagittal sinus (*arrowheads*). (*E*) Gadolinium-enhanced T1-weighted MR imaging of the brain dem-onstrates enhancing brain metastases (*arrows*) and the superior sagittal sinus (*arrowhead*). (*F*) Axial fused PET/computed tomography (CT), CT, and PET images 8 days after ^{89}Zr-pertuzumab administration demonstrate avidity in the brain metastases (*arrows*) and minimal residual avidity in the superior sagittal sinus (*arrowhead*). (*From* Ulaner GA, Lyashchenko SK, Riedl C, et al. First-in-human HER2-targeted imaging using 89Zr-pertuzumab PET/CT: Dosimetry and clinical application in patients with breast cancer. J Nucl Med 2017. [Epub ahead of print]; with permission.)

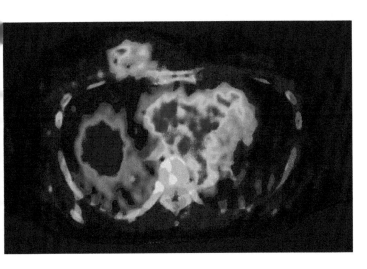

Fig. 4. Visualization of HER2-specific intratumoral heterogeneity (IHC 1⁺ and 2⁺) with ^{64}Cu-trastuzumab. (*From* Sasada S, Kurihara H, Kinoshita T, et al. Visualization of HER2-specific breast cancer intratumoral heteroge-neity using 64Cu-DOTA-trastuzumab PET. Eur J Nucl Med Mol Imaging 2017;44(12):2146; with permission.)

cancer. Women with biopsy-confirmed metastatic breast cancer and not given trastuzumab for 2 months underwent complete staging, including ^{18}F-FDG PET/CT. Although ^{18}F-FDG has been shown to be avid for some cancers, it does not fully address the heterogeneity in breast cancer.[5,49–51] Patients were classified as HER2$^+$ or HER2$^-$ based on fluorescence in situ hybridization and IHC of biopsied tumor tissue (**Fig. 5**). Eighteen patients underwent ^{64}Cu-trastuzumab injection, preceded in 16 cases by trastuzumab infusion (45 mg). PET/CT was performed on 1 and 2 days after hours after injection with ^{64}Cu-trastuzumab (**Fig. 6**).

The observations made by Mortimer and coworkers show that most tumors are well visualized with PET and uptake is indicative of binding to HER2 within 1 day after injection, even in patients classified as HER2$^-$, which indicates that trastuzumab uptake in metastatic breast cancer

is sufficiently rapid, and does not require longer lived isotopes or lag times. This finding is significant for PET imaging of trastuzumab with respect to both patient radiation dose and clinical applicability.

^{177}Lu-Trastuzumab

Bhusari and coworkers[52] developed a ^{177}Lu-trastuzumab tracer for radioimmunotherapy of HER2 expressing breast cancer and also explored its potential as an imaging agent. This study demonstrated that the development, characterization, and radiolabeling of ^{177}Lu-trastuzumab can be efficiently achieved in house and that this radiotracer is safe to be administered to the patients. The HER2$^+$ primary and metastatic breast lesions specifically take up ^{177}Lu-trastuzumab with 2 patient examples shown in **Fig. 7** (day 1 and day 7 time points) and **Fig. 8** (day 5). This

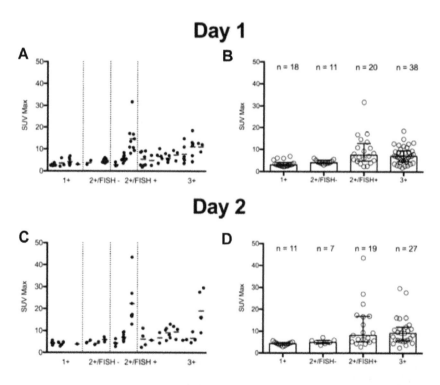

Fig. 5. Tumor uptake (maximum standardized uptake value [SUV$_{max}$]) of ^{64}Cu-DOTA-trastuzumab versus patient immunohistochemistry (IHC)/fluorescence in situ hybridization (FISH) score from biopsied tumor. Data are from ^{64}Cu-DOTA-trastuzumab PET/CT scans acquired 1 day (*A, B*) and 2 days (*C, D*) after injection. In A and C, the data for individual tumors (*black dots*) are grouped by patient and IHC/FISH score. Intrapatient means are represented by red horizontal lines. In B and D, the SUV$_{max}$ values for individual lesions (*open circles*) are combined across patients and grouped by IHC/FISH score (n = number of tumors per group). Intragroup medians are represented as amplitudes of rectangular overlays; errors bars denote the first and third quartiles. In both analyses, tumor uptake is generally higher for the HER2$^+$ subgroups (3$^+$ or 2$^+$/FISH$^+$; P<.005). The relative variability of uptake was greater for the HER2$^+$ than the HER2$^-$ group, both among (P<.001) and within (P<.05 on day 2) patients. (*From* Mortimer JE, Bading JR, Park JM, et al. Tumor uptake of 64Cu-DOTA-Trastuzumab in patients with metastatic breast cancer. J Nucl Med 2018;59(1):41; with permission.)

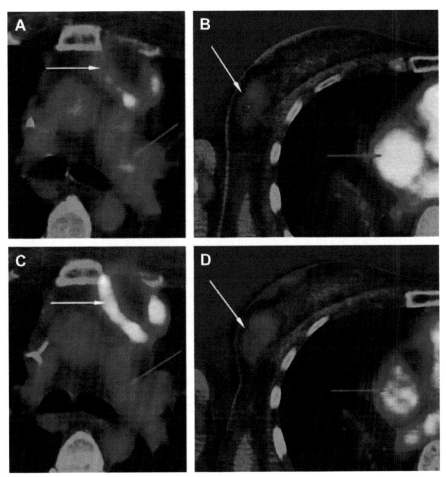

Fig. 6. Examples of increased tumor uptake and tumor-to-nontumor contrast between 1 and 2 days after injection of ⁶⁴Cu-DOTA-trastuzumab. White and red arrows, respectively, denote tumors and blood pool as seen in transaxial PET/computed tomography fusion images. The images on the left are from a HER2⁺ (IHC2⁺/fluorescence in situ hybridization positive) patient. A (day 1) and C (day 2) show a large metastasis in a prevascular lymph node for which uptake was concentrated at the tumor surface. The upper intensity threshold (*white color*) corresponds with a standardized uptake value (SUV) of 22 g/mL. At the times of the 2 scans (24 and 48 hours), measured the maximum SUV (SUV$_{max}$) for the tumor was 17 and 27 g/mL, respectively, whereas the SUV for blood was 15 and 11 g/mL. The right-hand column depicts a metastatic mass in the right breast of a HER2-negative patient (IHC1⁺). The upper intensity threshold for the images (*white color*) was set at an SUV of 10 g/mL. The SUV$_{max}$ for the tumor increased from 2.6 to 5.0 g/mL between (*B*) the day 1 (25 hour after injection) and the (*D*) day 2 (49 hours after injection) scan, whereas the SUV for blood decrease from 12.0 to 8.8 g/mL. (*From* Mortimer JE, Bading JR, Park JM, et al. Tumor uptake of 64Cu-DOTA-Trastuzumab in patients with metastatic breast cancer. J Nucl Med 2018;59(1):42; with permission.)

strategy can be considered as an agent for palliative treatment in combination to other conventional treatments for treatment of HER2 metastatic breast cancer.

NANOPARTICLES IN HUMAN EPIDERMAL GROWTH FACTOR RECEPTOR 2-TARGETED IMAGING AND THERANOSTICS

Nanoparticles and other nanomaterials have also been embellished with the HER2 target in mind.

Therapeutic nanoparticles are designed to deliver their drug payloads through enhanced permeability and retention in solid tumors. The extent of enhanced permeability and retention and its variability in human tumors is a controversial issue in the field, because it may be the reason for variable responses to therapeutic nanoparticles in clinical studies. This issue was addressed by Lee and colleagues[53] in an imaging study in metastatic breast cancer with ⁶⁴Cu-MM-302, a radiolabeled HER2-targeted

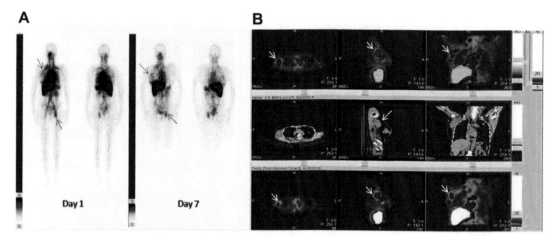

Fig. 7. (*A*) Whole body image of a 60-year-old patient with breast HER2 (2$^+$) at cancer day 1 and day 7 after administration of 370 MBq ^{177}Lu-trastuzumab (5 mg, coadministered with 20 mg cold trastuzumab). Tracer uptake can be observed in primary breast tumor (*black arrows*) with a T/N = 2.9 and 3.2 at day 1 and day 7, respectively. The bone metastasis in the acetabulum region was visualized at day 1 (T/N = 1.2) and day 7 (T/N = 2.5; *blue arrows*). (*B*) Single photon emission computed tomography (SPECT)/computed tomography (CT), CT, and SPECT images showing lymph node metastases (T/N = 2.4) that could not be localized on whole body scan (*white arrows*). (*From* Bhusari P, Vatsa R, Singh G, et al. Development of Lu-177-trastuzumab for radioimmunotherapy of HER2 expressing breast cancer and its feasibility assessment in breast cancer patients. Int J Cancer 2017;140(4):943; with permission.)

PEGylated liposomal doxorubicin. Nineteen patients with HER2$^+$ metastatic breast cancer underwent 2 to 3 PET/CT scans after administration of ^{64}Cu-MM-302 as part of a clinical trial of MM-302 plus trastuzumab with and without cyclophosphamide.[54–56] Tumor accumulation of ^{64}Cu-MM-302 at 24 to 48 hours varied from 0.52% to 18.5% ID/kg (**Fig. 9**), including

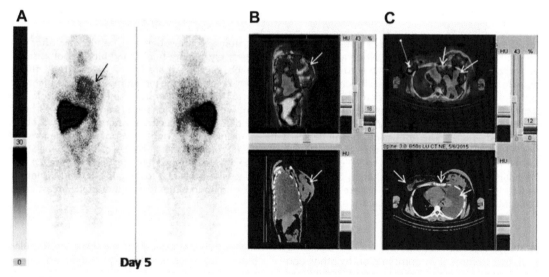

Fig. 8. (*A*) Whole body images of a 30-year-old woman patient with HER2 (3$^+$) breast cancer showing ^{177}Lu-trastuzumab (445 MBq) uptake in primary breast tumor (*black arrow*; T/N = 3.1). (*B*) Single photon emission computed tomography (SPECT)/computed tomography (CT) and CT sagittal sections of the primary breast tumor showing localization of ^{177}Lu-trastuzumab (T/N = 3.6; *white arrows*). (*C*) SPECT/CT and CT images showing ^{177}Lu-trastuzumab localization at the metastatic sites: lymph node (T/N = 3.4) and lesion in the sternum (T/N = 1.3; *white arrows*) and lung metastases (T/N = 1.5) at day 5 after the administration of 444 MBq ^{177}Lu-trastuzumab. (*From* Bhusari P, Vatsa R, Singh G, et al. Development of Lu-177-trastuzumab for radioimmunotherapy of HER2 expressing breast cancer and its feasibility assessment in breast cancer patients. Int J Cancer 2017;140(4):945; with permission.)

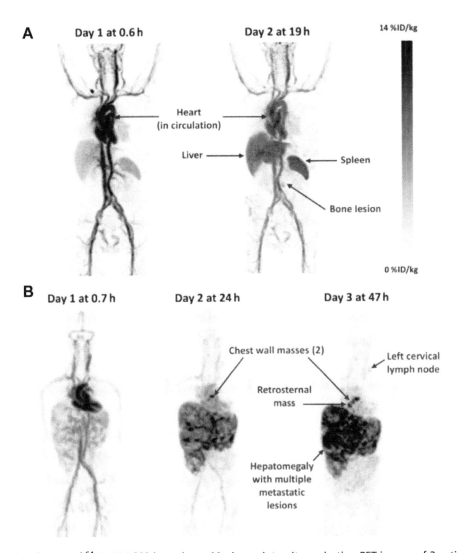

A

Day 1 at 0.6 h   Day 2 at 19 h   14 %ID/kg

Heart
(in circulation)

Liver   Spleen

Bone lesion

0 %ID/kg

B

Day 1 at 0.7 h   Day 2 at 24 h   Day 3 at 47 h

Chest wall masses (2)   Left cervical
lymph node

Retrosternal
mass

Hepatomegaly
with multiple
metastatic
lesions

Fig. 9. Biodistribution of ^{64}Cu-MM-302 in patients. Maximum intensity projection PET images of 2 patients with HER2$^+$ breast cancer injected with 30 mg/m^2 of MM-302 and a tracer dose of ^{64}Cu-MM-302 (400 MBq). PET/ computed tomography (CT) images were acquired at 0.6 and 19.0 hours after injection in patient 2 (*A*), and 0.7, 24.0, and 47.0 hours after injection in patient 6 (*B*). Immediately after administration, ^{64}Cu-MM-302 activity was primarily confined in the blood pool because of the extended circulation property of liposomes. On days 2 and 3, ^{64}Cu-MM-302 uptake was evident in normal spleen and liver, as well as in various tumor lesions. (*Reproduced from* Lee H, Shields AF, Siegel BA, et al. Cu-MM-302 positron emission tomography quantifies variability of enhanced permeability and retention of nanoparticles in relation to treatment response in patients with metastatic breast cancer. Clin Cancer Res 2017;23(15):4195; with permission.)

deposition in bone and brain lesions, along with significant background uptake of ^{64}Cu-MM-302 in the liver and spleen. Peak liposome circulation was found to be between 24 and 48 hours based on computational analysis, and high ^{64}Cu-MM-302 deposition was associated with more favorable treatment outcomes. These findings deliver key evidence and quantification of the enhanced permeability and retention effect in HER2$^+$ metastatic tumors, supporting the use of nanoparticle

imaging as a tool to stratify patients that would benefit from such therapy.

Other nanoparticles on the preclinical end that show promise include studies with ^{99m}Tc-nano-silica[57] and superparamagnetic nanoparticles[58] for detection of HER2$^+$ breast cancer. This emerging realm will bridge the gap between therapies and imaging in the field of nanomedicine, allowing for new subsets of targeted molecules.

PET AND SINGLE PHOTON EMISSION COMPUTED TOMOGRAPHY IMAGING WITH MONOCLONAL ANTIBODIES IN HUMAN EPIDERMAL GROWTH FACTOR RECEPTOR 3$^+$ BREAST CANCER

As there are emerging strategies with monoclonal antibodies to diagnosis disease, assess progression, and interpret specific biomarkers within breast cancer, an up and coming area of this strategy is developing with HER3-targeted antibodies. One of the latest treatments incorporated into clinical trials is patritumab, which binds the extracellular domain of HER3 and promotes receptor internalization, leading to the inhibition of basal and ligand-induced HER3 activation and downstream signaling. Patritumab was labeled with ^{64}Cu and imaging studies were done in patients with multiple tumor types (including breast) that were HER3$^+$, in a recent publication from Lockhart and coworkers.[16] Dosimetry, safety, and receptor occupancy were the main objectives of this clinical trial. The tumor maximum standardized uptake values were 5.6 ± 4.5, 3.3 ± 1.7, and 3.0 ± 1.1 at 3, 24, and 48 hours, respectively, in the dosimetry cohort. The liver was the dose-limiting organ, with a critical dose of 0.46 ± 0.086 mGy/MBq. In the cohort of patients undergoing receptor occupancy assessment, the tumor-to-blood ratio decreased from 1.00 ± 0.32 at baseline to 0.57 ± 0.17 after patritumab treatment, corresponding with a receptor occupancy of 42.1 ± 3.9%. Future studies are needed to improve the characterization of HER3 receptor occupancy by patritumab and its relationship with serum patritumab levels. Additional trials will likely incorporate reduced the time between ^{89}Zr-labeled and unlabeled antibody dosing to reduce liver uptake of the labeled product.

Another antibody-based radiotracer was developed by Bensch and colleagues[17] with ^{89}Zr-lumretuzumab PET to assess therapy response with lumretuzumab in patients with solid tumors. Lumretuzumab is a humanized monoclonal antibody directed against the extracellular domain of HER3, displacing its ligand and inhibiting heterodimerization and downstream signaling. Furthermore, it has been shown that lumretuzumab can cause cell death through antibody-dependent cellular cytotoxicity. A phase I study in patients with solid tumors showed that lumretuzumab monotherapy was well-tolerated and clinically useful, leading to an imaging study with ^{89}Zr-lumretuzumab. This trial recruited 20 patients with histologically confirmed HER3-expressing tumors who underwent ^{89}Zr-lumretuzumab PET. In 1 arm of the trial, ^{89}Zr-lumretuzumab was given alongside escalating doses of unlabeled lumretuzumab and scans were performed 2, 4, and 7 days after injection to determine optimal imaging conditions. In another arm of the trial, patients were scanned after tracer injection before (baseline) and after a pharmacodynamic-active lumretuzumab dose to determine saturation. HER3 expression was determined via immunohistochemical analysis of skin biopsies.

Optimal PET conditions were found to be 4 and 7 days after administration of ^{89}Zr-lumretuzumab with 100 mg of unlabeled antibody. At baseline, after administration of "cold" lumretuzumab (100 mg), the tumor SUV$_{max}$ was 3.4 ± 1.9 at 4 days after injection of ^{89}Zr-lumretuzumab. Tumor uptake decreased by 11.9 ± 8.2%, 10.0 ± 16.5%, and 24.6 ± 20.9% after lumretuzumab administration (escalating doses of 400, 800, and 1600 mg respectively) when compared with baseline. HER3 expression was also downregulated in concurrent skin biopsies at the lowest dose of lumretuzumab (400 mg). Overall, this study with ^{89}Zr-lumretuzumab PET showed promising biodistribution and tumor specificity. Despite the correlative trend between increased doses of lumretuzumab and decreased ^{89}Zr-lumretuzumab uptake, the tumor uptake never plateaued, indicating a lack of tumor saturation. Therefore, it is possible that the dosing of the radiotracer will need further optimization to have optimal delineation.

Although there are a number of preclinical tracers to target HER3 that are increasing, few have yet to reach the clinic to drive the relevance of this protein in breast cancer imaging. Some of the more recent antibody developments include those that are not only relevant for diagnosis,[59–6] but also assessing therapy response,[62–64] some of which were actually used in the clinical trials described herein. Affibodies are also an up and coming strategy that has been more embellished upon with the HER2 target, but is also slowly increasing with regard to HER3.[65–68] Radiotracers that are successful for both diagnostic purposes and predicting therapy are particularly useful from a breast cancer standpoint, because many chemotherapeutic and targeted therapy options can be toxic and have harmful side effects. The use of a specific, biologically relevant radiotracer to detect changes in HER3 expression and assess therapy response serves to improve breast cancer treatment.

SUMMARY

HER receptor status, namely HER2 and HER3, encompass a subset of critical biomarkers in patients with breast cancer, and can be essential to making treatment decisions and finalizing prognosis. The heterogeneous expression of HER proteins both intratumorally and between primary and metastatic disease limits the value of tumor biopsies and demonstrates a need for accurate, whole body assessment, which is where targeted molecular imaging arises as a valuable tool to solve this clinical issue. Antibodies, antibody fragments, affibodies, and nanoparticles targeted to HER2 and HER3 can be radiolabeled for PET and SPECT imaging to target HER2 and HER3 lesions and metastases and therapy response. These clinical tools are necessary to make the push toward precision medicine and will serve to improve the outcomes for patients with breast cancer everywhere.

ACKNOWLEDGMENTS

The authors acknowledge the National Institute of Health R01CA204167 (J.S. Lewis, G.A. Ulaner), the Department of Defense BC132676 (G.A. Ulaner), and the MSKCC Radiochemistry and Molecular Imaging Probe Core (NIH grant P30 CA008748). K.E. Henry gratefully acknowledges the Center for Molecular Imaging and Technology Tow Fellowship.

REFERENCES

1. World Health Organization (WHO). Breast Cancer: prevention and control. Available at: http://www.who.int/cancer/detection/breastcancer/en/. Accessed September 29, 2017.

2. Beca F, Polyak K. Intratumor heterogeneity in breast cancer. Adv Exp Med Biol 2016;886:169–89.

3. Scully OJ, Bay BH, Yip G, et al. Breast cancer metastasis. Cancer Genomics Proteomics 2012; 9(5):311–20.

4. Mardamshina M, Geiger T. Next-generation proteomics and its application to clinical breast cancer research. Am J Pathol 2017;187(10):2175–84.

5. Henry KE, Dilling TR, Abdel-Atti D, et al. Non-invasive 89Zr-transferrin PET shows improved tumor targeting compared to 18F-FDG PET in MYC-overexpressing human triple negative breast cancer. J Nucl Med 2018;59(1):51–7.

6. Vercher-Conejero JL, Pelegrí-Martinez L, Lopez-Aznar D, et al. Positron emission tomography in breast cancer. Diagnostics (Basel) 2015;5(1):61–83.

7. Chudgar A, Clark A, Mankoff D. Applications of PET/CT in breast cancer, NCCN guidelines and beyond. J Nucl Med 2016;57(supplement 2):1304.

8. Dunnwald LK, Rossing MA, Li CI. Hormone receptor status, tumor characteristics, and prognosis: a prospective cohort of breast cancer patients. Breast Cancer Res 2007;9(1):1–10.

9. Ulaner GA, Hyman D, Ross D, et al. Detection of HER2-positive metastases in patients with HER2-negative primary breast cancer using the 89Zr-DFO-trastuzumab PET/CT. J Nucl Med 2016; 57(10):1523–8.

10. Ulaner GA, Riedl CC, Dickler MN, et al. Molecular imaging of biomarkers in breast cancer. J Nucl Med 2016;57(Supplement 1):53S–9S.

11. Kol A, Terwisscha van Scheltinga AGT, Timmer-Bosscha H, et al. HER3, serious partner in crime: therapeutic approaches and potential biomarkers for effect of HER3-targeting. Pharmacol Ther 2014;143(1):1–11.

12. Pool M, de Boer HR, Hooge MNL, et al. Harnessing integrative omics to facilitate molecular imaging of the human epidermal growth factor receptor family for precision medicine. Theranostics 2017;7(7): 2111–33.

13. Tolmachev V. Imaging of HER-2 overexpression in tumors for guiding therapy. Curr Pharm Des 2008; 14(28):2999–3019.

14. Elias SG, Adams A, Wisner DJ, et al. Imaging features of HER2 overexpression in breast cancer: a systematic review and meta-analysis. Cancer Epidemiol Biomarkers Prev 2014;23(8):1464–83.

15. Henry KE, Ulaner GA, Lewis JS. HER2-targeted PET/SPECT imaging of breast cancer: non-invasive measurement of a biomarker integral to tumor treatment and prognosis. PET Clin 2017;12(3): 269–88.

16. Lockhart AC, Liu Y, Dehdashti F, et al. Phase 1 evaluation of (64)Cu-DOTA-Patritumab to assess dosimetry, apparent receptor occupancy, and safety in subjects with advanced solid tumors. Mol Imaging Biol 2016;18(3):446–53.

17. Bensch F, Lamberts LE, Smeenk MM, et al. Zr-lumretuzumab PET imaging before and during HER3 antibody lumretuzumab treatment in patients with solid tumors. Clin Cancer Res 2017;23(20):6128–37.

18. Bénard F, Turcotte É. Imaging in breast cancer: single-photon computed tomography and positron-emission tomography. Breast Cancer Res 2005; 7(4):153–62.

19. Warram JM, de Boer E, Sorace AG, et al. Antibody based imaging strategies of cancer. Cancer Metastasis Rev 2014;33(2–3):809–22.

20. Lamberts LE, Williams SP, Terwisscha van Scheltinga AGT, et al. Antibody positron emission tomography imaging in anticancer drug development. J Clin Oncol 2015;33(13):1491–504.

21. Boerman OC, Oyen WJ. Immuno-PET of cancer: a revival of antibody imaging. J Nucl Med 2011; 52(8):1171–2.

22. van Dongen GA, Visser GW, Lub-de Hooge MN, et al. Immuno-PET: a navigator in monoclonal antibody development and applications. Oncologist 2007;12(12):1379–89.

23. Capala J, Bouchelouche K. Molecular imaging of HER2-positive breast cancer - a step toward an individualized "Image and Treat" strategy. Curr Opin Oncol 2010;22(6):559–66.

24. Deri MA, Zeglis BM, Francesconi LC, et al. PET imaging with (89)Zr: from radiochemistry to the clinic. Nucl Med Biol 2013;40(1):3–14.

25. Kurihara H, Hamada A, Yoshida M, et al. 64Cu-DOTA-trastuzumab PET imaging and HER2 specificity of brain metastases in HER2-positive breast cancer patients. EJNMMI Res 2015;5(1):1–8.

26. Tamura K, Kurihara H, Yonemori K, et al. 64Cu-DOTA-trastuzumab PET imaging in patients with HER2-positive breast cancer. J Nucl Med 2013; 54(11):1869–75.

27. Mortimer JE, Bading JR, Colcher DM, et al. Functional imaging of human epidermal growth factor receptor 2–positive metastatic breast cancer using 64Cu-DOTA-trastuzumab PET. J Nucl Med 2014; 5(1):23–9.

28. Sandström M, Lindskog K, Velikyan I, et al. Biodistribution and radiation dosimetry of the anti-HER2 affibody molecule 68Ga-ABY-025 in breast cancer patients. J Nucl Med 2016;57(6):867–71.

29. Sörensen J, Sandberg D, Sandström M, et al. First-in-human molecular imaging of HER2 expression in breast cancer metastases using the 111In-ABY-025 affibody molecule. J Nucl Med 2014;55(5):730–5.

30. Tolmachev V, Velikyan I, Sandström M, et al. A HER2-binding affibody molecule labelled with 68Ga for PET imaging: direct in vivo comparison with the 111In-labelled analogue. Eur J Nucl Med 2010;37(7):1356–67.

31. Sörensen J, Velikyan I, Sandberg D, et al. Measuring HER2-receptor expression in metastatic breast cancer using [(68)Ga]ABY-025 Affibody PET/CT. Theranostics 2016;6(2):262–71.

32. Wong JY, Raubitschek A, Yamauchi D, et al. A pretherapy biodistribution and dosimetry study of indium-111-radiolabeled trastuzumab in patients with human epidermal growth factor receptor 2-overexpressing breast cancer. Cancer Biother Radiopharm 2010;25(4):387–94.

33. Gebhart G, Lamberts LE, Wimana Z, et al. Molecular imaging as a tool to investigate heterogeneity of advanced HER2-positive breast cancer and to predict patient outcome under trastuzumab emtansine (T-DM1): the ZEPHIR trial. Ann Oncol 2016;27(4): 619–24.

34. Baselga J. Phase I and II clinical trials of trastuzumab. Ann Oncol 2001;12(suppl 1):S49–55.

35. Swain SM, Baselga J, Kim SB, et al. Pertuzumab, trastuzumab, and docetaxel in HER2-positive metastatic breast cancer. N Engl J Med 2015;372(8): 724–34.

36. Oude Munnink TH, Korte MA, Nagengast WB, et al. 89Zr-trastuzumab PET visualises HER2 downregulation by the HSP90 inhibitor NVP-AUY922 in a human tumour xenograft. Eur J Cancer 2010;46(3):678–84.

37. Gaykema SB, Brouwers AH, Hovenga S, et al. Zirconium-89-trastuzumab positron emission tomography as a tool to solve a clinical dilemma in a patient with breast cancer: a case report. J Clin Oncol 2012; 30(6):e74–5.

38. Dijkers EC, Oude Munnink TH, Kosterink JG, et al. Biodistribution of 89Zr-trastuzumab and PET imaging of HER2-positive lesions in patients with metastatic breast cancer. Clin Pharmacol Ther 2010; 87(5):586–92.

39. Washington University School of Medicine, National Cancer Institute (NCI). 89Zr-trastuzumab breast imaging with positron emission tomography. St Louis (MO): Washington University School of Medicine (US), ClinicalTrials.gov; 2016 [cited Nov 3, 2016]. NLM Identifier: NCT02065609. Available at: https:// clinicaltrials.gov/ct2/show/NCT02065609. Accessed September 29, 2017.

40. Jules Bordet Institute. Pilot imaging study with 89Zr-trastuzumab in HER2-positive metastatic breast cancer patients (IJBMNZrT003). In: [Internet]. Brussels, Belgium: Institut Jules Bordet. ClinicalTrials; 2016 [cited Nov 3, 2016]. NLM Identifier: NCT01420146. Available at: https://clinicaltrials.gov/ct2/show/NCT01420146.

41. Ulaner GA, Hyman DM, Lyashchenko SK, et al. 89Zr-trastuzumab PET/CT for detection of human epidermal growth factor receptor 2-positive metastases in patients with human epidermal growth factor receptor 2-negative primary breast cancer. Clin Nucl Med 2017;42(12):912–7.

42. Cornelis FH, Durack J, Pandit-Taskar N, et al. Long half-life 89Zr labeled radiotracers can guide in suite percutaneous molecular imaging PET/CT-guided biopsies without reinjection of radiotracer. J Nucl Med 2017. https://doi.org/10.2967/jnumed.117.194480.

43. Laforest R, Lapi SE, Oyama R, et al. [89Zr]trastuzumab: evaluation of radiation dosimetry, safety, and optimal imaging parameters in women with HER2-positive breast cancer. Mol Imaging Biol 2016; 18(6):952–9.

44. Dijkers EC, Kosterink JG, Rademaker AP, et al. Development and characterization of clinical-grade 89Zr-trastuzumab for HER2/neu ImmunoPET imaging. J Nucl Med 2009;50(6):974–81.

45. Hudis CA. Trastuzumab — mechanism of action and use in clinical practice. N Engl J Med 2007;357(1): 39–51.

46. Ulaner GA, Lyashchenko SK, Riedl C, et al. First-in-human HER2-targeted imaging using 89Zr-pertuzumab PET/CT: dosimetry and clinical application in patients with breast cancer. J Nucl Med 2017. [Epub ahead of print].

47. Sasada S, Kurihara H, Kinoshita T, et al. Visualization of HER2-specific breast cancer intratumoral

heterogeneity using 64Cu-DOTA-trastuzumab PET. Eur J Nucl Med Mol Imaging 2017;44(12):2146–7.

48. Mortimer JE, Bading JR, Park JM, et al. Tumor uptake of 64Cu-DOTA-trastuzumab in patients with metastatic breast cancer. J Nucl Med 2018;59(1):38–43.

49. Scheidhauer K, Scharl A, Pietrzyk U, et al. Qualitative [18F]FDG positron emission tomography in primary breast cancer: clinical relevance and practicability. Eur J Nucl Med 1996;23(6):618–23.

50. Moon D, Maddahi J, Silverman DH, et al. Accuracy of whole-body FDG PET for the detection of recurrent or metastatic breast carcinoma. J Nucl Med 1998;39(3):431–5.

51. Shreve PD, Anzai Y, Wahl RL. Pitfalls in oncologic diagnosis with FDG PET imaging: physiologic and benign variants. Radiographics 1999;19(1):61–77.

52. Bhusari P, Vatsa R, Singh G, et al. Development of Lu-177-trastuzumab for radioimmunotherapy of HER2 expressing breast cancer and its feasibility assessment in breast cancer patients. Int J Cancer 2017;140(4):938–47.

53. Lee H, Shields AF, Siegel BA, et al. Cu-MM-302 positron emission tomography quantifies variability of enhanced permeability and retention of nanoparticles in relation to treatment response in patients with metastatic breast cancer. Clin Cancer Res 2017;23(15):4190–202.

54. University of California, San Francisco. 64-Cu labeled brain PET/MRI for MM-302 in advanced HER2+ cancers with brain METs. San Francisco (CA): University of California, San Francisco (US). ClinicalTrials.gov; 2016 [cited 2016, Nov 3]. NLM Identifier: NCT02735798. Available at: https://clinicaltrials.gov/ct2/show/NCT02735798. Accessed September 29, 2017.

55. Merrimack Pharmaceuticals. MM-302 plus trastuzumab vs. chemotherapy of physician's choice plus trastuzumab in HER2-positive locally advanced/metastatic breast cancer patients (HERMIONE). Cambridge (MA): ClinicalTrials.gov. Merrimack Pharmaceuticals (US); 2016 [cited Nov 3, 2016]. NLM Identifier: NCT02213744. Available at: https://clinicaltrials.gov/ct2/show/NCT02213744. Accessed September 29, 2017.

56. Merrimack Pharmaceuticals. Safety and pharmacokinetic study of MM-302 in patients with advanced breast cancer. Cambridge (MA): Merrimack Pharmaceuticals (US); 2016 [cited Nov 3, 2016]. NLM Identifier: NCT01304797. 2016. Available at: ClinicalTrials.gov https://clinicaltrials.gov/ct2/show/NCT01304797. Accessed September 29, 2017.

57. Rainone P, Riva B, Belloli S, et al. Development of (99m)Tc-radiolabeled nanosilica for targeted detection of HER2-positive breast cancer. Int J Nanomedicine 2017;12:3447–61.

58. Li DL, Tan JE, Tian Y, et al. Multifunctional superparamagnetic nanoparticles conjugated with fluorescein-labeled designed ankyrin repeat protein as an efficient HER2-targeted probe in breast cancer. Biomaterials 2017;147:86–98.

59. Terwisscha van Scheltinga AGT, Lub-de Hooge MN, Abiraj K, et al. ImmunoPET and biodistribution with human epidermal growth factor receptor 3 targeting antibody 89Zr-RG7116. MAbs 2014;6(4):1051–8.

60. Warnders FJ, Terwisscha van Scheltinga AGT, Knuehl C, et al. Human epidermal growth factor receptor 3–specific tumor uptake and biodistribution of 89Zr-MSB0010853 visualized by real-time and noninvasive PET imaging. J Nucl Med 2017;58(8):1210–5.

61. Wehrenberg-Klee E, Turker NS, Chang B, et al. Development of a HER3 PET probe for breast cancer imaging. J Nucl Med 2014;55(supplement 1):550.

62. Wehrenberg-Klee E, Turker NS, Heidari P, et al. Differential receptor tyrosine kinase PET imaging for therapeutic guidance. J Nucl Med 2016;57(9):1413–9.

63. Pool M, Kol A, de Jong JR, et al. 89Zr-mAb3481 PET for HER3 tumor status assessment during lapatinib treatment. MAbs 2017;9(8):1370–8.

64. Alsaid H, Skedzielewski T, Rambo MV, et al. Non invasive imaging assessment of the biodistribution of GSK2849330, an ADCC and CDC optimized anti HER3 mAb, and its role in tumor macrophage recruitment in human tumor-bearing mice. PLoS One 2017;12(4). e0176075.

65. Orlova A, Malm M, Rosestedt M, et al. Imaging of HER3-expressing xenografts in mice using a 99mTc(CO)3-HEHEHE-ZHER3:08699 affibody molecule. Eur J Nucl Med 2014;41(7):1450–9.

66. Rosestedt M, Andersson KG, Mitran B, et al. Affibody-mediated PET imaging of HER3 expression in malignant tumours. Sci Rep 2015;5:15226.

67. Andersson KG, Rosestedt M, Varasteh O, et al. Comparative evaluation of 111In-labeled NOTA-conjugated affibody molecules for visualization of HER3 expression in malignant tumors. Oncol Rep 2015;34(2):1042–8.

68. Da Pieve C, Allott L, Martins CD, et al. Efficient [18F] AIF Radiolabeling of ZHER3:8698 affibody molecule for imaging of HER3 positive tumors. Bioconjug Chem 2016;27(8):1839–49.

Amino Acid Metabolism as a Target for Breast Cancer Imaging

Gary A. Ulaner, MD, PhD[a,b,]*, David M. Schuster, MD[c]

KEYWORDS

- Breast cancer • PET/CT • Amino acid • Methionine • Fluciclovine

KEY POINTS

- Amino acids are an alternate energy source to glucose, and amino acid metabolism is up-regulated in multiple malignancies, including breast cancers.
- Multiple amino acid radiotracers have been used to image breast cancer with unique strengths and weaknesses.
- ^{11}C-methionine uptake correlates with S-phase fraction in breast cancer and may be useful for evaluation of treatment response.
- Invasive lobular breast cancers may demonstrate greater ^{18}F-fluciclovine avidity than ^{18}F-fluorodeoxyglucose. Thus, different histologic subtypes of breast cancer may utilize diverse metabolic pathways and may be better imaged by different tracers.

INTRODUCTION

Cellular metabolism has been a major target of nuclear imaging, with the glucose analog fludeoxyglucose F 18 (^{18}F-FDG) serving as the prototype metabolic imaging radiotracer. This successful ^{18}F-FDG paradigm has focused on the increased metabolism of glucose in malignancy.[1] ^{18}F-FDG PET has led to important advances in the care of patients with breast cancer (See Dhritiman Chakraborty and colleagues' article, "Diagnostic Role of FDG PET in Breast Cancer: A History to Current Application," and David Groheux's article, "Role of FDG in Breast Cancer: Treatment Response," in this issue). ^{18}F-FDG has multiple limitations, however, including difficulty distinguishing malignant from benign primary breast lesions,[2] limited utility in the evaluation of the breast and axilla compared with other imaging methods,[3–5] and variable sensitivity and specificity of breast cancer lesions, depending on tumor and patient characteristics.[6–10] In particular, invasive lobular carcinoma (ILC) is a histologic subtype of breast cancer with lower FDG avidity than the more common invasive ductal carcinoma (IDC) in both primary and metastatic lesions.[11–14] Therefore, multiple opportunities remain for novel metabolic imaging agents in breast malignancies.

Although glucose metabolism is recognized as a key metabolic pathway for imaging, less well known to imaging specialists are the multiple other intermediary metabolic pathways of cellular metabolism.[15] In addition to glycolysis, the citric acid cycle, amino acid metabolism, and lipid metabolism are also altered during neoplasia.[15] This can be demonstrated at the genomic level as well as at

[a] Department of Radiology, Memorial Sloan Kettering Cancer Center, 1275 York Avenue, Box 77, New York, NY 10065, USA; [b] Department of Radiology, Weill Cornell Medical School, 525 East 68th Street, New York, NY 10065, USA; [c] Division of Nuclear Medicine and Molecular Imaging, Department of Radiology and Imaging Sciences, Emory University Hospital, Room E152, 1364 Clifton Road, Atlanta, GA 30322, USA
* Corresponding author. Memorial Sloan Kettering Cancer Center, 1275 York Avenue, Box 77, New York, NY 10065.
E-mail address: ulanerg@mskcc.org

PET Clin 13 (2018) 437–444
https://doi.org/10.1016/j.cpet.2018.02.009
1556-8598/18/© 2018 Elsevier Inc. All rights reserved.

the level of messenger ribosomal nucleic acid transcription, protein expression, and metabolic phenotypes.[16] Exploiting these metabolic pathways for imaging malignancy has been a focus of research over the past 2 decades. In particular, multiple radiotracers have been designed and tested for imaging of amino acid metabolism with initial successes and potential future opportunities.

This review focuses on basic amino acid metabolism, the radiotracers that have thus far been central to amino acid metabolism imaging in patients with breast cancer, and possibilities for future development of these agents.

BASICS OF AMINO ACID METABOLISM IN NORMAL CELLS AND MALIGNANCY

Although hundreds of amino acids have been described, 20 are encoded in the human genome and serve as the basic building blocks for proteins.[16] These amino acids are the components of multiple metabolic pathways that are essential for cellular maintenance. Amino acids are transported into the interior of the cell by amino acid transporters in the cell membrane. There are more than 20 amino acid transporter families, including the major amino acid transport systems L, alanine-serine-cysteine (ASC), and A.

Increased levels of methionine, glutamine, cystine, tryptophan, tyrosine, and other amino acids have been noted in many malignancies, including breast cancers.[16–20] Cancer cells with up-regulation of amino acid metabolism stimulate increased transport of amino acids into the cell.[16,21] The increased consumption of amino acids and overexpression of amino acid transporters in malignancies make radiolabeled amino acids attractive oncologic imaging agents.[22]

Multiple amino acid transporter families have been demonstrated to be up-regulated in breast cancer cells, including L-type amino acid transporter (LAT1), ASC transporter 2 (ASCT2), ATB$^{0,+}$, SNAT1, and x_c^-.[18,23–27] LAT1 is essential for the transport of large neutral amino acids[21] and is overexpressed in multiple malignant tumor types, including breast cancer.[21,24] Furuya and colleagues[28] have described LAT1 transporter expression with CD98 as an independent prognostic factor in triple-negative breast cancer. The ASCT2 and system A component SNAT1 have been shown up-regulated in a tissue microarray of 702 breast malignancies.[26,27] Expression of ASCT2 also has prognostic associations in breast cancer.[29] The system x_c^- transporter, which mediates cystine uptake, is up-regulated in some breast cancer tumors, as demonstrated by the PET radiotracer (4S)-4-(3-[^{18}F]fluoropropyl)-L-glutamate (^{18}F-FSPG).[18]

METHIONINE IMAGING

11C-methionine was an early agent for amino acid metabolic imaging. Methionine is a natural large neutral amino acid that is, readily radiolabeled with 11C. 11C-methionine serves as a metabolic marker for methionine uptake by L-type amino acid transporters. Initial work has demonstrated that both primary and metastatic sites of breast malignancy are visualized by 11C-methionine PET.[17] In addition, 11C-methionine uptake correlated with the fraction of cells in mitosis in these lesions, suggesting that amino acid uptake may correlate with proliferation rate in breast malignancies.

Subsequent work with 11C-methionine extended to imaging of breast cancer treatment response.[30–32] Uptake of 11C-methionine decreased in patients before clinical objective response or regression of tumor size and provided early evidence that radionuclide metabolic imaging could predict treatment response earlier than other methods. 11C-methionine could distinguish responders from nonresponders of endocrine or combination endocrine and chemotherapy after as little as 1 cycle of treatment.[30,32] In some cases, 11C-methionine even outperformed ^{18}F-FDG.[31] These studies included only a small number of patients—51 patients among the 4 studies[17,30–32]—limiting the conclusions that can be drawn from the data.

Physiologic sites of uptake of 11C-methionine include the liver and bone marrow, which could limit evaluation of breast cancer metastases. Other limitations of 11C-methionine include its relatively short (20-min) half-life and nonprotein metabolites, which may interfere with imaging. More recently, 99m-technetium-labeled methionine has been developed and used with dedicated breast scintigraphy equipment for the detection of primary breast malignancies.[33] This radiotracer, 99mTc-DTPA-bis-methionine, could be produced with high efficiency from a single vial kit, and has demonstrated high sensitivity in the initial clinical trial.[33]

^{18}F-FLUCICLOVINE

^{18}F-fluciclovine (*anti*-1-amino-3-18F-fluorocyclobutane-1-carboxylic acid) is a synthetic amino acid initially developed at Emory University as a leucine analog for imaging brain malignancies,[34] and subsequently developed as a valuable radiotracer for prostate malignancies.[35,36] In 2016, ^{18}F-fluciclovine was approved by the United States Food and Drug Administration for PET imaging of patients with suspected prostate cancer recurrence based on elevated PSA levels after prior treatment.

[18]F-fluciclovine is transported into the cell primarily by the ASCT2 transporter with additional involvement of LAT1 in certain conditions, such as dense acidic tumor environments.[37,38] Uptake into cells is most similar to that of the naturally occurring amino acid glutamine.[38,39] Preclinical work has demonstrated uptake of fluciclovine into breast cancer cell lines and mouse orthotopic tumor xenografts.[21] A recent preliminary in vitro study reported that fluciclovine uptake into breast cancer cells occurred mostly via ASCT2 transporters.[40] Because amino acid transporters, including ASC-type transporters,[26] are upregulated in breast cancer cells, investigators have extended clinical trials with ^{18}F-fluciclovine to patients with breast lesions and breast cancer.[41–43]

In a study of 12 women, ^{18}F-fluciclovine uptake in malignant breast lesions was more than 4-fold greater than in benign lesions.[42] The greatest uptake of ^{18}F-fluciclovine was found in the highest-grade malignancies. In another study of 27 women with breast cancer, the primary breast malignancy was visualized in all patients and in 20 of 21 pathologically confirmed axillary nodal metastases.[41] In addition, ^{18}F-fluciclovine detected histologically confirmed extra-axillary nodal metastases that were previously undetected. Both of these studies identified an interesting correlation between ^{18}F-fluciclovine avidity and histologic subtypes of breast malignancy. Although IDC demonstrated equal or inferior fluciclovine avidity compared with FDG avidity, the ILC histology tumors demonstrated greater fluciclovine avidity than FDG avidity[41,42] (**Fig. 1**). This suggests a varying dependence of metabolic pathways between histologic subtypes of breast cancer, raising an interesting question: Could radiotracers targeting different metabolic pathways be suited for imaging specific breast cancer histologic subtypes?

A separate study evaluated the ability of ^{18}F-fluciclovine avidity to determine neoadjuvant therapy response, using histology after definitive surgical management as the gold standard.[43] Changes in ^{18}F-fluciclovine avidity strongly correlated with the percentage of reduction of tumor seen on pathology (**Fig. 2**). Although as reported with ^{18}F-FDG, histologic complete response could not be accurately distinguished from noncomplete responses, because small-volume residual malignancy in patients with greater than 90% tumor reduction on histology could not be readily appreciated by ^{18}F-fluciclovine PET/CT (**Fig. 3**).

These initial studies emphasized ^{18}F-fluciclovine avidity in local disease, with only 1 distal (osseous) metastasis visualized. Of importance will be future trials evaluating ^{18}F-fluciclovine avidity in patients with distant metastatic disease, where the advantages of whole body metabolic imaging will likely be greatest. Preclinical studies have demonstrated substantial success of ^{18}F-fluciclovine in the detection of osseous metastases.[44,45] Physiologic fluciclovine avidity is seen in the liver, pancreas, and skeletal muscle. The physiologic avidity in the liver will likely limit detection of hepatic metastases, a common site of metastatic disease in patients with breast cancer. In one of the trials, hepatic breast metastases were relatively photopenic to background liver.[42]

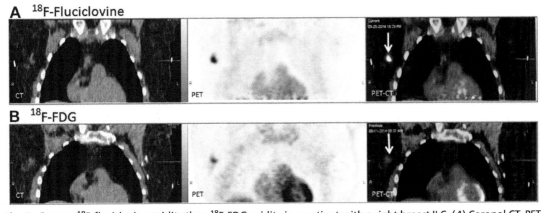

Fig. 1. Greater ^{18}F-fluciclovine avidity than ^{18}F-FDG avidity in a patient with a right breast ILC. (*A*) Coronal CT, PET, and fused PET/CT images from a ^{18}F-fluciclovine PET/CT demonstrate a ^{18}F-fluciclovine–avid right breast ILC ([*arrow*] SUV 7.1). (*B*) Coronal CT, PET, and fused PET/CT images from an ^{18}F-FDG PET/CT on the same patient demonstrate lower FDG avidity ([*arrow*] SUV 3.5). (*Adapted from* Tade FI, Cohen MA, Styblo TM, et al. Anti-3-18F-FACBC (^{18}F-Fluciclovine) PET/CT of breast cancer: an exploratory study. J Nucl Med 2016;57(9):1362; with permission.)

A ^{18}F-Fluciclovine at initial staging

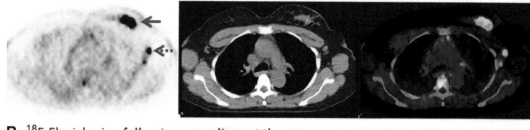

B ^{18}F-Fluciclovine following neoadjuvant therapy

Fig. 2. Reduction in ^{18}F-fluciclovine avidity after neoadjuvant therapy in a 52-year-old woman with breast cancer (*A*) Axial PET, CT, and fused images from a ^{18}F-fluciclovine PET/CT at baseline demonstrate the ^{18}F-fluciclovine-avid primary breast mass (*arrow*) and ^{18}F-fluciclovine–avid axillary nodal metastases (*dashed arrow*). (*B*) Axia PET, CT, and fused PET/CT images from a ^{18}F-fluciclovine PET/CT after neoadjuvant therapy demonstrate decrease ^{18}F-fluciclovine avidity of all lesions to background. On pathology, there was a complete pathologic response, with no residual tumor. (*Adapted from* Ulaner GA, Goldman DA, Corben A, et al. Prospective clinical trial o ^{18}F-fluciclovine PET/CT for determining the response to neoadjuvant therapy in invasive ductal and invasive lobular breast cancers. J Nucl Med 2017;58(7):1040; with permission.)

Breast malignancies with ILC histology have a propensity to metastasize to nodes and bone, where ^{18}F-fluciclovine background is lower, as well as a greater propensity to metastasize to the genitourinary and gastrointestinal tracts than IDC, where background avidity with ^{18}F-FDG is

more problematic. A direct comparison of ^{18}F-fluciclovine and FDG for metastatic ILC could provide evidence of where ^{18}F-fluciclovine may improve staging in ILC.

Given that amino acid transporters mediate both uptake and efflux of amino acids in cells,

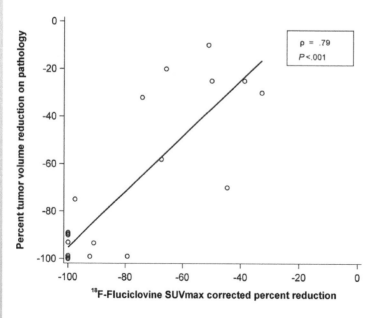

Fig. 3. Scatterplot demonstrating a strong correlation between ^{18}F-fluciclovine SUVmax and percent tumor volume reduction on pathology in 24 patients with breast cancer after neoadjuvant therapy. Note that a 100% reduction in SUV on PET correlated with a 90% to 100% reduction in tumor reduction. Thus, although the correlation was strong, a 100% reduction in ^{18}F-fluciclovine SUV could not distinguish a pathologic complete response from a pathologic noncomplete response. ρ, Spearman rho. (*Adapted from* Ulaner GA, Goldman DA, Corben A, et al. Prospective clinical trial of ^{18}F-fluciclovine PET/CT for determining the response to neoadjuvant therapy in invasive ductal and invasive lobular breast cancers. J Nucl Med 2017;58(7):1041; with permission.)

and ^{18}F-fluciclovine is not intracellularly metabolized and trapped like ^{18}F-FDG, the dynamics of ^{18}F-fluciclovine uptake are different from ^{18}F-FDG. Although longer uptake times tend to increase ^{18}F-FDG uptake, ^{18}F-fluciclovine uptake peaks within the first 20 minutes and then often demonstrates slow washout from breast tumors.[41,42] This phenomenon makes proper protocoling of ^{18}F-fluciclovine PET/CT studies of great importance, with radiotracer administration followed by imaging when the patient is already positioned on the PET/CT scanner.

CYSTEINE TRANSPORTER IMAGING

The amino acid transporter system x_c^- mediates cellular uptake of cystine with concurrent efflux of glutamate. Amino acid analog radiotracers have been designed to examine x_c^- activity and provide PET/CT imaging of tumors. ^{18}F-FSPG is 1 such novel amino acid analog radiotracer that has demonstrated tumor visualization in small animal models[46] and in patients with lung and breast cancer,[18] although uptake in breast cancer lesions was lower and not appreciated in all breast tumors. Histologic or molecular subtypes of breast cancer may influence x_c^- activity and ^{18}F-FSPG uptake. Standardized uptake value (SUV) of ^{18}F-FSPG on PET/CT correlated significantly with extent of immunohistochemical staining for x_c^- transporter on pathology.[18] More recent preclinical studies of a cystine/glutamate analog, ^{18}F-fluoroaminosuberic acid,[47] demonstrated tumor uptake in multiple breast cancer cell lines and breast cancer tumor-bearing mice[48] and may soon be seen in clinical trials.

OTHER AMINO ACID ANALOGS FOR IMAGING

Multiple radiolabeled tyrosine analogs have been developed for tumor imaging, including L-[1–11C]tyrosine.[20] L-[1–11C]tyrosine successfully demonstrated uptake in breast malignancies and had lower uptake than ^{18}F-FDG in a limited number of benign lesions.[20] Technetium 99m Technetium–labeled tyrosine analogs have also been synthesized with high yield and distinguish breast malignancies from benign breast tissues.[49,50] Propanoic acid amino acid analogs, primarily dependent on system A transport, have been developed by the same group at Emory University that synthesized ^{18}F-fluciclovine.[51] In preclinical studies, multiple propanoic acid derivatives demonstrated good tumor uptake in human-derived breast cancer cells as well as in mouse tumor xenografts.[51]

Tryptophan analogs, primarily using L-type amino acid transport, have been developed by multiple research groups and have also demonstrated uptake in breast cancer cells and in small animal studies.[19,52] Recently, a newer leucine analog, 5-^{18}F]fluoroleucine, was synthesized, with primary transport via LAT1.[53] Both cell lines and breast cancer xenografts demonstrate 5-^{18}F]fluoroleucine uptake. As opposed to ^{18}F-fluciclovine, 5-^{18}F]fluoroleucine uptake progressively increases over time.[53] The glutaminolysis pathway is highly active in many malignancies, including triple-negative breast cancers.[54] Preclinical work with the glutamine analog [^{18}F](2S,4 R)4-fluoroglutamine[55,56] has demonstrated the ability of this tracer to track changes in the cellular glutamine pool size and the glutaminolysis pathway following glutaminase inhibition.[54]

FUTURE APPLICATIONS

There is substantial interest in the synthesis of novel amino acid metabolic radiotracers and the application of promising agents for tumor imaging, with the goal of developing molecular imaging biomarkers that predict the most efficacious therapies or successfully measure response to therapy.[57] Visualization of primary breast tumors is usually the first hurdle when promising agents are translating into human studies; however, this is unlikely to be where clinical benefit will be derived. As has been shown with ^{18}F-FDG, whole-body PET/CT is not sensitive for the primary breast malignancy compared with other available imaging modalities, such as mammography, ultrasound, and MRI. Truly remarkable sensitivity of a novel amino acid tracer would be required to supplant these imaging modalities for the primary breast malignancy. Rather, PET/CT has, to date, demonstrated unparalleled utility in the evaluation of distant metastases (and to a lesser extent, extra-axillary nodal metastases) with ^{18}F-FDG as the radiotracer.

The clinical impact of amino acid analog radiotracers could be determined by identifying niches where they outperform ^{18}F-FDG, such as the potential of ^{18}F-fluciclovine in lobular breast cancer. A thorough analysis of ^{18}F-fluciclovine for the detection of unsuspected distant metastases in patients with ILC, as well as its ability to monitor ILC treatment response, seems warranted. Because LAT1- mediated and ASCT2-mediated amino acid transport are involved in mTOR tumor signaling, therapy directed against this pathway could potentially be studied with amino acid transport imaging. Another interesting possibility is that, relative to indiscriminate ^{18}F-FDG uptake in inflammation, ^{18}F-fluciclovine is more selectively taken up by T cells and B cells, which could prove useful in imaging of immunomodulatory therapies.[58] Although the ultimate goal of a highly sensitive and specific radiotracer for breast cancer likely lies in targeted biomarker imaging directed to the breast cancer cell, metabolic agents, such as amino acid analogs, are ripe for nearer-term applications in specific scenarios of breast cancer.

SUMMARY

Amino acids are central to multiple metabolic processes in the cell. Amino acid transporters and amino acid metabolism are up-regulated in multiple malignancies, including breast cancers. Multiple amino acid analog radiotracers have been used to image breast cancer with unique strengths and weaknesses. Early work with ^{11}C-methionine demonstrated tracer uptake, which correlates with S-phase fraction in breast cancer and may be useful for evaluation of treatment response. Invasive lobular breast cancers may demonstrate greater ^{18}F-fluciclovine avidity than ^{18}F-FDG avidity, and thus evaluation of this tracer at initial ILC staging for the detection of unsuspected distant metastases, as well as for evaluation of treatment response in metastatic ILC, is warranted. There continues to be substantial research into the development and application of novel amino acid radiotracers.

ACKNOWLEDGMENTS

Dr G.A. Ulaner acknowledges the Department of Defense Breast Cancer Research Program Breakthrough Award BC132676 and the Memorial Sloan Kettering Cancer Center Radiochemistry and Molecular Imaging Probe Core (National Institutes of Health/National Cancer Institute (NIH/NCI) Cancer Center Support Grant P30 CA008748). Dr D.M. Schuster acknowledges support from the Glenn Family Breast Cancer Center, Winship Cancer Institute, Emory University, and has also participated in Emory University's Office of Sponsored Projects research supported in part by Blue Earth Diagnostics, Ltd, and Nihon Medi-Physics Co. Ltd.

REFERENCES

1. Gambhir SS, Czernin J, Schwimmer J, et al. A tabulated summary of the FDG PET literature. J Nucl Med 2001;42(5 Suppl):1S–93S.
2. Kang BJ, Lee JH, Yoo Ie R, et al. Clinical significance of incidental finding of focal activity in the breast at 18F-FDG PET/CT. AJR Am J Roentgenol 2011;197(2):341–7.
3. Fletcher JW, Djulbegovic B, Soares HP, et al. Recommendations on the use of 18F-FDG PET in oncology. J Nucl Med 2008;49(3):480–508.
4. Wahl RL, Siegel BA, Coleman RE, et al. Prospective multicenter study of axillary nodal staging by positron emission tomography in breast cancer: a report of the staging breast cancer with PET Study Group. J Clin Oncol 2004;22(2):277–85.
5. Peare R, Staff RT, Heys SD. The use of FDG-PET in assessing axillary lymph node status in breast cancer: a systematic review and meta-analysis of the literature. Breast Cancer Res Treat 2010;123(1):281–90.
6. Avril N, Menzel M, Dose J, et al. Glucose metabolism of breast cancer assessed by 18F-FDG PET: histologic and immunohistochemical tissue analysis. J Nucl Med 2001;42(1):9–16.
7. Buck A, Schirrmeister H, Kuhn T, et al. FDG uptake in breast cancer: correlation with biological and clinical prognostic parameters. Eur J Nucl Med Mol Imaging 2002;29(10):1317–23.
8. Gourin CG, Williams HT, Seabolt WN, et al. Utility of positron emission tomography-computed tomography in identification of residual nodal disease after chemoradiation for advanced head and neck cancer. Laryngoscope 2006;116(5):705–10.
9. Heudel P, Cimarelli S, Montella A, et al. Value of PET-FDG in primary breast cancer based on histopathological and immunohistochemical prognostic factors. Int J Clin Oncol 2010;15(6):588–93.
10. Riedl CC, Slobod E, Jochelson M, et al. Retrospective analysis of 18F-FDG PET/CT for staging asymptomatic breast cancer patients younger than 40 years. J Nucl Med 2014;55(10):1578–83.
11. Avril N, Rose CA, Schelling M, et al. Breast imaging with positron emission tomography and fluorine-18 fluorodeoxyglucose: use and limitations. J Clin Oncol 2000;18(20):3495–502.
12. Bos R, van Der Hoeven JJ, van Der Wall E, et al. Biologic correlates of (18)fluorodeoxyglucose uptake in human breast cancer measured by positron emission tomography. J Clin Oncol 2002;20(2):379–87.
13. Dashevsky BZ, Goldman DA, Parsons M, et al. Appearance of untreated bone metastases from breast cancer on FDG PET/CT: importance of histologic subtype. Eur J Nucl Med Mol Imaging 2015;42(11):1666–73.
14. Hogan MP, Goldman DA, Dashevsky B, et al. Comparison of 18F-FDG PET/CT for systemic staging of newly diagnosed invasive lobular carcinoma versus invasive ductal carcinoma. J Nucl Med 2015;56(11):1674–80.
15. Harrelson JP, Lee MW. Expanding the view of breast cancer metabolism: promising molecular targets and therapeutic opportunities. Pharmacol Ther 2016;167:60–73.

16. Haukaas TH, Euceda LR, Giskeodegard GF, et al. Metabolic portraits of breast cancer by HR MAS MR spectroscopy of intact tissue samples. Metabolites 2017;7(2) [pii: E18].

17. Leskinen-Kallio S, Nagren K, Lehikoinen P, et al. Uptake of 11C-methionine in breast cancer studied by PET. An association with the size of S-phase fraction. Br J Cancer 1991;64(6):1121–4.

18. Baek S, Choi CM, Ahn SH, et al. Exploratory clinical trial of (4S)-4-(3-[18F]fluoropropyl)-L-glutamate for imaging xC- transporter using positron emission tomography in patients with non-small cell lung or breast cancer. Clin Cancer Res 2012;18(19): 5427–37.

19. Xin Y, Cai H. Improved radiosynthesis and biological evaluations of L- and D-1-[18F]Fluoroethyl-tryptophan for PET imaging of IDO-mediated kynurenine pathway of tryptophan metabolism. Mol Imaging Biol 2017;19(4):589–98.

20. Kole AC, Nieweg OE, Pruim J, et al. Standardized uptake value and quantification of metabolism for breast cancer imaging with FDG and L-[1-11C]tyrosine PET. J Nucl Med 1997;38(5):692–6.

21. Liang Z, Cho HT, Williams L, et al. Potential biomarker of L-type amino acid transporter 1 in breast cancer progression. Nucl Med Mol Imaging 2011;45(2):93–102.

22. Jager PL, Plaat BE, de Vries EG, et al. Imaging of soft-tissue tumors using L-3-[iodine-123]iodo-alpha-methyl-tyrosine single photon emission computed tomography: comparison with proliferative and mitotic activity, cellularity, and vascularity. Clin Cancer Res 2000;6(6):2252–9.

23. Fuchs BC, Bode BP. Amino acid transporters ASCT2 and LAT1 in cancer: partners in crime? Semin Cancer Biol 2005;15(4):254–66.

24. Shennan DB, Thomson J. Inhibition of system L (LAT1/CD98hc) reduces the growth of cultured human breast cancer cells. Oncol Rep 2008;20(4): 885–9.

25. Karunakaran S, Ramachandran S, Coothankandaswamy V, et al. SLC6A14 (ATB0,+) protein, a highly concentrative and broad specific amino acid transporter, is a novel and effective drug target for treatment of estrogen receptor-positive breast cancer. J Biol Chem 2011;286(36): 31830–8.

26. Kim S, Kim DH, Jung WH, et al. Expression of glutamine metabolism-related proteins according to molecular subtype of breast cancer. Endocr Relat Cancer 2013;20(3):339–48.

27. Wang K, Cao F, Fang W, et al. Activation of SNAT1/SLC38A1 in human breast cancer: correlation with p-Akt overexpression. BMC Cancer 2013; 13:343.

28. Furuya M, Horiguchi J, Nakajima H, et al. Correlation of L-type amino acid transporter 1 and CD98 expression with triple negative breast cancer prognosis. Cancer Sci 2012;103(2):382–9.

29. van Geldermalsen M, Wang Q, Nagarajah R, et al. ASCT2/SLC1A5 controls glutamine uptake and tumour growth in triple-negative basal-like breast cancer. Oncogene 2016;35(24):3201–8.

30. Huovinen R, Leskinen-Kallio S, Nagren K, et al. Carbon-11-methionine and PET in evaluation of treatment response of breast cancer. Br J Cancer 1993;67(4):787–91.

31. Jansson T, Westlin JE, Ahlstrom H, et al. Positron emission tomography studies in patients with locally advanced and/or metastatic breast cancer: a method for early therapy evaluation? J Clin Oncol 1995;13(6):1470–7.

32. Lindholm P, Lapela M, Nagren K, et al. Preliminary study of carbon-11 methionine PET in the evaluation of early response to therapy in advanced breast cancer. Nucl Med Commun 2009;30(1): 30–6.

33. Sharma S, Singh B, Mishra AK, et al. LAT-1 based primary breast cancer detection by ^{99m}Tc-labeled DTPA-bis-methionine scintimammography: first results using indigenously developed single vial kit preparation. Cancer Biother Radiopharm 2014;29(7):283–8.

34. Shoup TM, Olson J, Hoffman JM, et al. Synthesis and evaluation of [18F]1-amino-3-fluorocyclobutane-1-carboxylic acid to image brain tumors. J Nucl Med 1999;40(2):331–8.

35. Schuster DM, Nanni C, Fanti S. Evaluation of prostate cancer with radiolabeled amino acid analogs. J Nucl Med 2016;57(Suppl 3):61S–6S.

36. Savir-Baruch B, Zanoni L, Schuster DM. Imaging of prostate cancer using fluciclovine. PET Clin 2017; 12(2):145–57.

37. Okudaira H, Shikano N, Nishii R, et al. Putative transport mechanism and intracellular fate of trans-1-amino-3-18F-fluorocyclobutanecarboxylic acid in human prostate cancer. J Nucl Med 2011;52(5): 822–9.

38. Okudaira H, Nakanishi T, Oka S, et al. Kinetic analyses of trans-1-amino-3-[18F]fluorocyclobutanecarboxylic acid transport in Xenopus laevis oocytes expressing human ASCT2 and SNAT2. Nucl Med Biol 2013; 40(5):670–5.

39. Oka S, Okudaira H, Ono M, et al. Differences in transport mechanisms of trans-1-amino-3-[18F] fluorocyclobutanecarboxylic acid in inflammation, prostate cancer, and glioma cells: comparison with L-[methyl-11C]methionine and 2-deoxy-2-[18F]fluoro-D-glucose. Mol Imaging Biol 2014; 16(3):322–9.

40. Teoh E, Morotti M, Bridges E, et al. Fluciclovine (18F) is a marker for high-affinity glutamine transporter ASCT2-mediated amino acid transport in breast cancer. J Nucl Med 2017;58(supplement 1):1028.

41. Ulaner GA, Goldman DA, Gonen M, et al. Initial results of a prospective clinical trial of 18F-fluciclovine PET/CT in newly diagnosed invasive ductal and invasive lobular breast cancers. J Nucl Med 2016; 57(9):1350–6.

42. Tade FI, Cohen MA, Styblo TM, et al. Anti-3-18F-FACBC (18F-Fluciclovine) PET/CT of breast cancer: an exploratory study. J Nucl Med 2016;57(9): 1357–63.

43. Ulaner GA, Goldman DA, Corben A, et al. Prospective clinical trial of 18F-fluciclovine PET/CT for determining the response to neoadjuvant therapy in invasive ductal and invasive lobular breast cancers. J Nucl Med 2017;58(7):1037–42.

44. Oka S, Kanagawa M, Doi Y, et al. PET tracer 18F-fluciclovine can detect histologically proven bone metastatic lesions: a preclinical study in rat osteolytic and osteoblastic bone metastasis models. Theranostics 2017;7(7):2048–64.

45. Oka S, Kanagawa M, Doi Y, et al. Fasting enhances the contrast of bone metastatic lesions in 18F-fluciclovine-PET: preclinical study using a rat model of mixed osteolytic/osteoblastic bone metastases. Int J Mol Sci 2017;18(5) [pii: E934].

46. Koglin N, Mueller A, Berndt M, et al. Specific PET imaging of xC- transporter activity using a (1)(8)F-labeled glutamate derivative reveals a dominant pathway in tumor metabolism. Clin Cancer Res 2011;17(18):6000–11.

47. Webster JM, Morton CA, Johnson BF, et al. Functional imaging of oxidative stress with a novel PET imaging agent, 18F-5-fluoro-L-aminosuberic acid. J Nucl Med 2014;55(4):657–64.

48. Yang H, Jenni S, Colovic M, et al. 18F-5-fluoroaminosuberic acid as a potential tracer to gauge oxidative stress in breast cancer models. J Nucl Med 2017; 58(3):367–73.

49. Kong FL, Ali MS, Zhang Y, et al. Synthesis and evaluation of amino acid-based radiotracer 99mTc-N4-AMT for breast cancer imaging. J Biomed Biotechnol 2011 2011:276907.

50. Kong FL, Ali MS, Rollo A, et al. Development o tyrosine-based radiotracer 99mTc-N4-Tyrosine fo breast cancer imaging. J Biomed Biotechnol 2012 2012:671708.

51. Yu W, McConathy J, Olson JJ, et al. System a amin acid transport-targeted brain and systemic tumo PET imaging agents 2-amino-3-[(18)F]fluoro-2 methylpropanoic acid and 3-[(18)F]fluoro-2-methyl 2-(methylamino)propanoic acid. Nucl Med Bic 2015;42(1):8–18.

52. Michelhaugh SK, Muzik O, Guastella AR, et al Assessment of tryptophan uptake and kinetics usinς 1-(2-18F-fluoroethyl)-l-tryptophan and alpha-11C methyl-l-tryptophan PET imaging in mice implanted with patient-derived brain tumor xenografts. J Nuc Med 2017;58(2):208–13.

53. Chin BB, McDougald D, Weitzel DH, et al. Synthesis and preliminary evaluation of 5-[18F]fluoroleucine Curr Radiopharm 2017;10(1):41–50.

54. Zhou R, Pantel AR, Li S, et al. [18F](2S,4R)4-fluoro glutamine PET detects glutamine pool size change in triple-negative breast cancer in response to gluta minase inhibition. Cancer Res 2017;77(6):1476–84.

55. Qu W, Zha Z, Ploessl K, et al. Synthesis of opticalĺ pure 4-fluoro-glutamines as potential metabolic im aging agents for tumors. J Am Chem Soc 2011 133(4):1122–33.

56. Lieberman BP, Ploessl K, Wang L, et al. PET imaginς of glutaminolysis in tumors by 18F-(2S,4R)4-fluoro glutamine. J Nucl Med 2011;52(12):1947–55.

57. Ulaner GA, Riedl CC, Dickler MN, et al. Molecula imaging of biomarkers in breast cancer. J Nuc Med 2016;57(Suppl 1):53S–9S.

58. Teoh EJ, Tsakok MT, Bradley KM, et al. Recurren malignant melanoma detected on 18F-fluciclovine PET/CT imaging for prostate cancer. Clin Nucl Mec 2017;42(10):803–4.

Imaging Tumor Proliferation in Breast Cancer
Current Update on Predictive Imaging Biomarkers

Azadeh Elmi, MD, Elizabeth S. McDonald, MD, PhD,
David Mankoff, MD, PhD*

KEYWORDS

- Breast cancer • PET imaging • Radiotracer • Tumor proliferation • Targeted therapies

KEY POINTS

- Imaging cell proliferation can provide an early measure of treatment response that can be used to guide personalized treatment.
- Imaging biomarkers of proliferation is especially beneficial in the setting of regimens exploiting cell cycle–targeted chemotherapies in combination with endocrine therapy.
- FLT uptake can quantify the S-phase fraction of cycling cancer cells.
- ISO-1 uptake can measure overall proliferative status of the tumor.

INTRODUCTION

Breast cancer is one of the most common cancers and the second leading cause of cancer-related death among women in the United States. Up to 6% of breast cancers are advanced or metastatic at the time of diagnosis, requiring chemotherapy.[1,2] Accelerated growth is a hallmark of cancer,[3] including breast cancer. The rapid expansion of treatments targeted to aberrant cell growth (eg, cell cycle–targeted chemotherapies for the treatment of metastatic breast cancer) allows for precise targeting of specific alterations in tumor cell proliferation pathway with the goal of reducing tumor cellular proliferation and increasing tumor cell death while minimizing toxicities associated with chemotherapy. The growing application of these targeted therapies motivates cell proliferation imaging techniques that can reflect the treatment response from cell cycle inhibition before morphologic and anatomic changes.

Evaluation of Ki-67 expression on biopsy samples is currently considered the gold standard for evaluating cell proliferation. A major drawback for clinical use of Ki-67 is that it requires serial biopsies of the primary tumor sites and/or metastatic lesions to assess changes in cell proliferation in response to therapy. Therefore, this technique is invasive and also prone to sampling errors and underestimation of tumor heterogeneity.[4,5] An

This work was supported in part by the Susan G. Komen Foundation (Dr E.S. McDonald CCR16376362 and Dr D. Mankoff SAC130060, Department of Energy Grant DE-SC0012476, and NIH Grant 5T32EB004311-13 for radiology research track residency). Dr E.S. McDonald is also the 2016–2018 American Roentgen Ray Society/Philips Healthcare Scholar. Grants support related research and support, in part, the effort of the coauthors.
Department of Radiology, Perelman School of Medicine, University of Pennsylvania, 3400 Spruce Street, Philadelphia, PA 19104, USA
* Corresponding author. Hospital of the University of Pennsylvania, 3400 Spruce Street, 1 Donner, Philadelphia, PA 19104.
E-mail address: david.mankoff@uphs.upenn.edu

PET Clin 13 (2018) 445–457
https://doi.org/10.1016/j.cpet.2018.02.007

imaging biomarker is an attractive noninvasive alternative that can provide spatial data of primary and metastatic disease. Imaging cell proliferation can provide an early noninvasive indicator of cancer therapeutic response that is used to guide personalized treatment with identifying patients that benefit from those that might not need or benefit from the therapy, early in the course of treatment to avoid toxicity and additional costs.

This review focuses on currently investigational cell proliferation imaging PET radiotracers to evaluate tumor proliferation in the setting of cell cycle–targeted chemotherapy and endocrine therapy for metastatic breast cancer. We review the underlying biology associated with cancer proliferation and cell cycle–targeted drugs, followed by a review of the mechanistic underpinnings of cell proliferation tracers, and finally, their application to therapy targeted to aberrant breast cancer proliferation.

CELL CYCLE AND PROLIFERATION CONTROL: ENHANCING ENDOCRINE THERAPY WITH CELL CYCLE–TARGETING AGENTS

Proliferating cells must progress through four phases of cell cycle (G1, S, G2, and M); however, they may exit the cell cycle and enter quiescence (G0) when stressed or deprived of biologic stimuli (eg, in breast cancer with estrogen deprivation).[6,7] Cyclin-dependent kinases (CDKs) play a key role in controlling cell cycle progression. Among these kinases, CDK4/6 is the key regulator of G1 to S transition by controlling transcription of genes necessary for cell cycle progression. This kinase is activated on binding to cyclin D, leading to expression of genes required for S-phase entry.[8] The tightly regulated cyclin D-CDK4/6 complex is frequently disrupted in breast cancer, with subsequent inactivation of the G1-S checkpoint, which can lead to aberrant growth and ultimately tumor formation.[8,9]

Another important player in breast cancer is estrogen pathway. Estrogen stimulates the proliferation of estrogen receptor (ER)-positive cancer cells via activation of cyclin D (**Fig. 1**).[10] Approximately 70% to 75% of breast cancers express hormone receptors and most of these cancers depend on estrogen signaling for their growth and survival.[11] Endocrine therapy has been the mainstay of treatment in patients with metastatic ER-positive disease and when compared with conventional chemotherapy, it is primarily cytostatic.[12] Endocrine therapy–induced growth inhibition traps cancer cells at the G0/G1 phase of the cell cycle.[13] Subsequently, the apoptotic pathway is activated for some of these cells resulting in cell death. However, fractions of the cells might remain in quiescence and evidence suggests that these cells may play an important role in recurrences of hormone-responsive breast cancer, reflecting underlying tumor dormancy.[14]

Tamoxifen is a selective ER modulator and is used to treat early and advanced ER-positive breast cancer. In breast tissue, tamoxifen is a selective ER down-regulator resulting in blockade of the estrogen-signaling pathway.[15] Prior studies demonstrated clear survival benefits in patients with ER-positive breast cancer. For example, the EBCTCG study reported approximately 30% reduction in breast cancer mortality for 15 years after diagnosis along with substantial reduction in cancer recurrence in patients reviving tamoxifen.[16] Fulvestrant is another ER modulator, approved for the treatment of ER-positive metastatic breast cancer after standard antiestrogen

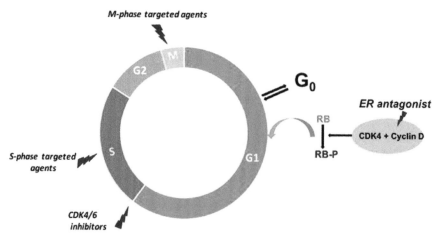

Fig. 1. Cell cycle–targeted chemotherapeutics and estrogen modulators.

therapy.[17] This agent inhibits estrogen signaling and tumor proliferation by competing with estradiol binding to the ER, and by down-regulating ER receptor with subsequent reduction in tumor proliferation.[18]

Additional cancer therapies that target ER pathway deplete the agonist ligand, estradiol. Aromatase inhibitors work by blocking aromatase enzyme activity resulting in reduction of circulating and local estrogen levels. Several meta-analyses underscore clear advantage of third-generation aromatase inhibitors (anastrozole and letrozole) compared with tamoxifen[19,20] for postmenopausal patients, for whom the lack of ovarian synthesis makes aromatase inhibition an effective strategy.

Despite efficacy of various ER antagonists, eventual resistance to such therapies unfortunately can occur,[21] sometimes leading to relapse and death. Several mechanisms of resistance to endocrine therapy have been described including the cross-talk between the ER pathway and cell cycle and growth factors, such as high cyclin D1 expression and Rb phosphorylation.[22] Changes in these key cell cycle check points result in dysregulated cell cycle progression contributing to loss of endocrine responsiveness.[23] Different strategies have been used to delay acquired resistance and improve the outcome of patients with ER-positive metastatic breast cancer. One of the emerging treatments is combining endocrine therapy with a cell cycle–targeted agent.

CDK4/6 inhibitors have recently become an important tool for breast cancer treatment. CDK4/6 inhibitors work by blocking the phosphorylation of Rb, inducing G1 arrest and halting proliferation and resulting in tumor cell senescence.[24] Because ER-positive tumors usually retain Rb activity and can have cyclin-D1 amplification, they are good targets for CDK4/6 inhibitors. ER signaling upregulates cyclin D1 levels and potentiate multiple signaling pathways largely culminating in upregulation of CDK4/6 activity.[25,26] One main outcome of such treatment is the arrest of the cancer cells at G1, so when combined with other agents, such as ER selective modulators, they synergistically inhibit cancer growth.[27] Three CDK4/6 inhibitors have been evaluated in clinical trials in patients with hormone receptor–positive early and metastatic breast cancer: palbociclib, ribociclib, and abemaciclib. Palbociclib recently received Food and Drug Administration (FDA) approval as the first-line treatment of metastatic ER-positive breast cancer in combination with endocrine therapy, in women with prior endocrine-resistant cancer.[28] Ribociclib also has been approved by the FDA as a combination therapy with aromatase inhibitor as initial therapy in postmenopausal women with ER-positive HER2-negative breast cancer.[29]

Response to endocrine therapy has been evaluated using conventional anatomic imaging and fluorodeoxyglucose (FDG)-PET. Metabolic response assessed by [18F]FDG-PET in patients with metastatic breast cancer undergoing endocrine therapy has been shown to be predictive of progression-free survival.[30] Recently [18F]F-fluoroestradiol PET, which is a specific ER-targeted molecular probe for PET for evaluation of ER expression, has successfully been used for quantifying in vivo ER expression in patients with breast cancer. Numerous clinical studies evaluated the role of [18F]F-fluoroestradiol PET as a predictive biomarker for assessing in vivo pharmacodynamic response to endocrine therapy.[31] Although clinical studies have shown efficacy of different PET imaging biomarkers in predicting the response to endocrine therapy,[32] increasing application of combination cell cycle–targeted therapies raises the need for imaging targeting cell proliferation and the cell cycle to evaluate response to targeted treatments.

TISSUE PROLIFERATION ASSAYS

Numerous techniques have been used as measures of cell proliferation using patients' blood/tissue samples. These techniques mainly focus on evaluation of cells in S-phase after tissue biopsy. Mitotic index was one of the initial techniques, which is still widely used and often integrated into tumor grading systems. Historically, thymidine labeling index was used to measure the S-phase fraction, requiring incubation of fresh tissue section with tritiated thymidine (3HTdR) in vitro followed by autoradiography of the slides.[33] However, flow cytometric analysis of cell cycle by evaluating cell DNA content is another common method for measuring proliferation in the clinical setting. Expression of a nuclear protein during the cell cycle, Ki-67, is currently the standard technique for assessing cell proliferation. Studies have confirmed that the Ki67 index correlates with the results of mitotic index and flow cytometry.[34,35] Inwald and colleagues[36] studied the associations between Ki-67 and common histopathologic parameters in a large cohort of 3658 patients. They demonstrated an association between Ki-67 expression and tumor grading. In multivariable analysis, Ki-67 was a prognostic parameter for disease-free survival and overall survival, independent of clinical and histopathologic factors. Clinical application of the tissue-based proliferation assays is largely limited by the heterogeneity of the proliferation process in tumors and the invasive nature of these methods.

IMAGING CELL PROLIFERATION: TRACER DEVELOPMENT
Early Tracers

PET imaging has been used to evaluate in vivo tumor proliferation. Much of the work on proliferation imaging has focused on radiotracers that are precursors for DNA synthesis, such as [11]C- and [18]fluorine-labeled nucleosides. Nucleoside-based imaging enables assessment of tumor proliferation by rapid incorporation of radiolabeled nucleosides into newly synthesized DNA. Thymidine has been the main target for such imaging because it is a nucleotide that is exclusively incorporated into DNA and not RNA.[37] Briefly, thymidine from the bloodstream enters the biochemical pathway to DNA synthesis via the "salvage" pathway, where it is transported into the cell, phosphorylated by thymidine kinase, and incorporated into DNA.[38]

Historically, tritiated thymidine was used to evaluate tumor proliferation[38,39]; quantitative autoradiography of the animal tissues to record emissions from the tritium was correlated to pathologic measures of thymidine incorporation. Although this technique can quantify the fraction of the cells at the S phase, it cannot provide information about the cells in other phases of cell cycle, and the pace of cell proliferation. Another important pitfall was the limitation of this technique for clinical application, such as the need for tumor biopsy and radiation exposure, because of long-lived tracer.

Early studies paved the road for development of thymidine-based radiotracers for PET imaging using short-lived tracers with minimal radiation burden. [11C]thymidine was one of the first PET proliferation radiotracers used in the setting of cancer imaging, in analogy with early work using [14C]thymidine as an in vitro marker of cellular proliferation.[38] The most successful version of [11C]thymidine was labeled with ^{11}C at the C2-position in the pyrimidine ring or at the 5-methyl position. Preclinical and clinical studies demonstrated good correlation between this radiotracer, DNA synthesis, and proliferation.[40] Shields and colleagues[37] performed one of the early studies to investigate the ability of [11C]thymidine to measure early response to chemotherapy after 1 week of therapy and compared the findings with metabolic changes in the tumor as measured by FDG-PET. They reported significant decrease in radiotracer uptake in the responder group; although these differences were present in the FDG-PET, the changes in [11C]thymidine-PET uptake were better correlated with response. Despite the early promising result, this probe was not practical for the clinical setting because of the short half-life (half-life, 20 minutes) and rapid metabolism.[40] Another drawback was the complexity of imaging interpretation needing mathematical modeling and accurate measurements of the circulating metabolites.[41]

Subsequent studies investigated the pyrimidine probes labeled with ^{18}F with the goal of longer half-life (half-life, 110 minutes) and less catabolism to enable clinical imaging with these tracers. 3'-deoxy-3'[18F]fluorothymidine (FLT) and 2'-fluoro-5-([11C]-methyl)-1-beta-D-arabinofuranosyluracil (FMAU) are the more favorable radiotracers that have been used in preclinical and clinical settings. Conti and colleagues[42] reported FMAU as a promising radiotracer for cellular proliferation. They suggested that this radiotracer shares some important in vivo features of thymidine such as phosphorylation by kinase, incorporation into DNA, and limited catabolism. Thus, FMAU has potential for providing simplified kinetic models for determination of cellular proliferation using PET imaging. However, because FMAU also takes part in cytosolic DNA synthesis along with the nuclear DNA, this might be a limitation because this background incorporation into mitochondrial DNA leads to nonspecific FMAU retention, making this radiotracer less sensitive than FLT for assessment of changes in cell proliferation.[43]

3'-Deoxy-3'[18F]Fluorothymidine-PET

3'-Deoxy-3'[18F]fluorothymidine is a metabolized thymidine analogue that can serve as a surrogate of proliferation by targeting the activity of thymidine salvage pathway of DNA synthesis.[44] This radiotracer has better metabolic stability when compared with prior labeled thymidine analogues, such as IUdR and [11C]thymidine. FLT enters tissue by Na^+-dependent active transporters dominated by human equilibrative nucleoside transporter 1. The level of this transporter increases as proliferating cells enter the cell cycle; accordingly, the expression is upregulated in the setting of cancer[45] and this might influence radiotracer uptake and signal in the in vivo setting.[46] [18F]FLT is phosphorylated in the cells by thymidine kinase-1 resulting in intracellular trapping and accumulation of this tracer; but unlike thymidine, FLT is not incorporated into the DNA structure. Thymidine kinase-1 activity is a rate limiting factor in the salvage pathway of DNA synthesis; thus, its activity is closely correlated with DNA synthesis.[38] Concentration of this enzyme increases almost 10-fold during the S-phase of cell cycle and subsequently [18F]FLT-PET uptake increases, which can indirectly quantify the S-phase fraction of cycling cancer cells, reflecting cell proliferation.[47] Semi-routine production of [18F]FLT has been established in many centers, including some commercial suppliers, and it has been widely studied in clinical trials for imaging cell proliferation of various tumor types, such as lung, head and neck, and breast cancer.[48]

3'-Deoxy-3'[18F]fluorothymidine uptake in primary breast cancer as a prognostic factor

[18F]FLT uptake has been shown to correlate with cell proliferation in untreated patients with breast cancer. Smyczek-Gargya and coworkers[49] used [18F]FLT-PET in the setting of primary breast cancer and compared its performance with [18F]FDG-PET and reported uptake of both radiotracers in cancer tissues. The standardized uptake values (SUVs) of primary tumors and axillary lymph node metastases were lower in FLT-PET when compared with FDG study (SUV_{FLT}, 3.2 vs SUV_{FDG}, 4.7 in primary tumors; SUV_{FLT}, 2.9 vs SUV_{FDG}, 4.6 in lymph node metastases). However, given very low background FLT uptake in the mediastinum, the tumor-to-mediastinum ratio was significantly higher in [18F]FLT-PET studies.[49] Of note, however, the high level of [18F]FLT uptake in the liver (caused by hepatic clearance) and proliferating bone marrow makes visualization and quantification of uptake in liver and bone metastases challenging.

Kenny and colleagues[50] demonstrated [18F]FLT accumulation in primary tumor, nodal disease, and lung metastases in patients with breast cancer. They also noted heterogeneity of radiotracer uptake, which was related to heterogeneity of cell proliferation within and between disease sites.[50] The delivery and retention of [18F]FLT was shown to be higher when compared with normal breast tissue ($P<.0001$), and FLT retention correlated with Ki-67 labeling index from tumor biopsies.

Tumor expression of Ki-67 has been established as a marker of proliferation and a prognostic marker in breast cancer. A meta-analysis explored the correlation between FLT uptake and Ki-67 expression and showed a correlation, independent of cancer type. Additionally, subgroup analysis supported a correlation between FLT uptake and expression in breast cancer.[51]

3'-Deoxy-3'[18F]fluorothymidine-PET for early treatment response prediction to chemotherapy

[18F]FDG-PET/computed tomography has been widely used for assessing response to chemotherapy, targeted therapy, and endocrine treatment in breast cancer[52,53]; however, this imaging technique does not capture changes in

proliferation in response to therapy. Contractor and colleagues[54] evaluated the early changes in [18F]FLT-PET uptake after 2 weeks of initiating the first or second cycle of docetaxel in a prospective study in 20 patients with breast cancer. They demonstrated a significant decrease in SUVmax and SUVmean at 60 minutes, which was significantly different in responders when compared with the nonresponders (40% vs 11%). This reduction in tumor SUV was associated with target lesion size changes mid-therapy (after three cycles). Another study of [18F]FLT-PET in the neoadjuvant setting failed to demonstrated any significant association between baseline, postchemotherapy, or change in SUVmax and pathologic response, despite sizable reduction in SUVmax in most of the cases. However, the baseline SUVmax was significantly associated with Ki-67, confirming the role of FLT-PET as a proliferation biomarker.[55] A prospective cohort pilot study of patients with potentially operable, locally advanced T2/T3 breast cancer undergoing anthracycline/taxane-based neoadjuvant chemotherapy followed by surgical resection of cancer evaluated the role of [18F]FLT-PET in predicting treatment response before, after the first cycle, and at the end of neoadjuvant therapy (**Fig. 2**).[56] After the first cycle of chemotherapy, changes in the SUVmax of primary tumor demonstrated a good predictive power for identifying complete and near complete responders with overall accuracy of 93.3%, sensitivity of 83.3%, the specificity of 100.0%, and the positive and negative predictive values of 100.0% and 90.0%, respectively.[56]

Data from these single-center studies have been promising with good sensitivity of [18F]FLT-PET for assessing changes in tumor proliferation after chemotherapy to predict subsequent treatment response; however, they all came from single centers and included small patient populations, suggesting the need for further validation. The American College of Radiology Imaging Network (ACRIN) study 6688 performed a nonrandomized, multicenter phase II study with the aim of correlating changes of [18F]FLT-PET approximately 1 week after chemotherapy with pathologic response at the end of treatment in patients with primary breast cancer who were undergoing neoadjuvant therapy.[57] Fifty-one patients underwent FLT-PET/CT at baseline, after one cycle and after completion of neoadjuvant therapy. Complete pathologic response was reported in nine patients (18%) with significant but modest difference when comparing changes in SUVmax between those with complete pathologic response and other patients (P value = .05). They also assessed the correlation

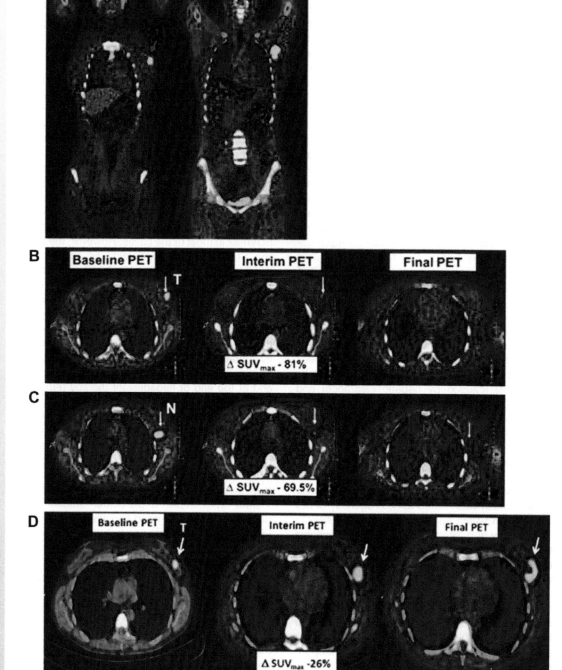

Fig. 2. FLT-PET for prediction of early treatment response. (*A*) Coronal fused PET/computed tomography (CT) slices show abnormal areas of FLT uptake corresponding to a primary breast tumor (T) and a dominant axillary metastatic node (N). (*B, C*) Transaxial CT, PET, and fused PET/CT images in an neoadjuvant chemotherapy (NCT) responding patient show FLT uptake changes in the primary breast tumor (*B*) and in the dominant axillary metastatic node (*C*). Postsurgery histology revealed a complete pathologic response in the mammary gland and in the removed axillary nodes (0/10 nodes). (*D*) Axial fused PET/CT slices in a nonresponding patient. In the interim PET image, the abnormal area of FLT uptake corresponding to the primary cancer (*arrow*) is larger than in the baseline PET image, despite a partial reduction in tracer accumulation (ΔSUVmax = −26%). In the final PET image, there is a further increase in the area of FLT uptake with appearance of a photopenic central area, attributable to tumor necrosis. (*Adapted from* Crippa F, Agresti R, Sandri M, et al. ^{18}F-FLT PET/CT as an imaging tool for early prediction of pathological response in patients with locally advanced breast cancer treated with neoadjuvant chemotherapy: a pilot study. Eur J Nucl Med Mol Imaging 2015;42(6):822; with permission.)

between baseline and post-treatment SUVmax with Ki-67 and reported strong correlation only between SUVmax and Ki-67 after completion of neoadjuvant therapy. Although this was a multi-center study, results need further validation because there were a small number of patients. In addition, the chemotherapy regimen was variable among centers and treatment variation was not considered in the analysis. This study supports the potential of FLT-PET, but thus far, has not provided sufficient evidence to support FDA approval of FLT-PET as an early biomarker of treatment response in breast cancer.

A recent meta-analysis of four articles including 46 patients and 54 tumors evaluated the diagnostic performance of [18F]FLT-PET for assessing response to chemotherapy in patients with breast cancer and reported a pooled sensitivity of 77.3% and pooled specificity of 68% predicting response for this modality and concluded that this imaging technique is useful to predict response with reasonable diagnostic profile.[58] The result of this review is limited because of the pooled small studies and patient number and using different chemotherapy regimens, imaging techniques, and reference standard across different studies.

3'-Deoxy-3'[18F]fluorothymidine-PET for predicting treatment response to endocrine therapy

To commit a patient with breast cancer to endocrine therapy alone, it would be ideal to determine which tumors will respond to such therapy early in the course of treatment. Serial biopsy and Ki-67 analysis demonstrated potential for assessing endocrine therapy response early in the course of treatment, predicting long-term outcome after neoadjuvant endocrine therapy in several clinical trials.[59,60] ACOSOG Z1031 trial also tested Ki-67-based algorithms to identify patients who are poorly responsive to neoadjuvant endocrine therapy.[61] Previous imaging studies supported the ability of FDG-PET, as an indirect measure of cell proliferation, to evaluate early treatment response to endocrine therapy,[52] in line with Ki-67-based studies. The results from tissue assay studies, however, motivate the evaluation of more direct imaging measures of proliferation, such as FLT-PET. Roberts and colleagues evaluated the associations between parametric analysis of dynamic [18F]FLT-PET and Ki-67 at baseline and following 2 weeks of endocrine monotherapy in patients with early stage ER-positive breast cancer, before definitive surgery. SUVmax declined in all 26 patients except for one, whereas Ki-67 declined in all lesions. An average decline of 27% in SUVmax after 2 weeks of treatment was reported correlating to an average of 68% decrease in Ki-67.[62] This study, still at an early stage of evaluation, motivates investigations of the possible role of [18F]FLT-PET as an early noninvasive biomarker of response in the setting of endocrine therapy.

Further support for FLT as a marker of endocrine therapy response is found in published preclinical literature. Whisenant et al. evaluated FLT-PET as an early marker of trastuzumab response in HER2-overexpressing xenografts of breast cancer. This was further investigated in xenograft model of breast cancer by comparing the changes in tumor-to-muscle FLT uptake ratio both in trastuzumab-sensitive and -resistant before and after treatment with trastuzumab. They concluded [18F]FLT-PET is a sensitive modality for predicting early molecular changes in trastuzumab-sensitive breast cancer xenografts. They suggested that [18F]FLT-PET may be able to distinguish nonresponders from responders earlier during the course of treatment.[63]

[18F]FLT-PET has been also used in the setting of treatment with investigational drug, steroid sulfatase inhibitor. Steroid sulfatase targets aromatase pathway for estrogen synthesis by converting estrone sulfate to estrone. Irosustat is a first-generation, irreversible steroid sulfatase inhibitor that has been recently evaluated in clinical trials.[64] A presurgical window of opportunity study used [18F]FLT-PET in postmenopausal women with ER-positive breast cancer at baseline and after 2 weeks of therapy with irosustat to demonstrate proof of concept data that suggest that steroid sulfatase inhibition is effective in reducing tumor proliferation as measured by FLT-PET, in vivo. They reported significant reduction in FLT uptake and Ki-67 after 2 weeks of treatment.[65]

Limitation of 3'-deoxy-3'[18F]fluorothymidine-PET for cancer proliferation imaging

Overall, lower uptake of FLT is an inherent limitation of this imaging technique. This could result in low sensitivity for assessment of changes in the small metastatic lesions and regional lymph node metastases with more false-negative findings compared with [18F]FDG-PET. Another drawback is related to high background [18F]FLT uptake in liver and bone marrow, which has been attributed to glucuronidation of [18F]FLT in liver and high level of cellular proliferation and kinetics of FLT in bone marrow.[50,55,66] This physiologic uptake limits evaluation of extent of disease in these organs that are in fact common sites of metastatic breast cancer.

Tumors are heterogeneous, growing asynchronously with tumor cells in different phases of cell cycle. Thus, measuring only S-fraction as obtained by FLT-PET underestimates the pool of proliferating cells because it cannot differentiate between proliferating cells in G1, G2, and M phases versus quiescent cells at G0. This may have important implications for determining appropriate treatment regimen. For example, cell cycle–targeted chemotherapies are effective in tumors with a high index of cell proliferation, whereas other agents should be used in the setting of low-proliferating tumors.[67] McKinley and coworkers[68] addressed the mixed results about accuracy of [18F]FLT in quantification of changes in proliferation by assessing the quantitative relationships between [18F]FLT-PET and cellular metrics of proliferation in human breast cancer model. They demonstrated that the de novo pathway of thymidine synthesis is one of the causes of decoupling of [18F]FLT uptake from Ki-67 expression in the tumors that mainly depend on this de novo thymidine synthesis pathway.[68]

Alternative Approach to Imaging Proliferation: [2-(2-[18F]fluoroethoxy)-N-(4-(3,4-dihydro-6,7-dimethoxyisoquinolin-2(1H)-yl)butyl)-5-methylbenzamide PET

Proliferative status is one of the principal measures of cell proliferation and is defined as the ratio of proliferating cells (in G1, S, G2, or M phases) to quiescent cells (P:Q ratio). Estimation of S-fraction by [18F]FLT is insufficient to provide a comprehensive estimate of proliferative status as it measures DNA synthesis, which happens primarily in the S-phase. An alternative approach targets the σ-receptors, which has been investigated as a biomarker of proliferative status.[69] This marker originally was classified as opiate receptors with two subtypes: σ_1 and σ_2. The σ_2-receptor subtype been shown to be unregulated during transition from quiescent state to G1 and it has been reported to be overexpressed in some tumors, including breast cancer.[70] Accordingly, the expression is higher in proliferating cells making it a particularly appealing receptor-based biomarker of cell proliferation in breast cancer. Mach and colleagues[69] compared the density of σ_2-receptors between proliferating and quiescent mouse mammary adenocarcinoma cell line 66 and showed that it is approximately 10 times higher in the proliferating breast cancer cells.

[11]C labeled σ_2 receptor ligands were developed initially. Mach and colleagues[71] reported four ^{11}C-labeled benzamide analogues with high affinity and selectivity for σ_2 versus σ_1-receptors. They suggested one of these compounds ((2-methoxy-^{11}C)-N-(4-(3,4-dihydro-6,7-dimethoxy-isoquinolin-2(1H)-yl)butyl)-5-methylbenzamide) has potential for imaging the breast tumors proliferation given the high tumor uptake and suitable tumor to background ratio.[72] They also established comparison of this compound with [18F]FLT-PET, which is currently performed as a measure of cell proliferation and demonstrated similar tumor/lung and tumor/fat ratios for both imaging markers, whereas their radiotracer for imaging σ_2 receptor had a higher tumor/blood and tumor/muscle ratio.

[18]F-radiolabeled σ_2-receptor was also validated in a variety of cancer animal models such as pancreatic cancer and breast cancer.[7] Correlative analysis of the tissue using micro-PET imaging revealed preferential expression of σ_2 in tumor as opposed to normal tissues. A ^{18}F-radiolabeled σ_2-receptors were synthesized and analysis of the chemistry and biodistribution data showed two fluorine-containing benzamide analogues that can be used for proliferation imaging.[74]

Preclinical data: 2-(2-[18F]fluoroethoxy)-N-(4-(3,4-dihydro-6,7-dimethoxyisoquinolin-2(1H)-yl)butyl)-5-methylbenzamide for imaging the proliferative status of tumors

One of the early preclinical studies evaluated the treatment response to bexarotene in mouse mammary tumor 66 with σ_2 receptor ligand 2-(2-[18F]fluoroethoxy)-N-(4-(3,4-dihydro-6,7-dimethoxyisoquinolin-2(1H)-yl)butyl)-5-methylbenzamide, ([18F]ISO-1) and findings were compared with [18F]FDG micro-PET and MR imaging.[75] This imaging finding was also correlated with P:Q ratio as determined by flow cytometric cell cycle analysis. [18F]ISO-1 revealed good contrast with high tumor to background uptake ratio when compared with [18F]FDG-PET. Accordingly, [18F]ISO-1 imaging demonstrated a strong linear correlation between the radiotracer uptake ratio and P:Q ratio ($R = 0.87$), although this correlation was poor for [18F]FDG-PET ($R = 0.37$). Using another model of breast cancer (N-methyl-N-nitrosourea (MNU-induced tumors) they assessed tumor growth rate in relation to [18F]ISO-1 uptake. The changes of [18F]ISO-1 uptake significantly correlated with relative changes in tumor volume as defined by changes in tumor volume based on MR imaging (**Fig. 3**).[75] One important clinical implications of this study was to provide evidence for the potential role of [18F]ISO-1 as a predictive measure of tumor growth rate.

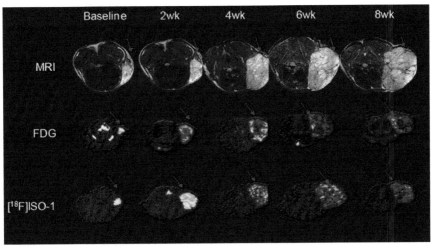

Fig. 3. Three modalities for treatment response assessment. Representative time course imaging of MNU-induced tumors at baseline, 2 weeks, 4 weeks, 6 weeks, and 8 weeks with MR imaging, FDG, and [^{18}F]ISO-1. *Arrows* depicting tumor. (*Adapted from* Shoghi KI, Xu J, Su Yi, et al. Quantitative receptor-based imaging of tumor proliferation with the sigma-2 ligand [18F]ISO-1 PLoS One 2013;8(9):e74188; with permission.)

Early clinical data: 2-(2-[^{18}F]fluoroethoxy)-N-(4-(3,4-dihydro-6,7-dimethoxyisoquinolin-2(1H)-yl)butyl)-5-methylbenzamide safety and feasibility studies

The first study evaluating [^{18}F]ISO-1 in humans was performed in 30 adult patients with different cancers, including 13 patients with newly diagnosed breast cancer.[76] The primary aim of the study was to evaluate the safety and dosimetry of [^{18}F]ISO-1. [^{18}F]ISO-1 uptake was assessed semi-quantitatively by obtaining SUVmax, tumor to normal tissue, and tumor to muscle, and relative distribution volume ratios. Significant correlation between tumor SUVmax and tumor-to-muscle ratio with Ki-67 was reported ($P = .04$ and $P = .003$, respectively). They also suggested that [^{18}F]ISO-1 uptake is helpful in stratification of the tumor sites to high- and low-proliferative tumors and this information can be potentially used in treatment planning to provide personalized treatment.

Preliminary results of an ongoing pilot phase I trial study using [^{18}F]ISO-1 as a σ_2 selective PET radiotracer demonstrated increased [^{18}F]ISO-1 uptake in primary breast cancer and nodal metastatic sites, suggesting this is a feasible technique for assessing σ_2-receptor expression in vivo.[77] Preliminary analysis demonstrated that [^{18}F]ISO-1 uptake in ER-positive tumors significantly correlates with expression levels of Ki-67.[77] Apart from the early clinical data on imaging σ_2-receptors, these receptors have been also evaluated as therapeutic targets for different disease processes. The suggested oncologic implication mainly focuses on the role of σ_2 ligands in inducing apoptosis in tumor cells.[78] The potentials

of this biomarker hold promise for a targeted diagnostic and therapeutic radiotracer in breast cancer.

SUMMARY OF CURRENT STATUS AND FUTURE DIRECTIONS

The ongoing development of new chemotherapeutic regimens with the goal of combining agents with different mechanism of actions to enhance response and at the same time reduce the toxicity profile challenges current imaging modalities for assessing treatment response. One emerging application is the increasing use of cell cycle–targeted chemotherapeutics, such as CDK4/6 inhibitors, in combination with previously established regimens, such as endocrine therapy, which motivates the need for clinically applicable noninvasive techniques for assessing early changes to therapy.

The promising results of ACRIN 6688 and the prospective studies pave the road for future multicenter trials exploring the role of the previously mentioned imaging techniques as a prognostic biomarker and an early indicator of cancer therapeutic response that can be used to guide personalized treatment in patients with breast cancer. An ongoing clinical trial in our institution is using [^{18}F]FLT-PET as a noninvasive tool to assess the impact of the CDK4/6 inhibitor and combined CDK4/6 inhibitor and chemotherapy on breast cancer proliferation in patients with recurrent or metastatic breast cancer following a phase II activity and safety study in 37 patients.[79] The need to synchronize the cell cycle agents with the timing of cytotoxic chemotherapy in this approach suggests a potential role for FLT-PET to track the pharmacodynamic effect of CDK4/6 inhibitors and its impact on cell cycle arrest. The capability of [^{18}F]ISO-1 to predict proliferative status is especially well-matched to cell cycle–specific chemotherapeutics, such as CDK4/6 inhibitors, and may also be applicable to their approved use as a component of first-line treatment of metastatic ER-positive breast cancer in combination with endocrine therapy. Ongoing and future preclinical studies are needed to validate this biomarker before clinical application.

REFERENCES

1. Lu J, Steeg PS, Price JE, et al. Breast cancer metastasis: challenges and opportunities. Cancer Res 2009;69(12):4951–3.
2. Brewster AM, Hortobagyi GN, Broglio KR, et al. Residual risk of breast cancer recurrence 5 years after adjuvant therapy. J Natl Cancer Inst 2008;100(16): 1179–83.
3. Hanahan D, Weinberg RA. Hallmarks of cancer: the next generation. Cell 2011;144(5):646–74.
4. Sorbye SW, Kilvaer TK, Valkov A, et al. Prognostic impact of CD57, CD68, M-CSF, CSF-1R, Ki67 and TGF-beta in soft tissue sarcomas. BMC Clin Pathol 2012;12:7.
5. Ishihara M, Mukai H, Nagai S, et al. Retrospective analysis of risk factors for central nervous system metastases in operable breast cancer: effects of biologic subtype and Ki67 overexpression on survival. Oncology 2013;84(3):135–40.
6. Mellor HR, Ferguson DJ, Callaghan R. A model of quiescent tumour microregions for evaluating multicellular resistance to chemotherapeutic drugs. Br J Cancer 2005;93(3):302–9.
7. Shackney SE, Shankey TV. Cell cycle models for molecular biology and molecular oncology: exploring new dimensions. Cytometry 1999;35(2): 97–116.
8. Choi YJ, Anders L. Signaling through cyclin D-dependent kinases. Oncogene 2014;33(15):1890–903.
9. Musgrove EA, Caldon CE, Barraclough J, et al. Cyclin D as a therapeutic target in cancer. Nat Rev Cancer 2011;11(8):558–72.
10. Quelle DE, Ashmun RA, Shurtleff SA, et al. Overexpression of mouse D-type cyclins accelerates G1 phase in rodent fibroblasts. Genes Dev 1993;7(8): 1559–71.
11. Nadji M, Gomez-Fernandez C, Ganjei-Azar P, et al. Immunohistochemistry of estrogen and progesterone receptors reconsidered: experience with 5,993 breast cancers. Am J Clin Pathol 2005; 123(1):21–7.
12. Schneider PG, Jackisch C, Brandt B. Endocrine management of breast cancer. Int J Fertil Menopausal Stud 1994;39(Suppl 2):115–27.
13. Kilker RL, Planas-Silva MD. Cyclin D1 is necessary for tamoxifen-induced cell cycle progression in human breast cancer cells. Cancer Res 2006;66(23): 11478–84.
14. Telli ML, Sledge GW. The future of breast cancer systemic therapy: the next 10 years. J Mol Med (Berl) 2015;93(2):119–25.
15. Osborne CK, Zhao H, Fuqua SA. Selective estrogen receptor modulators: structure, function, and clinical use. J Clin Oncol 2000;18(17): 3172–86.
16. Davies C, Godwin J, Gray R, et al. Relevance of breast cancer hormone receptors and other factors to the efficacy of adjuvant tamoxifen: patient-level meta-analysis of randomised trials. Lancet 2011; 378(9793):771–84.
17. Lumachi F, Luisetto G, Basso SM, et al. Endocrine therapy of breast cancer. Curr Med Chem 2011; 18(4):513–22.
18. Di Leo A, Jerusalem G, Petruzelka L, et al. Results of the CONFIRM phase III trial comparing fulvestrant 250 mg with fulvestrant 500 mg in postmenopausal women with estrogen receptor-positive advanced breast cancer. J Clin Oncol 2010; 28(30):4594–600.
19. Mauri D, Pavlidis N, Polyzos NP, et al. Survival with aromatase inhibitors and inactivators versus standard hormonal therapy in advanced breast cancer: meta-analysis. J Natl Cancer Inst 2006;98(18): 1285–91.
20. Dowsett M, Cuzick J, Ingle J, et al. Meta-analysis of breast cancer outcomes in adjuvant trials of aromatase inhibitors versus tamoxifen. J Clin Oncol 2010; 28(3):509–18.
21. Yeo B, Turner NC, Jones A. An update on the medical management of breast cancer. BMJ 2014;348: g3608.
22. Thangavel C, Dean JL, Ertel A, et al. Therapeutically activating RB: reestablishing cell cycle control in endocrine therapy-resistant breast cancer. Endocr Relat Cancer 2011;18(3): 333–45.
23. Murphy CG, Dickler MN. Endocrine resistance in hormone-responsive breast cancer: mechanisms and therapeutic strategies. Endocr Relat Cancer 2016;23(8):R337–52.
24. Choi YJ, Li X, Hydbring P, et al. The requirement for cyclin D function in tumor maintenance. Cancer Cell 2012;22(4):438–51.
25. Foster JS, Henley DC, Bukovsky A, et al. Multifaceted regulation of cell cycle progression by estrogen: regulation of CDK inhibitors and Cdc25A independent of cyclin D1-CDK4 function. Mol Cell Biol 2001;21(3):794–810.

6. Watts CK, Sweeney KJ, Warlters A, et al. Antiestrogen regulation of cell cycle progression and cyclin D1 gene expression in MCF-7 human breast cancer cells. Breast Cancer Res Treat 1994;31(1): 95–105.

27. Dean JL, McClendon AK, Knudsen ES. Modification of the DNA damage response by therapeutic CDK4/6 inhibition. J Biol Chem 2012;287(34): 29075–87.

28. Finn RS, Crown JP, Lang I, et al. The cyclin-dependent kinase 4/6 inhibitor palbociclib in combination with letrozole versus letrozole alone as first-line treatment of oestrogen receptor-positive, HER2-negative, advanced breast cancer (PALOMA-1/TRIO-18): a randomised phase 2 study. Lancet Oncol 2015; 16(1):25–35.

29. Shah A, et al. FDA Approval: Ribociclib for the Treatment of Postmenopausal Women with Hormone Receptor-Positive, HER2-Negative Advanced or Metastatic Breast Cancer. Clin Cancer Res 2018.

30. Mortazavi-Jehanno N, Giraudet AL, Champion L, et al. Assessment of response to endocrine therapy using FDG PET/CT in metastatic breast cancer: a pilot study. Eur J Nucl Med Mol Imaging 2012;39(3): 450–60.

31. Liao GJ, Clark AS, Schubert EK, et al. 18F-Fluoroestradiol PET: current status and potential future clinical applications. J Nucl Med 2016;57(8): 1269–75.

32. Kurland BF, Peterson LM, Lee JH, et al. Estrogen receptor binding (18F-FES PET) and glycolytic activity (18F-FDG PET) predict progression-free survival on endocrine therapy in patients with ER+ breast cancer. Clin Cancer Res 2017;23(2): 407–15.

33. Livingston RB, Johnson P, Goormastic M, et al. Effects on labeling index as a predictor of response to chemotherapy in the 13762 adenocarcinoma. Cancer Chemother Pharmacol 1982; 10(1):47–50.

34. Barnard NJ, Hall PA, Lemoine NR, et al. Proliferative index in breast carcinoma determined in situ by Ki67 immunostaining and its relationship to clinical and pathological variables. J Pathol 1987;152(4): 287–95.

35. Parrado C, Falkmer UG, Hoog A, et al. A technique for automatic/interactive assessment of the proliferating fraction of neoplastic cells in solid tumors. A methodological study on the Ki-67 immunoreactive cells in human mammary carcinomas, including a comparison with the results of conventional S-phase fraction assessments by means of DNA cytometry. Gen Diagn Pathol 1996;141(3–4):215–27.

36. Inwald EC, Klinkhammer-Schalke M, Hofstadter F, et al. Ki-67 is a prognostic parameter in breast cancer patients: results of a large population-based cohort of a cancer registry. Breast Cancer Res Treat 2013;139(2):539–52.

37. Shields AF, Mankoff DA, Link JM, et al. Carbon-11-thymidine and FDG to measure therapy response. J Nucl Med 1998;39(10):1757–62.

38. Cleaver JC. Thymidine metabolism and cell kinetics. Amsterdam: North-Holland Publishing Company; 1967.

39. Livingston RB, Ambus U, George SL, et al. In vitro determination of thymidine-3H labeling index in human solid tumors. Cancer Res 1974;34(6): 1376–80.

40. Shields AF, Lim K, Grierson J, et al. Utilization of labeled thymidine in DNA synthesis: studies for PET. J Nucl Med 1990;31(3):337–42.

41. Mankoff DA, Shields AF, Graham MM, et al. Kinetic analysis of 2-[carbon-11]thymidine PET imaging studies: compartmental model and mathematical analysis. J Nucl Med 1998;39(6): 1043–55.

42. Conti PS, Bading JR, Mouton PP, et al. In vivo measurement of cell proliferation in canine brain tumor using C-11-labeled FMAU and PET. Nucl Med Biol 2008;35(1):131–41.

43. Chou TC, Kong XB, Fanucchi MP, et al. Synthesis and biological effects of 2'-fluoro-5-ethyl-1-beta-D-arabinofuranosyluracil. Antimicrob Agents Chemother 1987;31(9):1355–8.

44. Grierson JR, Schwartz JL, Muzi M, et al. Metabolism of 3'-deoxy-3'-[F-18]fluorothymidine in proliferating A549 cells: validations for positron emission tomography. Nucl Med Biol 2004;31(7): 829–37.

45. Belt JA, Marina NM, Phelps DA, et al. Nucleoside transport in normal and neoplastic cells. Adv Enzyme Regul 1993;33:235–52.

46. Plotnik DA, Emerick LE, Krohn KA, et al. Different modes of transport for 3H-thymidine, 3H-FLT, and 3H-FMAU in proliferating and nonproliferating human tumor cells. J Nucl Med 2010;51(9): 1464–71.

47. Rasey JS, Grierson JR, Wiens LW, et al. Validation of FLT uptake as a measure of thymidine kinase-1 activity in A549 carcinoma cells. J Nucl Med 2002; 43(9):1210–7.

48. Bollineni VR, Kramer GM, Jansma EP, et al. A systematic review on [(18)F]FLT-PET uptake as a measure of treatment response in cancer patients. Eur J Cancer 2016;55:81–97.

49. Smyczek-Gargya B, Fersis N, Dittmann H, et al. PET with [18F]fluorothymidine for imaging of primary breast cancer: a pilot study. Eur J Nucl Med Mol Imaging 2004;31(5):720–4.

50. Kenny LM, Vigushin DM, Al-Nahhas A, et al. Quantification of cellular proliferation in tumor and normal tissues of patients with breast cancer by [18F] fluorothymidine-positron emission tomography

imaging: evaluation of analytical methods. Cancer Res 2005;65(21):10104–12.

51. Chalkidou A, Landau DB, Odell EW, et al. Correlation between Ki-67 immunohistochemistry and 18F-fluorothymidine uptake in patients with cancer: a systematic review and meta-analysis. Eur J Cancer 2012;48(18):3499–513.

52. Dehdashti F, Flanagan FL, Mortimer JE, et al. Positron emission tomographic assessment of "metabolic flare" to predict response of metastatic breast cancer to antiestrogen therapy. Eur J Nucl Med 1999;26(1):51–6.

53. Duch J, Fuster D, Munoz M, et al. 18F-FDG PET/CT for early prediction of response to neoadjuvant chemotherapy in breast cancer. Eur J Nucl Med Mol Imaging 2009;36(10):1551–7.

54. Contractor KB, Kenny LM, Stebbing J, et al. [18F]-3'Deoxy-3'-fluorothymidine positron emission tomography and breast cancer response to docetaxel. Clin Cancer Res 2011;17(24):7664–72.

55. Woolf DK, Beresford M, Li SP, et al. Evaluation of FLT-PET-CT as an imaging biomarker of proliferation in primary breast cancer. Br J Cancer 2014;110(12):2847–54.

56. Crippa F, Agresti R, Sandri M, et al. (1)(8)F-FLT PET/CT as an imaging tool for early prediction of pathological response in patients with locally advanced breast cancer treated with neoadjuvant chemotherapy: a pilot study. Eur J Nucl Med Mol Imaging 2015;42(6):818–30.

57. Kostakoglu L, Duan F, Idowu MO, et al. A phase II study of 3'-deoxy-3'-18F-fluorothymidine PET in the assessment of early response of breast cancer to neoadjuvant chemotherapy: results from ACRIN 6688. J Nucl Med 2015;56(11):1681–9.

58. Deng SM, Zhang W, Zhang B, et al. Assessment of tumor response to chemotherapy in patients with breast cancer using (18)F-FLT: a meta-analysis. Chin J Cancer Res 2014;26(5):517–24.

59. Dowsett M, Smith IE, Ebbs SR, et al. Prognostic value of Ki67 expression after short-term presurgical endocrine therapy for primary breast cancer. J Natl Cancer Inst 2007;99(2):167–70.

60. Eiermann W, Paepke S, Appfelstaedt J, et al. Preoperative treatment of postmenopausal breast cancer patients with letrozole: a randomized double-blind multicenter study. Ann Oncol 2001;12(11):1527–32.

61. Ellis MJ, Suman VJ, Hoog J, et al. Ki67 proliferation index as a tool for chemotherapy decisions during and after neoadjuvant aromatase inhibitor treatment of breast cancer: results from the American College of Surgeons Oncology Group Z1031 trial (Alliance). J Clin Oncol 2017;35(10):1061–9.

62. Roberts TK, Peterson L, Kurland B, et al. Use of serial 18F-fluorothymidine (FLT) PET and Ki-67 to predict response to aromatase inhibitors (AI) women with ER+ breast cancer. J Clin Onc 2016;34(15 Suppl):12039.

63. Whisenant JG, McIntyre JO, Peterson TE, et al. Utility of [18 F]FLT-PET to assess treatment response trastuzumab-resistant and trastuzumab-sensitive HER2-overexpressing human breast cancer xenografts. Mol Imaging Biol 2015;17(1):119–28.

64. Palmieri C, Stein RC, Liu X, et al. IRIS study: phase II study of the steroid sulfatase inhibitor irosustat when added to an aromatase inhibitor ER-positive breast cancer patients. Breast Cancer Res Treat 2017;165(2):343–53.

65. Palmieri C, Szydlo R, Miller M, et al. IPET study an FLT-PET window study to assess the activity of the steroid sulfatase inhibitor irosustat in early breast cancer. Breast Cancer Res Treat 2017; 166:1–13.

66. Muzi M, Vesselle H, Grierson JR, et al. Kinetic analysis of 3'-deoxy-3'-fluorothymidine PET studies: validation studies in patients with lung cancer. J Nucl Med 2005;46(2):274–82.

67. Loddo M, Kingsbury SR, Rashid M, et al. Cell-cycle phase progression analysis identifies unique phenotypes of major prognostic and predictive significance in breast cancer. Br J Cancer 2009;100(6): 959–70.

68. McKinley ET, Ayers GD, Smith RA, et al. Limits of [18F]-FLT PET as a biomarker of proliferation in oncology. PLoS One 2013;8(3):e58938.

69. Mach RH, Smith CR, al-Nabulsi I, et al. Sigma 2 receptors as potential biomarkers of proliferation in breast cancer. Cancer Res 1997;57(1): 156–61.

70. Bem WT, Thomas GE, Mamone JY, et al. Overexpression of sigma receptors in nonneural human tumors. Cancer Res 1991;51(24):6558–62.

71. Mach RH, Huang Y, Freeman RA, et al. Conformationally-flexible benzamide analogues as dopamine D3 and sigma 2 receptor ligands. Bioorg Med Chem Lett 2004;14(1):195–202.

72. Tu Z, Dence CS, Ponde DE, et al. Carbon-11 labeled sigma2 receptor ligands for imaging breast cancer. Nucl Med Biol 2005;32(5):423–30.

73. Kashiwagi H, McDunn JE, Simon PO Jr, et al. Selective sigma-2 ligands preferentially bind to pancreatic adenocarcinomas: applications in diagnostic imaging and therapy. Mol Cancer 2007;6:48.

74. Tu Z, Xu J, Jones LA, et al. Fluorine-18-labeled benzamide analogues for imaging the sigma2 receptor status of solid tumors with positron emission tomography. J Med Chem 2007;50(14): 3194–204.

75. Shoghi KI, Xu J, Su Y, et al. Quantitative receptor-based imaging of tumor proliferation with the

sigma-2 ligand [(18)F]ISO-1. PLoS One 2013;8(9): e74188.

76. Dehdashti F, Laforest R, Gao F, et al. Assessment of cellular proliferation in tumors by PET using 18F-ISO-1. J Nucl Med 2013;54(3):350–7.

77. McDonald ES, Tchou J, Doot R, et al. Imaging proliferative status in primary breast cancer using the sigma-2 selective ligand, ^{18}F-ISO-1. J Nucl Med 2016;57(232 Suppl):32.

78. McDonald ES, Mankoff J, Makvandi M, et al. Sigma-2 ligands and PARP inhibitors synergistically trigger cell death in breast cancer cells. Biochem Biophys Res Commun 2017;486(3):788–95.

79. DeMichele A, Clark AS, Tan KS, et al. CDK 4/6 inhibitor palbociclib (PD0332991) in Rb+ advanced breast cancer: phase II activity, safety, and predictive biomarker assessment. Clin Cancer Res 2015; 21(5):995–1001.

Moving?

Make sure your subscription moves with you!

To notify us of your new address, find your **Clinics Account Number** (located on your mailing label above your name), and contact customer service at:

Email: journalscustomerservice-usa@elsevier.com

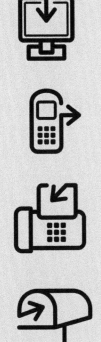

800-654-2452 (subscribers in the U.S. & Canada)
314-447-8871 (subscribers outside of the U.S. & Canada)

Fax number: 314-447-8029

Elsevier Health Sciences Division
Subscription Customer Service
3251 Riverport Lane
Maryland Heights, MO 63043

Printed and bound by CPI Group (UK) Ltd, Croydon, CR0 4YY

12/10/2024

01773370-0001